GASTROINTESTINAL ENDOSCOPY

Edited by **Oliviu Pascu**

Gastrointestinal Endoscopy
Edited by Oliviu Pascu

Published by InTech
Janeza Trdine 9, 51000 Rijeka, Croatia

Publishing Process Manager Masa Vidovic

Technical Editor Teodora Smiljanic

Cover Designer InTech Design Team

Additional hard copies can be obtained from orders@intechopen.com

Gastrointestinal Endoscopy, Edited by Oliviu Pascu
p. cm.
ISBN 978-953-307-385-9

For EU product safety concerns:
IN TECH d.o.o., Prolaz Marije Krucifikse Kozulić 3, 51000 Rijeka, Croatia,
info@intechopen.com or visit our website at intechopen.com.

Meet the editor

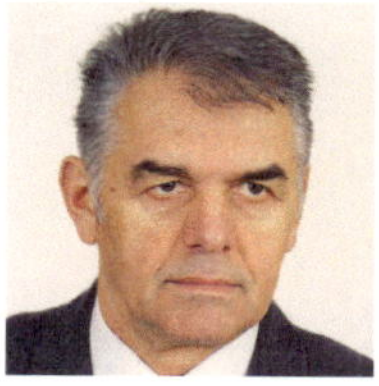

Dr. Oliviu Pascu graduated at the Faculty of General Medicine, Institute of Medicine &Pharmacy in 1963. He became professor of internal medicine and gastroenterology at the IIIrd Medical Clinic, University of Medicine and Pharmacy, Cluj-Napoca, Romania in 1990. From 1990 until 2000 he was dean (Faculty of Medicine) and then rector of the University of Medicine and Pharmacy in Cluj. Until 2009 he acted as president of the Romanian Society of Digestive Endoscopy and is presently honorary president). His first monograph on digestive endoscopy was published in Romania in 1982., while his first textbook on gastroenterology 1996-1997. He has practiced digestive endoscopy since 1969 and introduced hemostasis and polypectomy in Romania (1975). More than 150 of his articles have been published in Romanian and international medical journals. Dr. Pascu is member of the Academy of Medical Sciences Romania and many Romanian and European scientific societies.

Contents

Preface

Endoscopy has had a major impact in developing modern gastroenterology. By using different data it provided a better understanding of pathogenic mechanisms, described new entities and changed diagnostic and therapeutic strategies. Some examples such as the relationship esophagitis-Barrett, esophagus-esophageal adenocarcinoma, the description of early gastric cancer, the relationship helicobacteria-pylori-duodenal ulcer-gastric cancer and the affiliation colon adenoma-colon cancer remind us of the influence of endoscopy in gastroenterology. Moreover, endoscopy has surpassed its function as an examination tool and it became a rapid and efficient therapeutic tool of low invasiveness. We cannot imagine gastroenterology today without endoscopic hemostasis in variceal or non-variceal upper bleeding, gastric or colonic polypectomy, biliary sphincterotomy and endoscopic biliary stone removal, biliary or pancreatic endoscopic stenting or endoscopic drainage of abdominal fluid collection.

Meanwhile, taking benefit of many technical advances, endoscopy has had a spectacular development. New video-endoscopes, endoscopes with working channel, magnification endoscopes, confocal of narrow band imaging endoscopes emerged. Sophisticated devices for endoscopic ultrasound with the possibility of fine-needle aspiration or elastography, endoscopic capsules for exploring the small intestine as well as enteroscopes with single or double balloon and spiral enteroscopy are several examples of the evolution of the endoscopy field. At the same time many diagnostic techniques (vital staining, fluorescence) or treatment techniques (e.g. banding, metallic clips, laser use, plasma-argon coagulation, stenting, mucosectomies) recognized real improvement. .

The contributions in this book are diverse and very valuable. InTech Open Access Publisher selected several known names from all continents and countries with different levels of development. Multiple specific points of view, with respect to different origins of the authors were presented together with various topics regarding diagnostic or therapeutic endoscopy. As a result, the reader can take into consideration not only theoretical or practical knowledge in the field, but also the experience, point of view and local situation in a specific center of gastroenterology or in a specific country. This actually represents a valuable tool for formation and continuous medical education in endoscopy considering the performances or technical possibilities in different parts of the world.

My activity as editor was aided by the contribution of two exceptional endoscopists who accepted the statute of co-editors: associate professor Marcel Tantau MD, PhD and lecturer Andrada Seicean MD, PhD. I thank them sincerely for accepting to contribute to this publication, for the quality of their activity and their promptitude in editing chapters. Many thanks to InTech Open Access Publisher which offered me the possibility of editing this very attractive book. It was a real pleasure to read such interesting works by so many experts from all over the world. My sincere thanks to all my co-workers for the quality of the chapter editing. Not in the last turn, I thank Ms. Masa Vidovic and Ms. Mia Devic for their perfect, prompt and efficient co-operation.

Prof. Oliviu Pascu MD PhD Dr h.c. FRCP/Edin
3rd Medical Department
University of Medicine and Pharmacy 'Iuliu Hatieganu'
Cluj-Napoca
Romania

Part 1

General Aspects

1

Challenges of Gastrointestinal Endoscopy in Resource-Poor Countries

Nwokediuko Sylvester Chuks
Gastroenterology Unit, Department of Medicine,
University of Nigeria Teaching Hospital Ituku/Ozalla,
P.M.B. 01129 Enugu,
Nigeria

1. Introduction

Over the past 100 years, there has been a dramatic and explosive growth of information about and technology related to the science and practice of gastroenterology. Endoscopy services are the mainstay of diagnosis and treatment in gastroenterology. Endoscopies have undergone significant changes enabled by advances in information technology (IT). The ability to take video pictures onto the computer screen and to print them has enabled more effective image capture, image storage and retrieval as well as quality assessment.

The developed countries of the world have taken great advantage of these innovations and developments but the story is totally different for the developing or resource - poor countries. The developing countries are characterized by low measures of development such as income per capita, rate of literacy, life expectancy and other health indices. These countries have not achieved a significant degree of industrialization relative to their populations, and which have in most cases a low standard of living. Strictly speaking, the term developing implies mobility and does not acknowledge that development may be in decline or static in some countries, particularly African countries. It is for this reason that the World Bank classifies countries on the basis of Gross National Income (GNI) per capita (World Bank, 2010).

Digestive diseases impose a substantial burden on global health. In the United States, over 40 billion US Dollars was used for gastrointestinal disease in one year (Sandler et al 2002).Comparable information on the digestive health of people living in developing countries may not be available but it is known that diarrheal diseases account for 17.9% of deaths in low-income countries compared to 1.6% in high-income countries (World Health Organization, WHO 2008). Helicobacter pylori is a leading cause of gastrointestinal disease globally. Whereas the prevalence of this infection has declined considerably in the developed world, it is still very high in the developing countries (Torres et al 2000), with the majority of the global burden of infection found here (World Gastroenterology Organization, WGO 2006) because most of the risk factors for its transmission are rife in the developing countries. These include low socio-economic status, crowded living conditions, several children sleeping on one bed, large numbers of siblings and unclean water (Webb et al 1994, Malaty et al 1996, Lindkvist et al 1998, Dominici et al 1999, Nabwera et al 2000).

Because of the pivotal role of endoscopy in the teaching and practice of gastroenterology, various professional bodies in the developed countries have produced guidelines on what constitutes the minimum necessary facilities, equipment and staffing to deliver safe and effective endoscopy (Digestive Health Foundation, Australia, 2007, American Society of Gastrointestinal Endoscopy (ASGE) 2010). The training and qualification of endoscopists and nursing staff, the endoscopic equipment and accessories, the reprocessing of endoscopes, monitoring and resuscitation equipment must all be of globally accepted standards. Some of these standards will be highlighted in this article and compared with what obtains in developing countries using Nigeria as a typical example.

2. Location of services

An endoscopy unit may be hospital-based or free standing. For hospital-based endoscopy units, the location shall be in close proximity to acute emergency services. The location within the complex shall permit free access for out-patients and for the transport of in-patients by bed, trolley or wheel chair. Where the endoscopy unit is not located within the main hospital complex, provision for enclosed transfer of patients is advisable. Where the endoscopy service is in a free standing facility, it should be located within a 15 minute ambulance journey of an acute hospital that provides an intensive care or emergency service. There should be an agreed arrangement with this hospital to admit patients in a medical emergency.

The endoscopy services that are available in the developing countries do not meet the standards stated above. Very often there is a lot of improvisation in the siting of endoscopy suites. In some countries they are located in wards without any consideration for access to out-patients and transport of in-patients. The privately owned endoscopy services are even worse because in most cases, once the equipment is procured, it is installed in any existing facility. The absence of effective certification and accreditation of centres makes matters worse.

3. Facilities

An ideal endoscopy unit should posses the following areas as minimum requirements. (Digestive Health Foundation, Australia, 2007).

- Reception and Administration
- Waiting Area
- Procedure Room(s)
- Consulting/Interview Room
- Nurses' Station
- Storage Areas
- Separate Reprocessing Area
- Staff Room
- Toilets and Change Rooms
- Waste Disposal Area
- Recovery Room(s)

Each of these areas should have proper supply of consumables and necessary equipment. For instance; a recovery area should be situated adjacent to the procedure room(s) and must be freely accessible by a normal recovery room trolley. The recovery room should also have

an oxygen supply dedicated to this area. Oxygen outlets will need to be provided so that each recovery bay is supplied. Wall mounted suction is desirable, however where unavailable, at least one dedicated mobile suction unit shall be provided.
The endoscopy units in the developing countries are not in any way near the specifications listed above. It is common to have reception and administration, waiting area, consulting/interview room and staff room all housed in one room. In some instances, doctors and nurses share rooms. Some facilities may have only one toilet for male and female staff and patients. Suction machines and oxygen delivery are often in short supply. What you find in an average endoscopy unit in a developing country is a reflection of what is available in an average hospital.

3.1 Procedure room

The procedure room should be at least 4 meters by 5 meters. Larger rooms are required for video endoscopy and if endoscopic retrograde cholangiopancreatography (ERCP) procedures are performed, a larger room of not less than 35 square meters is required. The procedure room must be equipped with at least the following:

- Light source/video processor
- Medical grade monitor/video
- Suction x 2 (patient and instrument)
- Oxygen and accessory equipment
- Pulse oximeter
- Non-invasive blood pressure monitoring
- Hand washing facilities
- Emergency drugs
- Intercom or emergency call system.

3.2 Power supply

The problem of power supply is a major one in resource-poor countries. The Nigerian energy industry has been described as one of the most inefficient in the world in terms of meeting the needs of its customers. This has had a devastating effect on business to the extent that most businesses have to rely on generators, which are very expensive to run. Endoscopy procedures are often interrupted or cut short by power outages. Such incessant outages have deleterious effects on the endoscopy equipment with the result that there is frequent breakdown. The generators that serve as alternative may not be big enough to power air conditioners thus it is common to see the endoscopist, other support staff and the patient sweating profusely during endoscopic procedure. The quality of work done in this type of environment is bound to be substandard. The commonest cause of inconclusive endoscopic procedure in Nigeria is power failure.

4. Equipment

Minimum equipment required for gastrointestinal endoscopy includes:

- Endoscopic light source/video processor
- High resolution medical standard monitor (CRT or LCD)
- Fully immersible endoscopes
- Gastroscopes – not less than 2

- Colonoscopes – not less than 2
- Valve buttons, biopsy caps and adaptors
- Electrosurgical equipment
- Forceps
- Snares
- Sclerotherapy needles
- Dilators and guidewires

Ancillary equipment

- Recovery Trolley and Chairs
- Pulse Oximeter
- Non-invasive BP Monitoring
- Stethoscope
- Access to ECG Tracing
- Glucometer
- Transportable Oxygen Cylinder with Portable Suction
- Standard resuscitation equipment: which must be readily available, maintained in good working order, function checked daily and maintained and checked according to manufacturer's directions.

Permanently sited in the endoscopy facility will be the following items:

- Air viva – masks, bags, airways
- Adequate intravenous access equipment
- Plasma expander
- Intravenous fluids including Normal Saline, Dextrose etc
- Full range of emergency drugs
- Portable Oxygen and Suction

Rapid access (within 1-2minutes) to the following equipment is also mandatory.

- ECG machine
- Cardiac defibrillator
- Two laryngoscopes
- Appropriate range of endotracheal tubes and accessories

These minimum requirements are not even available in some of the surgical theatres and intensive care units of hospitals in the developing countries and therefore it will be unrealistic to expect endoscopy facilities to have them. Some teaching hospitals in resource-poor countries do not offer gastrointestinal endoscopy. In centres where the service is available, there may be only one functional gastroscope and/or one functional colonoscope. Often a lot of accessories are improvised. Again, using Nigeria as example, therapeutic endoscopy is still at its infancy. Majority of the teaching hospitals in the country have no facility for therapeutic endoscopy. One or 2 centres may be able to do band ligation of esophageal varices albeit in an unsustainable fashion. In one of the centres the doctors modified the normal variceal banding technique by cutting size 14 Folley's urethral catheters to size and reloading them on previously used caps, all in an attempt to reduce cost (Ladep et al 2008). Infection control remains a challenge in such ingenuity. It is also common to find non-immersible endoscopes in developing countries with obvious implication for cross-infection. The newer techniques in endoscopy like capsule endoscopy and endoscopic ultrasonography are yet to be available in most developing countries including Nigeria.

5. Staff requirements

5.1 Global distribution of medical personnel

In Nigeria, doctor to population ratio is 3 per 10,000 compared to US which stands at 26 per 10,000. The gap is even much wider when one considers the gastroenterologist to population ratio. Nigeria has only about 60 gastroenterologists (registered with the Society for Gastroenterology and Hepatology in Nigeria, SOGHIN). Out of this number, there are some who do not practice gastrointestinal endoscopy because they work in centres that do not have facilities for it. This number is grossly inadequate for a population of over 140 million. The anatomical pathologist plays an essential role in the diagnosis of numerous digestive disorders. The number of pathologists in Nigeria is equally abysmally low for the population and only very few of them are trained specially for gastrointestinal diseases.
Some high-income countries such as Austrialia, Canada, Saudi Arabia, the USA and the United Arab Emirates and the UK have sustained their relatively high physician – to population ratio by recruiting medical graduates from developing regions, including countries in sub-Saharan Africa (Labonte et al 2006, Mullan 2006, Pond et al 2006). In contrast, over half of the countries in sub-Saharan Africa do not meet the minimum acceptable physician to population ratio of one per 5000 (WHO 2007). Several recent reviews of health workers employed in Austrialia, Canada, the UK and the USA have shown the extent of brain drain. An estimated 13272 physicians trained in sub-Saharan Africa are practising in Australia, Canada, the UK and the USA (Mullan 2006). Around a third of medical graduates from Nigerian medical schools migrate within 10 years of graduation to Canada, the UK and the USA (Ihekweazu 2005). Nurses, who commonly bear the brunt of health-care delivery in sub-Saharan Africa are also not left out in the brain drain (Labonte 2006, Mandeville 2009)

5.2 Minimum staffing requirements

Staffing requirements for the performance of GI endoscopy should be based on what is needed to ensure safe and proficient performance of the individual procedure. Currently, staffing may vary as determined by local practice requirements, patient characteristics, and the type of endoscopic procedure being performed. While the physician is performing endoscopic procedure, the endoscopy suite staff will concentrate on patient monitoring, documentation and technical assistance. The level of education and training of the staff can vary, including qualified nurses with training in endoscopy and qualified nurses trainable on the job.
Because objective evidence pertaining to the relationship between endoscopy unit staffing levels and patient outcomes is lacking, it is difficult to make concrete recommendations to the developing countries where there is an acute shortage of medical staff including trained endoscopists and support staff.

5.3 Staff training

The World Gastroenterology Organization (WGO), a Federation of 110 National Societies and 4 regional associations of gastroenterology representing over 50,000 individual members worldwide focuses on the improvement of standards in gastroenterology training and education on a global scale. It has been christened the "global guardian of digestive health". In 2007 it published a document about the basic standards of a gastroenterology training program (WGO 2007). In drawing up the standards of training the WGO took into consideration the existing training programs in various countries. It is noteworthy that Egypt and Sudan were the only African countries that provided information about their existing training programs to the WGO Committee. The other countries in Africa, including Nigeria did not respond to the enquiry.

The WGO has training centres in the developing countries but these are very few and countries in the catchment areas of the centres have not taken adequate advantage of the institutions to develop their local digestive endoscopists. Prospective trainees usually find it difficult to secure funding from their countries.

5.4 Minimum training standards

The WGO proposes a minimum number of each procedure that must be completed by the trainees in the training centres. The body differentiates between level 1 and level 2 endoscopists with a remark that level 1 might be sufficient for some developing countries. A level 1 endoscopist is expected to be proficient in esophagogastroduodenoscopy, treatment of non-variceal bleeding, treatment of variceal bleeding, esophageal dilatation, flexible sigmoidoscopy, colonoscopy, polypectomy, placement of percutaneous endoscopic gastrostomy, liver biopsy, abdominal puncture and foreign body removal. It is a sad truth that most endoscopy centres in developing countries such as Nigeria do not carry out any form of therapeutic endoscopy. It therefore follows that trainees in these centres will not acquire the competences required of a level 1 endoscopist. Training of endoscopists takes place in the teaching hospitals that are grossly ill-equiped to perform the function. There are 2 postgraduate medical colleges in Nigeria: The West African College of Physicians or Surgeons and the National Postgraduate Medical College of Nigeria. These colleges supervise the training of residents and eventually certify them after passing the requisite examinations. The current practice does not ensure adequate exposure for the trainees who hardly complete the minimum number of procedures before they present themselves for examination. Furthermore, the method of evaluation is such that one can pass without having completed the prescribed procedures. Sometimes incessant industrial actions make it practically impossible for trainees to complete the procedures during the training period. The evaluation has no practical endoscopy component. In the developed countries, methods used in the evaluation of trainee competence vary from place to place and may include observation during procedure, formal assessment of clinical skills, using a patient-based examination, formal in-practice examination, use of log books, annual assessments, final assessment and feedback from trainees. These evaluation methods are largely absent in the developing countries. Where they exist, the regulations are often not applied strictly for economic, social and political reasons. The regulatory authorities are sometimes faced with a situation where they have to decide between closing a health facility because it lacks basic equipment and staff; and allowing it to continue to function at a substandard level because of political interests.

6. Infection control

Over the course of endoscopic examination, the external surface and internal channels of flexible endoscopes and accessory equipment are exposed to body fluids and contaminants. Disinfection of these reusable instruments poses special problems. Given their relatively delicate structure endoscopes cannot be autoclaved. Therefore processing is achieved by mechanical cleaning, followed by high level disinfection (HLD), rinsing and drying. Stringent guidelines are in place in most developed societies for the reprocessing of endoscopes (ASGE 2003 and the Gastgroenterological Society of Australia 2003). If these guidelines are followed, virtually no cases of infection transmission are encountered (Ciancio et al 2005, McDonald et al 1976, Hanson et al 1990).

The ability to reprocess equipment efficiently and safely is one of the most important functions of an endoscopy facility. An area dedicated to the cleaning and disinfection of endoscopic equipment must be available and should contain at least two (2) large sinks plus a tank/container of disinfecting solution or an automatic flexible endoscope reprocessing machine.

Reprocessing should commence immediately following use of an endoscope to prevent the drying of secretions within the channels. The cleaning and disinfection of endoscopes should only be performed by staff that have been fully trained and certified to do so. Inexperienced staff may not be aware of the specific design of the instrument and may cause severe damage or inadequately clean and disinfect the equipment.

Automated endoscope reprocessors have become available in developed countries. These automated brushless systems are an important step in raising the standard of care for flexible endoscope reprocessing (ASGE 2008, Society of Gastroenterology Nurses and Associates, SGNA 2008). This innovation also allows facilities to utilize valuable staff resources in other patient-related activities and reduce occupational health problems associated with reprocessing.

The situation in resource-poor countries is totally different. In the first place, there are no local guidelines for equipment reprocessing. Something as basic as potable water supply is a big challenge in many hospitals in resource-poor countries and that is bound to affect the cleaning of equipment. The acute shortage of trained endoscopy staff further worsens the picture. Supply of substandard disinfecting solution is a frequent occurrence in developing countries. Therefore, it is likely that infection transmission in endoscopy facilities may be substantial. Unfortunately, there are no data on the magnitude of this challenge.

Very often the recommended period of immersion of endoscopes in the disinfecting solution may be unwittingly shortened between procedures to reduce the waiting time of patients especially where there is only one endoscope that has to be reused on many patients the same day. This again has negative consequences for infection control.

Automated endoscope reprocessors are not yet available in most resource-poor countries. No centre in Nigeria has this equipment and I doubt if any is planning to acquire it soon. It may be more expedient for them to intensify adherence to the traditional methods of thorough manual washing, rinsing and drying.

7. Sedation

The provision of sedation and analgesia has been an important component of performing endoscopic procedure on the gastrointestinal tract. The different procedures can create pain and discomfort and are associated with anxiety for the patient. It is for this reason that sedation has become an essential component of endoscopy.

For routine diagnostic endoscopic procedures sedation is almost always used in North America and Australia. However in Europe, Asia and some African countries, the sedation

rate varies among countries and even among centres of the same country. The use of sedation improves the tolerance and acceptance of gastrointestinal endoscopy (Bell 2004) but increases the cost of the procedure and is responsible for about 50% of the GI endoscopy complication rates (Lazzaroni et al 2005).
Sedation for gastrointestinal endoscopy may induce central respiratory depression and/or airway obstruction. Early diagnosis and treatment of these complications is mandatory and this can only be accomplished by patient monitoring.

7.1 Monitoring
Current recommendations for monitoring include patient responsiveness, blood pressure, respiratory rate and oxygen saturation. Oxygen saturation is a critical vital sign, but there can be a significant delay between inadequate ventilation and desaturation. Supplemental oxygen can dangerously increase this disconnect. Thus one must monitor adequacy of ventilation by direct observation, auscultation and/or end-tidal CO_2 monitoring.

7.2 Training for sedation
Appropriate supervision and training is critical for developing skills necessary to perform conscious sedation. There is uniform agreement in the literature and all relevant societal guidelines agree that specific training is needed for both endoscopic procedure and any sedation associated with the procedure (America Society of Anaesthesiologists 2002, ASGE 2008, Cohen et al 2007).

7.3 Situation in developing countries
There are no published studies on the use of sedation in most African countries including Nigeria. This is partly because there are no guidelines in place to regulate the use of sedation in gastrointestinal endoscopy. Similarly the rate and type of sedation employed by endoscopists in these countries is not known. However, it is tempting to assume that endoscopists in developing countries either undersedate their patients or avoid sedation all together in order to avoid the attendant increase in cost and increase in complications.This is because the endoscopists do not have any special training in the use of sedatives and the centres where they work do not always have the basic facilities to monitor patients adequately during the procedures. One consequence of this situation is that patients who find the procedure seriously unpleasant because they were not sedated may not only refuse future examination but spread concern to others. A meta-analysis showed sedation to achieve better patient cooperation and satisfaction and willingness to have it repeated. (McQuaid et al 2008).

8. Quality assurance

8.1 Accreditation and certification
The development of quality assurance is a major task of the Health authorities in liaison with experts issued from the respective medical societies. It also applies to the hospital environment as well as to practitioners who have to be submitted to certification, after the report from expert visitors. Accreditation of gastroenterologists and certification of hospitals are done periodically to ensure that standards do not go below prescribed levels.
In Nigeria, the postgraduate medical colleges (West African College of Physicians/Surgeons and the National Postgraduate Medical College) undertake periodic accreditation visits to

the training institutions (Teaching Hospitals, Specialist Hospitals, Federal Medical Centres and some private hospitals). Because of funding constraints, these visits are not as regular as they should be. The Federal Government of Nigeria can make the regulatory colleges more efficient by improving the funding of their activities so that they do not depend on the hospitals being accredited for any financial assistance, a situation that may introduce conflict of interest.

8.2 Quality measurement

There are inherent difficulties of measuring quality in gastrointestinal endoscopic procedures. This is particularly so because complications are rare. Because mortality is negligible, rates do not vary greatly among physicians. Also there is a lack of surrogate measurable outcome measures in GI endoscopy. Measuring the process is the alternative but, again, there has not been any significant progress in process measurement.
Quality measurement is even more problematic in developing countries because of a general lack of baseline. There are no guidelines in place that reflect the peculiar economic realities in these countries.

9. Cost of endoscopic procedures

The cost of endoscopic procedures in developing countries is often out of the reach of many patients. Poverty is a major problem that militates against access to health care. Poverty exacerbates poor health while poor health makes it harder to get out of poverty. In Nigeria, most patients have to make out - of - pocket payments at the point of service and this has adversely affected service delivery. The Federal Government of Nigeria recently introduced the National Health Insurance Scheme but the coverage is still very low and does not cover all medical procedures and treatments. Catastrophic expenditure is more frequent when health care has to be paid for out - of - pocket at the point of service.

10. Conclusions and recommendations

The problems that face the teaching and practice of gastrointestinal endoscopy in developing countries are protean and generally reflect the low level of human and infrastructural development in these countries:

- There is an acute shortage of trained endoscopists, gastrointestinal pathologists, nurses and other support staff. This situation is daily compounded by the continuing brain-drain.
- Inadequate budgetary allocation to health and poor implementation of health programs and budgets.
- Inadequate and unsteady power supply.
- Lack of modern gastrointestinal endoscopic equipment and consumables for effective service delivery and training.
- Lack of guidelines for the practice and teaching of gastroenterology.
- Health service delivery is characterized by a high rate of out-of-pocket payments and a low rate of prepayment schemes, a situation that deprives many families of needed care because they cannot afford it.

The health care system in the developing countries needs a radical reorganization. The budgetary allocation to health and the implementation of policies related to health need radical improvement.

The governments should work in liaison with various medical societies to come out with firm guidelines that will take into account the financial capabilities of these obviously poorer countries without unduely compromising the health of their citizens and ensure strict compliance by all stakeholders.

It is no longer realistic to talk about global standards because of the problem of resource allocation. The available resources and technologies differ from country to country. For example, the ability to use narrow-band imaging, ERCP or procedures that are considered standard components of endoscopy in the United States may not be possible in developing countries and the guidelines must reflected these differences. It is essential to be cognizant of the local resources and to identify quality within their constraints.

The funding of health services should tend towards prepayment strategies rather than out-of-pocket payment and health insurance is a veritable tool for achieving this.

11. References

American Society of Anaesthesiologists (2002). Practice Guidelines for Sedation and Analgesia by Non-Anaesthesiologists. *Anaesthesiology* Vol. 94, pp. 1004-1017.

American Society of Gastrointestinal Endoscopy [ASGE] (2003). Multisociety guidelinefor reprocessing flexible gastrointestinal endoscopes. *Gastrointest Endosc* Vol. 58, pp.1-8.

ASGE (2008). Standards of Practice Committee. Sedation and anaesthesia in Gastrointestinal Endoscopy. *Gastrointest Endosc* 2008; Bol 68, pp 815-826.

ASGE (2010). Minimum staffing requirements for the performance of gastrointestinal endoscopy. *Gastrointest Endosc* Vol. 72, pp. 469-470.

Bell G.D. (2004). Preparation, premedication and surveillance. *Endoscopy* Vol. 36, pp. 23-31.

Ciancio A., Manzini P., Castagno F., D'Antico S., Reynaudo P., Coucourde L., Ciccone G., DelPiano M., Ballare M., Peyre S., Rizzi R., Barletti C., De Angelis C., Morgando A., Musso A., Repici A., Rizzetto M. & Saracco G. (2005). Digestive endoscopy is not a major risk factor for transmitting hepatitis C virus. *Ann Intern Med* Vol 142,No.11, (Jun2005) pp. 903-903. ISSN:0003-4819.

Cohen L.B., Delegge M.H., Aisenberg J., Brill J.V., Inadomi J.M., Kochman M.L., Piokowski J.D., Jr & AGA Institute (2007). AGA Institute review of endoscopic sedation. *Gastroenterology* Vol. 133, No.2, (August 2007) pp. 675-701. ISSN:0016-5058.

Digestive Health Foundation (2007). Standards for endoscopic facilities and services. *Gastrointestinal Society of Australia*. 3rd Edition.

Dominici P., Bellantani S., DiBiase A.R., Saccoccio G., Le Rose A., Massuti F., Viola L., Balli F., Tiribelli C., Grilli R., Fussilo M. & Grossi E. (1999). Familial clustering of Helicobacter pylori infection: population based study. *BMJ* Vol. 319, No. 7209, (August 1999) pp. 537-540. ISSN: 0959-8138.

Hanson P.J., Gor D., Jeffries D.J. & Collins J.V. (1990). Elimination of high titre HIV from fibreoptic endoscopes. *Gut* Vol. 31, No. 6, pp. 657-659, ISSN: 0017-5749.

Ihekweazu C., Anya J. & Anosike E. (2005).Nigerian Medical Graduates: where are they now? *Lancet* Vol. 365, No. 9474 pp. 1847-1848, ISSN: 0140-6736.

Labonte R., Packer C& Kalassen I.V. (2006). Managing health professional migration from sub-Saharan African to Canada: a stakeholder inquiry into policy options. *Hum Resour Health* Vol. 4, (August 2006) pp. 22, ISSN: 0160-4198.

Ladep N.G., Sule J., Umar S.M., Obienu O., Anyanechi C., & Okeke E.N. (2008). Oesophageal variceal band ligation using a saeed six-shooter multiband ligator, experience at Jos University Teaching Hospital, Nigeria: case report. *Niger J med* Vol. 17. No.1 (Jan-March 2008) pp. 110-111, ISSN: 1115-2613.

Lazzaroni M. & Poro G.B. (2005). Preparation, premedication, and surveillance. *Endoscopy* Vol. 37, No.2, (February 2005) pp. 101-109, ISSN: 1068-9249.

Lindkvist P., Enquselassie F., Asrat D., Muhe L., Nilson I., & Giesecke J. (1998). Risk factors for infection with Helicobacter pylori - a study of children in rural Ethiopia. *Scand J Infect Dis* Vol. 30, No. 4, pp. 371-376, ISSN: 0036-5548.

Malaty H.M., Paykov V., Bykova O., Ross A., Graham D.P., Anneger J.M. & Graham D.Y. (1996). Helicobacter and Socio-economic factors in Russia. *Helicobacter* Vol. 1, No.2, (June 1996) pp. 82-87, ISSN: 1083-4389.

Mandeville K.L., Krabahuis J., Ladep N.G., Mulder C.J., Quigley E.M. & Khan SA(2009). Gastroenterology in developing countries: issues and advances. *World J Gastroenterol* Vol. 15, No.23, (June 2009),pp. 2839-2854, ISSN: 1007-9327.

McDonald G.B. & Silverstain F.E. (1976) Can gastrointestinal endoscopy transmit hepatitis B to patients? *Gastrointest Endosc* Vol. 22, No. 3, (February 1976) pp. 168-170, ISSN: 0016-5107.

McQuaid K.R. & Laihe L. (2008). A systematic review ad meta-analysis of randomized controlled trials of moderate sedation for routine endoscopic procedures. *Gastrointest Endosc* Vol. 67, No. 6, pp. 910-923, ISSN: 0016-5107.

Mullan F. (2005). The metrics of the physician brain drain. *N Engl J Med* Vol. 353, No.17, pp. 1910-1818, ISSN: 1533-4406.

Nabwera H.M., Nguyen-van, Tam J.S., Logan R.F. & Logan R.P. (2000). Prevalence of Helicobacter pylori infection in Kenyan School Children aged 3-15 years and risk factors for infection. *Eur J Gastroenterol Hepatol* Vol. 12, No.5, (May 2000) pp. 483-487, ISSN: 0954-691X.

Pond B. & McPake B. (2006). The health migration crisis: the role of four organization for Economic Cooperation and Development Countries. *Lancet* Vol. 367, No.9520, (April 2006) pp. 1448-1455, ISSN: 0140-6736.

Sandler R.S., Everhart J.E., Donowitz M., Adams E., Cronin K., Goodman C., Gemmen E., Shah S., Avdic A. & Rubin R. (2002). The burden of selected digestive diseases in the United States. *Gastroenterology* Vol. 122, No.5, (May 2002) pp. 1500-1511, ISSN: 0016-5085.

Torres J., Perez-Perez G., Goodman K.J., Atherton J.C., Gold B.D., Harris P.R., La Garza Am, Guaner J. & Munoz O. (2000). A comprehensive review of the natural history of Helicobacter pylori infection in children. *Arch Med Res* Vol. 31, No.5, (September-October 2000) pp. 431-469, ISSN: 0188-4409.

Webb P.M., Knight T., Greaves S., Wilson A., Newel D.G., Elder J. & Forman D. (1994). Relation between infection with Helicobacter pylori and living conditions in Childhood: evidence for person to person transmission in early life *BMJ* Vol. 308,, No.6931, (March 1994), pp 750-753, ISSN: 0959-8183.

World Bank (2010). How we classify countries: Retrieved September 25, 2010.

World Gastroenterology Organization [WGO], (2006). Practice guidelines: Helicobacter pylori in developing countries. Available from

http://www.worldgastroenterology.org/helicobacter-pylori-in-developing-countries.html
WGO (2007). Standards in gastroenterology training.
WHO Geneva (2008). World Health Statistics. Available from
http://www.who.int/whosis/hostat/ 2008/en/index.html

2

Evidence Based Guidelines for Preparation Before Upper Gastrointestinal Endoscopy (UGIE)

Arjuna P. De Silva
Faculty of Medicine University of Kelaniya
Sri Lanka

1. Introduction

Current endoscopic guidelines advice a 6 hour fast for solids and a 4 hours fast for liquids before UGIE[1], while most anaesthesia guidelines advice a 6 hour fast for solids and a 2 hour fast for clear liquids[1,2]. The purpose for fasting before UGIE is two fold. The first is the same as in anaesthesia prior to surgery, to prevent the aspiration of food contents[3]. The second, which is specific for endoscopy, is to provide clear vision[4]. However, prolonged fasting may result in patient discomfort and undue stress[5]. Due to practical delays the fasting period for endoscopy can become much longer than the stipulated six hours, thus causing even more patient discomfort. This may become especially difficult to tolerate for patients with gastro-esophageal reflux disease (GERD). Physiological studies have shown that clear fluids leave the stomach rapidly[6], and several anesthetic guidelines now recommend a 2-hour pre-operative fast for clear fluids and a 6-h fast for solids before general anesthesia[2,7]. A pilot study done by us on 20 patients using real-time ultrasonography showed the time taken for a clear liquid (plain tea) or water to empty from the stomach was one hour.

The second issue with the guidelines was that these guidelines focus on a Western type diet[1]. Rice is the staple diet in many Asian countries which include more than half the worlds population. Rice consumption is also increasing in many western societies[8]. Normally, the proximal part of the stomach acts as a reservoir for food and the distal end acts as the grinder[9]. Gastric emptying in normal subjects is complicated process, and is affected by,various meal related factors like the fat content, consistency and the size of the meal[10]. However, patient dependant factors like age, sex and body mass index (BMI) have been shown to have no significant association with gastric emptying[11]. In a pilot study using real time ultrasound scanning we found that the time taken for complete gastric emptying after a standard rice meal was 10 hours. To the best of our knowledge there are no published guidelines on endoscopic preparation for a rice based diet. We therefore decided to investigate whether a six hour fast after a rice based meal was sufficient prior to UGIE.

2. Aims

The aim of the first study was to determine whether a 6-hour fast for solids and a one-hour fast for water prior to UGIE gives good endoscopic vision and less patient discomfort.

The aim of the second study was to determine whether a six hour fast after a standard rice based meal is sufficient to achieve good endoscopic vision during UGIE.

2.1 Methods (1)

Consecutive patients referred for UGIE to the Professorial Medical Unit of the Colombo North Teaching Hospital, Ragama, Sri Lanka, between the ages of 18 to 65 years, who were not pregnant, and had no alarm symptoms previous gastric surgery or clinically obvious motility problems were recruited from 2005 September to 2006 August. Patients on drugs known to affect gastrointestinal motility and acid secretion were requested to stop them for two weeks prior to endoscopy. Patients who could not / refused to comply were excluded from the study. All patients gave informed written consent.

All patients were given a standard meal consisting of two slices of bread and jam 6 hours before endoscopy. Patients were then randomized, using a computer generated random allocation table, to either nil by mouth for 6 hours (Group A) or no solids for six hours but allowed to drink water according to thirst for up to one hour prior to endoscopy (Group B). Patients in Group B were requested to keep a record of the amount of water they drank. Just prior to endoscopy patients were requested to indicate any discomfort due to fasting on a visual analog scale (0 - no discomfort, to 10 - severe discomfort). The endoscopist was blinded to the period of fasting but not to the indication for endoscopy. Endoscopies were performed in the afternoon because patients were given the standard meal in the morning. Commencing at 7 am meals were given to consecutive patients at twenty minute intervals, in order to maintain uniform periods of fasting. Before endoscopy, sterile water was aspirated through the suction channel and then drained dry. All patients had throat spray before endoscopy, and pulse-oxymetry during endoscopy. Endoscopies were performed by the same operator. Endoscopic vision was graded as good, average or poor. During endoscopy, any fluid in the gastric fundus was aspirated and the volume and pH of the aspirate were measured. Endoscopies were recorded on video, and two other endoscopists (ASD and HJdeS), independently assessed the adequacy of endoscopic vision. Patients were seen in the out-patient clinic one week later to detect any late complications.

2.1.1 Ethical clearance and trial registration

Ethical approval for this study was obtained from the Ethics Committee of the Faculty of Medicine, University of Kelaniya, Sri Lanka.

2.1.2 Statistics

We assumed that 50% of patients awaiting endoscopy will have discomfort due to fasting. By allowing them to drink water up to one hour prior to endoscopy we expected to reduce this to 20%. We calculated that a sample size of 80 was needed to give the study 80% power at $\alpha = 0.05$. The outcome variables were, endoscopic visibility, pH of gastric content, the number of patients with fluid in the gastric fundus, and the level of patient discomfort due to fasting. Statistical significance of the difference between the two groups was tested using the Mann-Whitney U test for continuous variables and Fisher's Exact Test for categorical variables. Kappa was used to calculate the degree of agreement between the endoscopist and the two independent assessors who viewed videos of the endoscopies. The p values are presented uncorrected for multiple testing.

2.2 Methods (2)

After informed written consent, consecutive patients referred for UGIE, to the Professorial Medical Unit of the Colombo North Teaching Hospital, Ragama, Sri Lanka, between the ages of 18 to 65 years, who were not pregnant, and had no alarm symptoms, previous gastric surgery or clinically obvious motility problems were recruited from September 2007 to June 2008 (Table 1).

Variables	R6	R10	P value
Number of patients Randomized	105(49.5%)	107(50.5%)	
Male : Female	47:58	56 :51	0.270*
Median age (Range) years	40(18 - 65)	44(18 - 65)	0.082*
GERD Symptoms	82	76	0.238*
Dyspeptic symptoms	20	27	0.278*
Non specific abdominal pain	3	4	0.072*

Table 1. Demographic and endoscopic findings of patients

Patients on drugs known to affect gastrointestinal motility and acid secretion were requested to stop them for two weeks prior to endoscopy. Patients who could not or refused to comply with this request were excluded from the study. Patients were then given a standard rice meal, which contained rice, dhal and an egg. All meals were isocaloric, and the caloric value of meals was calculated assuming a daily requirement of 2500 kcal (Table 2).

Standard Meal	Unit	Energy per unit (kcal)*	Total energy (kcal)
(Parboiled) White Rice 200g	per 100 g	371	742
Egg, whole, cooked, hard-boiled (one)	1 large = 50g	78	78
Lentils, mature seeds, cooked, boiled, with salt 100g	per 100 g	114	114
Total energy provided			934

Table 2. The standard rice based meal

U.S. Department of Agriculture, Agricultural Research Service (USDA:ARS) 1998 USDA Nutrient Database

The patients were then randomized into two groups in preparation for UGIE: fasting for 6 hours after the rice meal (R6) or fasting for 10 hours after the rice meal (R10). All patients were given the meal at 7 am and endoscopies were performed in the afternoon. Endoscopies were done using Olympus GIF 0145 video endoscopes. All endoscopies were performed by two operators (MN and UK). The endoscopists were blinded to the period of fasting, but not to the indication for endoscopy. Another endoscopist (JM), who was also blinded to the period of fasting, was present during all endoscopies and independently graded endosocopic vison. Endoscopic vision was graded as poor, average or good. If there was any discrepancy between the two endoscopist, grading the lower was taken. All patients were reviewed in the out-patient clinic one week later to detect any late complications.

2.2.1 Ethical clearance and trial registration

Ethical approval for this study was obtained from the Ethics Committee of the Faculty of Medicine, University of Kelaniya, Sri Lanka. Trial registration number: SLCTR/2008/004.

2.2.2 Statistics

We calculated that 105 subjects in each arm will give the study 80% power at an alpha of 0.05. We expected the percentage of subjects with good endoscopic vision to be 90% in R10 group compared to about 75% seen in our clinical practice (R6). The association between the different grades of endoscopic vision and period of fasting was assessed using the Extended Mantel-Haenszel X^2 test for trend in Winpepi (Abramson, J.H. WINPEPI (PEPI-for-Windows): computer programs for epidemiologists. Epidemiologic Perspectives & Innovations 2004, 1:6). Kappa was used to calculate the degree of agreement between the endoscopist and the independent assessor who viewed the endoscopies. The p values are presented uncorrected for multiple testing.

2.3 Results (1)

190 Patients were referred to us for endoscopy during the study period (Figure 1).

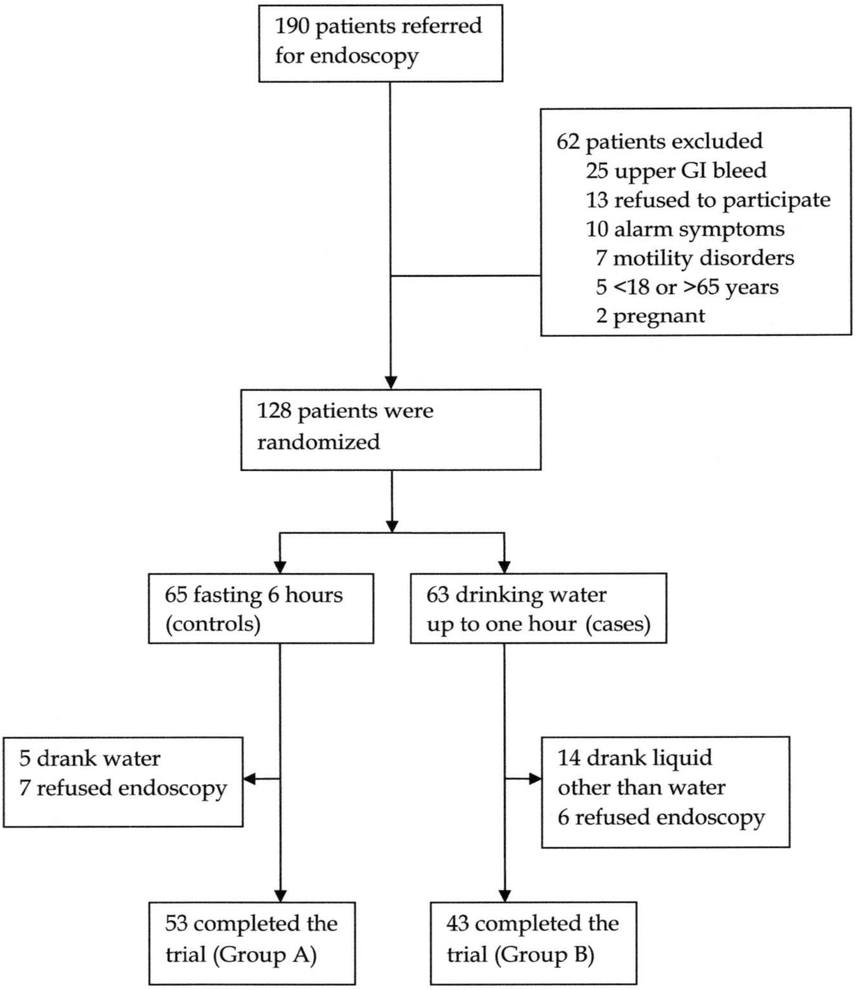

Fig. 1. Trial profile

62 were excluded. 128 were randomized to the two interventions, 65 to nil by mouth (Group A) and 63 to those allowed to drink water according to their thirst for up to one hour prior to endoscopy (Group B). The two groups were comparable for age and gender (Table 3).

32 patients (12 in group A and 20 in group B) did not complete the study; 19 had not followed instructions regarding pre-endoscopy preparation, 13 refused endoscopy after randomization (Figure 1). 96 patients completed the study; 53 in group and 43 in group B. All patients in group B had consumed at least 200 ml water (range 200 to 410) before endoscopy. Discomfort due to fasting was significantly lower in group B than in group A. According to the endoscopist, endoscopic vision was good in all 53 patients in group A and 40 patients in group B, and average in 3 patients in group B. None were graded as poor. There was good agreement between the endoscopist and independent assessors who viewed the videos of the endoscopies (Kappa= 0.64) (Table 3).

Fluid in the gastric fundus was noted in 11 patients in group A and 16 in group B. There were no significant differences in volume or pH of the gastric aspirate between the two groups. There were no complications attributable to the endoscopy in either group.

Variables	**Group A**	**Group B**	**P value**
Number of patients randomized	65	63	
Male : Female	32:33	31:32	0.9*
Median age (Range) years	48 (18-65)	49 (20-64)	0.9***
Indications of Endoscopy			
GERD Symptoms	35	33	0.88*
Dyspeptic symptoms	23	18	0.48*
Non specific abdominal pain	7	12	0.33*
Number of patients completed trial	53	43	
Male: Female	29:24	24:19	0.42*
Median age (Range) years	49(19-65)	48(20-64)	0.91**
Visual analog score [Median (IQR)] for discomfort	9.7(9.6-9.8)	5.6(4.3-8.5)	<0.0001**
Endoscopic vision			
Endoscopist	Good 53 Average 0	Good 40 Average 3	
Independent Assessor 1	Good 50 Average 3	Good 40 Average 3	0.00 $[1.1^{-19}]$***
Independent Assessor 2	Good 52 Average 1	Good 41 Average 2	
Number of Patients with fluid in the gastric fundus (%)	11(21%)	16(37%)	0.12*
Volume of gastric aspirate (ml) [Median (Range)]	8(0-65)	10 (0-78)	0.56**
pH of gastric aspirate[Median(Range)]	1.3(0.9-6.3)	2.9(0.9-5)	0.99**
Principal endoscopic diagnosis (%)			
GERD	18 (34%)	24 (56%)	0.04*
Gastritis	17 (32%)	6 (14%)	0.054*
Esophageal / gastric varices	6 (11%)	1 (2%)	0.13*
Gastric ulcer	2 (4%)		
Normal	10 (19%)	12 (28%)	0.33*

Table 3. Demography and indication for endoscopy in patients

2.4 Results (2)

A total of 335 patients were referred to us for endoscopy during the study period. Of these, 123 were excluded (61 had upper GI bleeding, 23 did not give consent, 15 had alarm symptoms, 6 had motility problems, 5 were <18 years or >65 years old, 8 not able to comply with the request for cessation of medication, 5 were pregnant). 212 patients were randomized to the two interventions: 107 to the R10 group and 105 to the R6 group. The two groups were comparable for age, gender and indications for enoscopy (Table 4). In the R10 group endoscopic vision was graded as poor in 2 (1.9%), average in 7 (6.5%), and good in 98 (91.5%), while in the R6 group it was graded as poor in 30 (28.6%), average in 19 (18.1%), good in 56 (53.3%). The observed difference of percentages among the two groups for endoscopic vision was significant (M-H Chi-Square for trend=25.67; df=1; P<0.001). There was good agreement between the endoscopists and the independent assessor who witnessed the endoscopies (Kappa = 0.97). There were no immediate or late complications due to endoscopy.

Variable	R6 (n=105)	R10 (n=107)	X^2	P value
Endoscopic vision				
Endoscopist	Good 56 (53.3%) Average 19 (18.1%) Poor 30 (28.6%)	Good 98 (91.6%) Average 7 (6.5%) Poor 2 (1.9%)	41.478	<0.0001**
Independent Assessor	Good 58 (55.2%) Average 19 (18.1%) Poor 28 (26.7%)	Good 99 (92.5%) Average 6 (5.6%) Poor 2 (1.9%)	39.985	<0.0001**
Number of Patients with fluid in the gastric fundus (%)	21 (20.0%)	25 (22.9%)	0.353	0.552*
Principal endoscopic diagnosis (%)				
GERD	22 (21.1%)	19 (17.8%)	0.347	0.556*
Gastritis	29 (27.6%)	36 (33.6%)	0.905	0.341*
Peptic Ulcers	12 (11.4%)	12 (11.2%)	0.002	0.961*
Bile reflux	1 (0.9%)	1 (0.9%)	0.000	0.989*
Any other pathology	3 (2.8%)	7 (6.5%)	1.601	0.206*
Normal	38 (36.2%)	32 (29.9%)	0.946	0.331*

*Based on Pearson Chi-square Value

**Based on Extended Mantel-Haenszel X^2 test for trend

Table 4. Endoscopic findings of patients

3. Conclusions

We have shown that a 6-hour fast for solids and one-hour fast for water prior to UGIE, gives good endoscopic vision and causes minimum patient discomfort. This confirms the results of an earlier study done more than 10 years ago[12,13]. Our study was designed mainly to assess the quality of endoscopic vision and patient discomfort. Even though we did not detect any complications, we admit that the numbers studied are too small to make firm conclusions regarding safety. As none of our patients were sedated, our results on safety may not be applicable to situations where sedation prior to endoscopy is routine.

Although the American Society for Gastrointestinal Endoscopy guidelines for UGIE advices fasting for at least 4 hours for liquids[1], we advised our controls to fast for 6 hours since this is the current practice in our unit, and some guidelines still advice 6 hours fasting for both solids and liquids. This may have had some effect on the degree of patient discomfort indicated by our controls. Another shortcoming in our study was the high drop out rate after randomization. Even though the instructions given were simple, several patients failed to follow them. Most patients who ultimately refused to undergo endoscopy expressed apprehension regarding the procedure.

Prolonged fasting for solids and clear liquids prior to endoscopy still remains in many guidelines[1]. Prolonged fasting for clear fluids is illogical because the stomach secretes up to 50ml of acidic fluid per hour even in the fasting state, and empties rapidly after ingestion of clear fluids[14]. This would explain why the volume and pH of gastric aspirate was similar in the two groups in our study; the fluid aspirated in Group B was more likely to be gastric secretion than any residual ingested water[15]. Endoscopic vision is affected when patients drink milk[16]. For this reason we allowed our patients to drink only water. To maximize practicalities we allowed them to drink water according to their thirst. As various types of food can affect the rate of gastric emptying we used a standard meal[11]. We also attempted to eliminate observer bias by having two other independent assessors.

In conclusion allowing patients to drink water for up to one hour prior to endoscopy together with a 6-hour fast for solids seems to be preferred by patients, and does not hamper endoscopic vision. Two studies done on two different populations more than ten years apart have now shown similar results[5].

We recommend that current guidelines on preparation for patients undergoing UGIE be reviewed.

Our second study shows that fasting for 6 hours after a rice based meal is inadequate to provide good vision during UGIE. Fasting for 10 hours significantly improves endoscopic vision. Our finding has several implications. Firstly, if patients consume a rice meal and fast for six hours they may be potentially at risk for aspiration. Although we did not encounter this complication, we admit that the numbers studied were too small to make firm conclusions regarding safety. Secondly, poor vision would hamper detection of lesions and would necessitate repeating the procedure. Thirdly, endoscopist may wrongly assume that these patients have slow gastric emptying and subject them to unnecessary and costly investigations. Our study also has implications for patients being prepared for general anaesthesia before surgery as none of the anaesthetic guidelines specify the period of fasting required after a rice based meal[17].

In an attempt to reduce individual bias as much as possible two operators performed all the endoscopies. We also attempted to reduce observer bias by having another independent assessor. The agreement between them was good, and whenever there was any disagreement on endoscopic vision grading between the endoscopist and the independent assessor, the lower grading was used. We did not attempt to measure the volume of left over food in the stomach.

In conclusion, patients consuming a rice based meal prior to UGIE need to fast for at least ten hours prior to the procedure in order to obtain good endoscopic vision Current guidelines need to be re-evaluated for populations where rice is the staple diet, and this is especially important in the Asian setting.

Based largely on the evidence of our studies we have suggested that the following guidelines be used before for preparation for upper GI endoscopy in the Asian setting.

1. Patients can eat two slices of bread with jam six hours before the procedure.
2. Clear liquids mainly water, plain tea, or king coconut water may be consumed according to thirst up to one hour before the procedure
3. Patients who consume a rice based meal will have to fast for at least ten hours.
4. Patients may take their medications before the procedure.
5. These guidelines apply to patients between 18 to 65 yr and who do not have any obvious motility disorders. Other patients may need longer fasting time.

4. References

[1] A SAGES Co endorsed ASGE guidelines. Preparation of patients for gastrointestinal endoscopy. 2006. http://www. asges.org.
[2] Canadian Anesthetists' Society's new guidelines for fasting in elective/emergency patients. Can J Anaesth 1990; 37: 905-6.
[3] Brady M, Kinn S, Stuart P. Preoperative fasting for adults to prevent perioperative complications. Cochrane Database Syst Rev; 2003:4CD004423.
[4] Faigel D, A SAGES Co Endorsed ASGE Guidelines. Preparation of patients for gastrointestinal endoscopy, 2006. Cited ** Available from URL: http//www.asges.org (Accessed 10 Jan 2009).
[5] Ljungqvist O, Soreide E. Preoperative fasting. Br J Surg 2003; 90: 400406.
[6] Hunt JN, Spurrell WR. The pattern of emptying of the human stomatch . J Physiol 1951; 113: 157-68.
[7] American Society of Anaethesiologist Task Force on Preoperative Fasting. Practice guidelines for preoperative fasting and the use of pharmacologic agents to reduce the risk of pulmonary aspiration:application to healthy patients undergoing elctive procedures. Anaesthesiology 1999;79:482-5.
[8] FAO. Food outlook. November 2008 page 15. URL: http//www.fao.org/docret/011/ai474e/ai474e05.htm (Accessed 10 January 2009).
[9] Minami II, MCallum RW. The physiology and pathophysiology of gastric emptying in humans. Gastroenterology 1984; 86: 1592-1610.
[10] Hunt JN. Mechanisms and disorders of gastric emptying. Annu Rev Med. 1983;34:219-29.
[11] Camilleri M. Integrated upper gastrointestinal response to food intake. Gastroenterology 2006;131:640-58.
[12] De Silva AP, Amarasiri L, Liyanage MN, Kottachchi D, Dassanayake AS, de Silva HJ. One-hour fast for water and six-hour fast for solids prior to endoscopy provides good endoscopic vision and results in minimum patient discomfort. J Gastroenterol Hepatol (in press).
[13] Webster GJ, Boling TE, Greenfield SM, Hallyburton E, Kuarn AM, Vicary FR, Beck ER. Assessment of residual gastric volume and thirst in patients who drink before gastroscopy. Gut 1996; 39: 360-2.
[14] Philips S, Hutchinson A, Davidson T. Preoperative drinking does not affect gastric contents. Br J Anaesth 1993; 70: 6-9.
[15] Hutchinson A, Maltby JR, Reid CRG. Gastric fluid volume and pH in elective inpatients. Part I: coffee or orange juice versus overnight fast. Can J Anaesth 1988; 35: 12-15.
[16] Webster GJ, Boling TE, Greenfield SM, Hallyburton E, Kuarn AM, Vicary FR, Beck ER. Drinking before endoscopy, milk or water? Gastrointest Endosc 1997; 45: 406-8.

3

Sedation Related to Gastrointestinal Endoscopy

Mitrut Paul, Mitrut Anca Oana,
Streba Liliana, Calina Daniela and Salplahta Daniel
University of Medicine and Pharmacy of Craiova
Romania

1. Introduction

In the last ten years the number of worldwide gastrointestinal endoscopic procedures has significantly increased; the majority are ambulatory endoscopies with appropriate intravenous sedation and analgesia which seems to be used more and more frequent.

By definition, sedation is a drug-induced depression in the level of consciousness. Moderate sedation current terminology replaces the previous terminology called conscious sedation (American Society of Anesthesiologists [ASA], 2002). Sedation and analgesia are being used in order to improve patient tolerance to endoscopic procedures by diminishing anxiety and discomfort. There are several sequent benefits: an adequate sedation allows the endoscopist to focus on the technical performance of the endoscopy, increases the rate of patients returning for follow-up examinations or for colonoscopic screening, prevents potentially harmful autonomic stress responses and improves the public reputation of the procedure. However, these benefits must be weighed against the complications (especially in the form of potential compromise of ventilatory function) and the added cost associated with the use of sedation and analgesia.

Patients with associated comorbidities address to the gastroscopist to perform an endoscopy without being evaluated for their pathologies that could influence the procedures used in sedation. In addition, in cases where the examination is more invasive or conducted in a larger time interval, the level of sedation should be optimized to achieve an ideal procedure (ASA, 2002; Faigel *et al.*, 2002).

The practice of sedation varies from country to country, determined by cultural differences in pain perception and expectations of patients and physicians. A recent international study of 21 centers in 10 European countries and in Canada reported that the use of sedation during endoscopy varies from 0% to 100% at different sites: it was used in 44% of all procedures in Asia, 56% in Europe, and 72% in Canada, Central America and South Latin America. In the United States, only flexible sigmoidoscopy is performed without sedation (Wang&Lin, 1999). Such diversity reflects social, cultural, regulatory and economic consideration.

Best practices for analgesia and sedation during gastrointestinal endoscopy are still debated. Ensuring an adequate sedation and analgesia influences some aspects of endoscopic procedures such as quality of examination, patient cooperation, patient and performing physician satisfaction (Bell, 2004).

There are several practical issues with implications for endoscopic sedation (Thomson *et al.*, 2010):

- gastrointestinal endoscopic procedures have short duration, there is no need of skin incisions, there are not associated with significant changes in body fluids and do not require medication to eliminate the post-exploratory discomfort
- most procedures are performed ambulatory, as cases of "single day admission"
- the level of sedation necessary to prevent discomfort during the procedure may be adjusted depending on the situation
- many patients are medically well, presenting only for screening
- during endoscopic procedures patients are not intubated, the airway remains open

There are also disadvantages: more time for post procedural patient's recovery, higher costs, does not allow patients to leave the endoscopy unit immediately after the procedure and return to work after the sedation or analgesia.

To obtain maximum benefit it is desirable for gastrointestinal endoscopy to have a building designed or adapted specifically for this purpose, so that patients can be treated safely, quickly and efficiently.

Medical clinics with "one day" profile, fit for the activity of digestive endoscopy, are usually self clinics (individual or collective), with one basic specialty, with individual financial assurance for the location, secured space, related facilities, personnel policy and independent accounting and financial management which enables maximum efficiency for development. These can also be clinics attached to the base hospital or ambulatory clinical departments.

These "one day" clinics have in general in the operational structure their own specialized diagnostic services through clinical, paraclinical and laboratory investigations designed to substantiate both gastrointestinal endoscopy indication and anesthetic-endoscopic protocol which is to be established by the anesthesiologist in collaboration with the physician and patient. On this occasion, the staff repeated contact with the patients creates an atmosphere of trust and mutual affection beneficial in relation to the gastrointestinal endoscopy which is expected to be made.

Endoscopy room should be equipped with: good lighting, air conditioning, centralized administration of medical fluids, modern equipment for anesthesia and monitoring, pulse oximeter, resuscitation equipment (Sitcai, 2005).

2. Technical specifications

2.1 Patient selection and appropriate investigation (Lytle, 2005)

In carrying out a gastrointestinal (GI) endoscopy under anesthesia is very important that gastroenterologists agree with anesthesiologist about GI exploration that follows and about patient selection criteria. The initial selection of patients is done by the gastroenterologist. To reduce the cancellation from the day of GI endoscopy is better for patients to be interviewed personally or by phone by the anesthesiologist a few days before the planned GI endoscopy. The check performed by the anaesthesiologist is very important to identify cases that require precautions or contraindications for a particular type of medicine used to sedate patients. To save time there are very useful questionnaires completed by the patients containing simple questions about general state of health.

In general, patients admitted for GI exploration are from ASA I class and ASA II class. Patients with chronic respiratory disease, hypertension or symptomatic cardiovascular disease have a higher risk of developing complications, but diabetes mellitus, bronchial asthma (AB), smoking and age are not necessarily problematic; biological age is more important than chronological age.

2.1.1 Selection criteria of patients for sedation in gastrointestinal endoscopy in an ambulatory unit (Lytle, 2005)

- ASA I and II
- Age 6 months – 70 years
- Patient weight – preferably BMI < 30
- - BMI = 31-34 – anesthesiologist decides if recommends sedation
- - BMI > 35: not recommended for sedation in ambulatory endoscopy, only in hospitals
- Good general condition (eg. the patient can safely climb two floors)

2.1.2 Exclusion criteria of patients for sedation in gastrointestinal endoscopy in an ambulatory unit (Lytle, 2005)

- Cardiovascular: history of heart attack, hypertension (diastolic arterial blood pressure > 100 mmHg), angina (angina crisis > 3 times/week or during effort), arrhythmias, cardiac insufficiency
- Respiratory: upper respiratory tract infection, corticodependent bronchial asthma or asthma that requires chronic beta 2 agonists treatment, COPD
- Metabolic disorders: chronic alcohol consumption, insulin-dependent diabetes, renal failure, liver disorders
- Neurological: stroke or transient ischemic attack, hard controlled epilepsy
- Drugs: steroids, MAOIs, anticoagulants, antiarrhythmics
- Blood: sickle cell anemia, hemophilia, anemia after gastrointestinal bleeding
- History of drug allergies or anesthesia problems

2.1.3 Minimum investigation required for sedation in ambulatory gastrointestinal endoscopy (Lytle, 2005)

- Weight
- Height
- Body mass index (BMI)
- Blood pressure measurement
- Hemoleucogram if indicated (eg in case of menorrhagia)
- Serum ionogram, after treatment with diuretics
- ECG in patients over 60 years

Patient preparation is very important for sedation in ambulatory gastrointestinal endoscopy. During the pre-endoscopic examination, patients receive an informed consent about the risks of intravenous sedation. They also receive information leaflets and get the opportunity to ask questions (Clarks, 2007).

Patients will initially be consulted and informed in writing about the medication which will be given, will be instructed not to drive vehicles and not to work with machinery 24 – 48 hours after the investigation, to avoid alcohol, to avoid the use of sedatives and to not sign official and financial documents. Antihypertensive medication should be continued with the morning dose, hypoglycemic medication instead should be omitted.

Attempting to improve the patient understanding of the procedure, the presentation of video movies is not recommended because it may increase anxiety and therefore need higher doses of analgesics, especially in women (Bytzer & Lindeberg, 2007).

2.2 Pharmacology of drugs for sedation and analgesia

There are four stages of sedation defined by the American Society for Anesthesiology (ASA) that range from minimal to moderate, deep and general anesthesia: minimal sedation or anxiolysis (a drug-induced relief of apprehension with minimal effect on consciousness), moderate sedation (a depression of consciousness in which the patient can respond purposely to verbal or light tactile stimuli and spontaneous ventilation and cardiovascular function are maintained), deep sedation (the patient may not be able to maintain airway reflexes or spontaneous ventilation, but cardiovascular function is usually maintained) and general anesthesia (airway intervention is often required and cardiovascular function is usually maintained) (ASA, 2002).

Ideally, the patient should be slightly sedated (eg. drowsiness, but able to be waked up), with no pain, keeping the airway open, maintaining respiratory reflexes, being able to cooperate but unable to remember the procedure, without feeling anxiety and fear (Thomson *et al*, 2010).

During endoscopic sedation, some complications that must be avoided may arise: eg. worsening of the patient, lack of physical and verbal response to stimuli, loss of protective airway reflexes, inability to maintain spontaneous breathing, hypoxemia/hypercapnia, cardiovascular instability (arrhythmias or hypotension) (Thomson *et al*, 2010).

2.2.1 Characteristics of ideal drug (Zuccaro, 2006) used for sedation in gastrointestinal endoscopy

- Anxiolisis
- Amnesia
- Analgesia
- Rapid onset of pharmacological effect
- Dose-proportional sedative predictable effects
- Safety on a wide range of therapeutic doses, hemodynamic stability
- No pain or irritation at the injection site
- Rapid recovery without residual sleepiness

No drug used alone has all these properties and to achieve these goals it is often used a combination of two or even three drugs. Sedation is often performed with benzodiazepines in combination with an opioid for pain relief; a barbiturate hypnotic agent can be added only if there is required a deeper sedation.

All pharmacological agents used produce temporary mild depression in lung and cardiopulmonary function, especially when they are used in combination. This justifies the need for appropriate monitoring by direct observation by the anesthesiologist and monitoring equipment in the endoscopy room.

2.2.2 Types of drugs currently used for sedation in gastrointestinal endoscopy

The choice of sedatives depends on the endoscopist's preference and the type of procedure, but generally benzodiazepines are used alone or in combination with an opiate (frequently used for synergism).

The most commonly used benzodiazepines are midazolam and diazepam. The efficacy of sedation with these two benzodiazepines is comparable. Midazolam is now the preferred benzodiazepine more than diazepam because of its short duration of action and improved safety profile. Benzodiazepines used in most endoscopic procedures produce sedation, amnesia, anxiolisis, have anticonvulsant effects and muscle relaxing effects but have no effect on pain. These actions are considered to be the result of binding to gamma-amino butyric acid (GABA) receptors in the central nervous system. Anxiolytic and muscle relaxing properties are not only mediated through GABA receptors, but also by glycine receptors in the spinal cord (Snyder *et al*, 1977). Respiratory depression is probably linked to a direct effect on the respiratory center in the brain, leading to hypoventilation and is an important side effect. Cardiovascular instability with decreased cardiac output and peripheral resistance and consequent hypotension usually occur only during deep sedation (Horn & Nesbit, 2004).

The benzodiazepine initially used in endoscopy was diazepam. However, for diazepam half-life was estimated between 24 and 57 hours, and its metabolites have also sedative properties. This means that it takes a long time to remove the effects, which often lasts until the next day. It is therefore an unsuitable agent for day procedures.

A new pharmacological sedative agent, midazolam, is now very commonly used in the practice of endoscopic sedation. This is a short-acting benzodiazepine; with good amnesic effect during the procedure (it does not cause amnesia before or after the endoscopic exploring). The half-life is less than one tenth compared to diazepam, and therefore, it is removed from the blood very quickly. Moreover, its metabolites have short-acting and do not have sedative properties. Dosages range from 1-5 mg (0.015-0.07 mg/kg).

Midazolam has few side effects and, if they occur are not serious. Respiratory depression is the most important adverse effect. It was also described a paradoxal response to midazolam with agitation instead of induced sedation (Yi&Shin, 2005) and is probably more common in the elderly (Horn&Nesbit, 2004). Pharmacological effects of midazolam may be antagonized by the administration of flumazenil, which competitively blocks GABA receptors. Other side effects: nasal itching, rash, dizziness, anxiety, irritability, dreams, seizures and unusual or involuntary muscle movements. Midazolam is contraindicated in patients with myasthenia gravis, acute glaucoma, in patients known to be allergic to this class of drugs. Caution should be exercised in patients with severe lung disease, COPD in particular (Horn & Nesbit, 2004).

From opioid class, fentanyl and meperidine are commonly used, endoscopic sedation with fentanyl being preferred by younger endoscopists. Endoscopic sedation with propofol is only made by the anesthesiologist (SAA, 2002, Faigel *et al*, 2002). Opioids have strong analgesic effect. In Australia, fentanyl is the most commonly used opiate, (Padmanabhan& Leslie, 2008; Clarke *et al*, 2002) and there is also significant use of pethidine. A London group showed a shorter recovery period for patients undergoing endoscopy if fentanyl and midazolam are used together, compared with the use of pethidine and midazolam, and there was no difference in pain perception (Hayee *et al*, 2009).

Fentanyl is a short acting opioid and is often used in combination with midazolam. The analgesic effect of fentanyl lasts about thirty minutes. These properties make it suitable for use in short-term exploration. The major side effect is respiratory distress and hypertension that may occur in one minute or less from the drug injection. It can also determine the decrease of heart rate (bradycardia). Hypovolemic patients and those with respiratory illnesses are particularly at risk of developing these complications (Horn &Nesbit, 2004). Fentanyl is contraindicated in patients taking first-generation MAOI drugs. Special precautions: pregnancy - safe use of fentanyl has not been established in the first three months of pregnancy, and therefore should be used only if potential benefits outweigh possible risks; lactation - not known whether fentanyl is excreted in breast milk, so fentanyl should be avoided in nursing mothers, although it has no clear contraindications (Qureshi *et al*, 2005).

Opioids and benzodiazepines are used for analgesia and anxiolisis. When they are used alone, the incidence of respiratory complications is quite low. In contrast, the rate of complications increases several times when both drugs are administered in combination. It should be noted that both pharmacological effects and side effects of benzodiazepines and opioids are synergistic, so that these drugs must be used carefully. Sedative effects are dose dependent and there is a substantial synergism between narcotics and benzodiazepines. Although traditional management was using progressive increasing doses, one study found that in healthy patients under the age of 65, colonoscopy could be initiated by the administration of a standardized dose expressed in mg/kg body weight, followed by endoscopic procedure performed 2 minutes later, with improved technical efficiency and without loss of patient satisfaction (Morrow *et al*, 2000).

Use of benzodiazepines and opioids provides some important benefits, including a long history of safety, effectiveness and widespread acceptance by non-anesthesiologists (Arrowsmithet al, 1991). In addition, the existence of specific pharmacological antagonists for benzodiazepines and opioids give these drugs a high level of safety compared with other classes of drugs.

Typically, recovery from sedation in GI endoscopy is gradual and pleasant. However, specific antagonist for benzodiazepine and opioid drugs should be available in the endoscopy room in an emergency (rare) for the rapid antagonizing of the sedative effects produced by the drug. For example, Flumazenil is a specific benzodiazepine receptor antagonist that acts within seconds while Naloxone is an opioid antagonist which antagonizes the respiratory depressant and analgesic effects of opioids. Naloxone is a competitive antagonist that binds μ-opioid receptors that prevents or reduces the above complications. Repeated administration may be necessary. Doses vary between 1 to 1.5 mg/kg, with lower doses in the elderly, in renal or hepatic failure. Lower doses may be necessary in patients with chronic heart and lung disease and in patients taking antidepressant MAOI of second generation.

Propofol is the recently appeared non-barbiturate intravenous anesthetic approved by FDA in 1989 as a pharmacological agent in induction and maintenance of anesthesia. Due to the rapid onset of action and short recovery period is ideal for sedation in gastrointestinal endoscopy. It increases the sedative effect of hypnotic agents, producing deep sedation depending on dose. Safe therapeutic range is narrower than of benzodizepines. It is a lipophilic drug that acts on GABA receptor subtype different from those that mediate the effects of benzodiazepines (Horn&Nesbit, 2004). Because in the propofol formulation are used soybean oil and egg lecithin, it is contraindicated in those with allergies to egg or soy protein. Propofol interacts with glycine, nicotinic and muscarinic receptors and has a direct effect on neuronal ion channels (Trapani *et al*, 2000). The duration of action is short, with the first phase of elimination usually at 2-3 minutes (Kanto&Gepts, 1989).

Propofol has a relatively small analgesic effect, and its effect is less amnesic than midazolam. In addition, it has a slightly antiemetic effect (Stark *et al*, 1985). Thus, it has a rapid onset of hypnotic action which usually occurs after a short lag time of 40 seconds (time for one arm-brain circulation). Waking up is relatively fast. It is rapidly metabolized by hepatic conjugation and excreted in urine. Its inactivation depends more on liver blood flow than

liver function. In patients with cirrhosis, the use of propofol for elective upper endoscopy does not precipitate the encephalopathy (Amoros *et al*, 2009).
Therapeutic plasma concentrations can only be estimated by the anesthesiologist, as there are no technical means besides the system called Diprifusor (injectomate), which distributes only plasma concentrations independent of the desired therapeutic effect.

POSITIVE EFFECTS	NEGATIVE EFFECTS
• Sedation • Hypnosis • Analgesia • Anticonvulsivant • Decreased intracranial pressure (reduces cerebral O_2 consumption and cerebral blood flow) • Good laryngeal relaxation	• Lowers BP during induction • Hallucinations, sexual fantasies • Respiratory depression with increased CO_2 and reduced centers sensitivity to hypoxia and hypercapnia (sleep apnea is common 1-2 min after administration – lasts a few seconds)

Table 1. Pharmacological effects of propofol

Among the effects of propofol listed in the table above (Table 1), there is to know that it produces pain when is administered into a vein in about 30% of cases, which then disappears within 1 minute. This can be controlled, if immediately before administration a mixed afentanil or lidocaine solution (1-2 ml) is used. It is contraindicated in children under 3 years both as a sedative and as an anesthetic and also during pregnancy and lactation. It should not be stored in the refrigerator and should not be used within hours of opening as it is a good medium for bacteria culture.

PROPOFOL SIDE EFFECTS				
CNS	**Cardiovascular**	**Respiratory**	**Gastrointestinal**	**Renal**
- headache - fever - dizziness - tremor - confusion - drowsiness - paresthesia - agitation - euphoria - fatigue - involuntary movements - modified dreams - vision problems	- bradycardia - hypotension - ventricular tachycardia - changes in ECG - ST segment flattening - asystole	- apnea - cough - hiccups - hypoventilation - wheezing - tachypnea - hypoxia	- nausea and vomiting - abdominal cramps - dry mouth - hypersalivation	- urinary retention - urine greenish hue

Table 2. Propofol side effects

In general, for the administration of propofol there are used two schemes:

- Combination - where a benzodiazepine and an opioid are administered intravenously (opioids may be omitted in some unstable patients and in elderly). After a pause, propofol can be administered as an infusion or by progressive increase doses.
- Propofol alone - administered as an infusion or by progressive increase doses.

If for the administration of the propofol is used the scheme, then the associated doses of fentanyl and midazolam are generally lower than if they were used without propofol. In general, if midazolam and fentanyl have been administered, the maximum dose of propofol should be 30 mg. In addition, once propofol administration started, the doses of fentanyl or midazolam should not be supplemented. In terms of approaching the "combination" scheme, an Australian study reported median total doses of 4 mg midazolam, 75 mg fentanyl and 60 mg propofol in a sample of 500 cases from a total of 28,472 patients undergoing ambulatory endoscopy. In all patients the three drugs were used (Qadeer *et al*, 2009).

In a Swiss study (Kulling *et al*, 2007) that included 27,061 patients undergoing ambulatory endoscopy, propofol was used as single agent for sedation. The initial dose of propofol was 0.5 mg/kg or 0.25 mg/kg in ASA III patients and those over 70 years, then were given additional 10-20 mg of propofol.

VanNatta and Rex from Indiana compared four schemes of sedation on a group of patients who received ambulatory colonoscopies (VanNatta & Rex, 2006). In each group the dose of propofol was increased under sedation requirements: (i) propofol alone (ii) fentanyl (50 micrograms with an optional add-on of 25 micrograms given for analgesia at the request of the endoscopist) and propofol (iii) midazolam (1 mg) and propofol and (iv) all three drugs: fentanyl (50 micrograms), midazolam (1mg) and propofol. When combination sedation was used, propofol was last administered. Those who received only propofol had the most profound sedation scores and received on average 215 mg of propofol compared with 82.5 mg in those who previously received midazolam and fentanyl. The doses of propofol in the other two groups were 140 mg (fentanyl alone group) and 125 mg (midazolam alone group). Those from the combination groups were sooner discharged from hospital. Patients from the group receiving the combination with fentanyl remembered the pain associated with the endoscopic procedure, compared with patients who received propofol alone and not remembered it. This study is important in highlighting the fact that the doses of propofol were reduced by almost 50% in association with only 1 mg of midazolam. Compared with the Australian study (Qadeer *et al*, 2009) the doses of fentanyl and midazolam were notably lower compared with higher doses in using propofol alone. In interpreting the Indiana trial one must take into account that in the study only a small number of patients (200 in total) were included.

To prevent complications related to propofol sedation in GI endoscopy, careful administration of appropriate doses is essential to avoid undesirable cardiorespiratory depression, especially in elderly and unstable patients. There is evidence that oxygen supplementation reduces the risk of hypoxemia during colonoscopy (Holm *et al*, 1999) but there are studies showing that when given supplemental oxygen, oxygen saturation levels do not reflect the ventilation function and may mask the CO_2 retention (Lazzaroni&Bianchi, 2001). However, a recent Australian study conducted by anesthesiologists showed that the use of supplemental oxygen was universal (Pena *et al*, 2005).

Preparing medical personnel in the management of airway obstruction and apnea is essential. Measures taken include: chin lift, jaw thrust, placing nasal tubes in airway and oral cavity, and for longer periods of respiratory depression, balloon and mask ventilation.

Pharmacological agents antagonizing with flumazenil and naloxone may occasionally be indicated.
Advanced respiratory ventilation measures, including the use of laryngeal masks and endotracheal intubation are rarely required in ambulatory (Rex&Deenadayalu, 2009). In patients who develop hypotension related to administration of sedative agents, intravenous fluids may be indicated.
For adults, several data suggest that sedation with propofol in endoscopic techniques may be sufficiently secure, without serious adverse events. Walker *et al* investigated the adverse events in 9,152 endoscopies (Walker *et al*, 2003). Seven patients had considerable respiratory complications and all were related to upper endoscopy, three had apnea, three had laryngospasm and one aspiration, five required assisted ventilation with face masks, but none were intubated. Rex *et al* collected data from two departments of endoscopy in the United States and one in Switzerland (Rex *et al*, 2005). Of 36,743 cases, of which about 50% were upper endoscopies, none required tracheal intubation and assisted ventilation was required in only one case from 500. There was no reported pulmonary aspiration. In all cases, propofol sedation was performed by non-anesthesiologists.
Who should administer propofol for sedation in GI endoscopy? Traditionally, the endoscopist themselves were administering sedative drugs, however recently it started being performed by a healthcare professional trained in this respect. In the U.S., 'nurse-anesthetists' have been used to manage a much selected range of sedative drugs in patients with decreased anesthetic risk in accordance to protocols. In the U.S., the use of the anesthesiologists for endoscopic sedation is very different between regions, ranging from less than 20% in most, to over 50% in states like New York and Florida (Brill, 2008). In recent years, in Australia, particularly in the private sector, the anesthesiologists were called to perform endoscopic sedation even in patients with low anesthesia risk.
Until recently, only anesthetists were allowed to administer propofol and their involvement measurably increased in performing sedated endoscopy. This fact allows the use of propofol in ambulatory and improves the quality of sedation without compromising patient safety. There is now evidence to suggest that propofol can be safely and effectively administered in ASA grade I, II and III patients by non-anesthesiologists. In a series of nearly 28,500 cases of sedated endoscopy, the sedative drugs were administered almost entirely by non-anesthetists (Qadeer *et al*, 2009) and there was no case of mortality and morbidity. In a multicenter trial (Rex&Deenadayalu, 2009) on 650,000 patients who received propofol sedation, given as unique pharmacological agent administered by a nurse under the direction of the endoscopist, there was only one death related to anesthesia. Whoever administered propofol sedation, there should be at least one properly trained individual whose sole function is to monitor the patient during the procedure. This person must possess the necessary skills and also to take necessary measures for the prevention and management of complications related to sedation.
Without being in contradiction with the above trials, the presence of anesthesiologists for sedated endoscopic procedures is mandatory in many cases, especially in the elderly and those with higher ASA classification, or if there were difficulties in intravenous sedation in the endoscopy history of the patient. In addition, complex procedures that require a longer time should not be undertaken without anesthesia support. In this regard, a recent Australian study showed that many Australian university hospitals have mentioned the presence of the anesthesiologist mandatory in sedated endoscopy (Louis *et al*, 2004).

In conclusion, propofol is a more "powerful" drug than midazolam in producing sedation, which makes it very useful in gastrointestinal endoscopic sedation, but requires a higher level of monitoring of vital functions.

Fospropofol is a pro-drug used for sedation in a variety of endoscopic procedures including colonoscopy (Fechner *et al*, 2004; Gibiansky *et al*, 2005). It is converted to propofol in a few minutes after intravenous injection and inactive metabolites: phosphate and formaldehyde (rapidly converted to formate). Therefore, the time for maximum plasma concentration is higher than for propofol and the elimination period is slower.This effect facilitates the administration, because for short-term endoscopic procedures such as upper endoscopy or colonoscopy, patients may require only one dose of fospropofol.

To improve pain control and to facilitate moderate sedation control, fospropofol is co-administered with a narcotic, typically fentanyl. Fospropofol is associated with slight increases in phosphorus serum levels after intravenous administration, but no significant clinical adverse effects are present as a result of these elevated levels of phosphorus (Fechner *et al*, 2004; Gibiansky *et al*, 2005). These apparent disadvantages were considered by the U.S. Food and Drug Administration (FDA) as "benefits" of this drug, and therefore recently approved (2008) for moderate sedation in gastroscopy. Any other requests for drugs approval to be used for deep sedation in gastroscopy were refused. FDA requires that fospropofol be used only by persons trained in general anesthesia (only anesthesist) and that all patients should be monitored continuously by the medical staff not involved itself in the endoscopic procedure.

Fospropofol does not cause pain at the injection site and is soluble in water. However, it has some side effects that are not described in propofol - particularly perineal pain or paresthesia (Fechner at al., 2004). Despite this, a preliminary report of a clinical trial indicates that patient satisfaction is very good (Pruitet al, 2005).

Droperidol is a neuroleptic butyrophenone used for conscious sedation in gastroscopy especially in the USA (Horn&Nesbit, 2004). It also has antiemetic action at low doses, explained by it occupying a GABA receptor. If it is used in the precursory period of endoscopic procedures, it can cause dysphoria, characterized by an apparent state of calm that masks in fact the anxiety generated by the endoscopic act. As a dopamine antagonist, droperidol may cause extrapyramidal side effects that can be countered by combination with promethazine or difenilhidramine. Droperidol determines cerebral vasoconstriction, but does not reduce cerebral metabolic rate, which may be detrimental to patients with cerebrovascular disease undergoing GI endoscopy. It does not produce amnesia and does not have anticonvulsant properties. Due to a weak alpha blocking action, may reduce blood pressure, significant effect in hypovolemic patients and Parkinson's disease. It protects the heart of the anti-arrhythmic effects of catecholamine release. One of the advantages of droperidol is that the response to the CO_2 does not change, moreover, given intravenously, stimulates the respiratory response to hypoxemia, which is recommended for patients with COPD premedication. Neuroleptanalgesia produced by droperidol is characterized by a similar trance state in which the patient is immobile and unresponsive to external stimuli. Analgesia is strong, allowing the endoscopic procedure. Combined with fentanyl it does not provide stronger analgesia, but extends its duration (Ionescu, 2005).

Promethazine is a powerful H1 antihistamine with antiemetic, anticholinergic, hypnotic, sedative/tranquilizing, analgesic and local anesthetic properties. It is used as an adjunct to endoscopic sedation and sedative in pediatrics.

The addition of diphenhydramine on narcotics and benzodiazepines has shown to improve sedation quality (Tu *et al*, 2006).

3. Current approaches to sedation for GI endoscopy

3.1 Unsedated endoscopy

Trials have shown that a substantial proportion of the patients from Asia, Europe and Canada are subjected to digestive endoscopic exploration without any sedation (Wang&Lin, 1999). This practice is not common in the United States of America and Australia. There is evidence that the low prevalence of endoscopy without sedation is due more to patient reserves, rather than physician preference (Faulx *et al*, 2005).

In terms of patient tolerance, a Finn double-blind trial compared intravenous midazolam alone with each of three other groups: one group without any sedation, a group that used a local pharynx anesthetic and a third control group (Ristikankare *et al*, 2004). Patients in the Midazolam group could not remember the procedure and reported desire to return to repeat the procedure. The effects were more pronounced in younger patients. Regarding the assessment of the endoscopist, patients in the Midazolam group were assessed as being easier to intubate by the endoscopist compared with placebo group, but there was no difference between Midazolam group and pharyngeal anesthesia group or control group. Interestingly, Midazolam group had a higher difficulty rating at endoscopy and retching during the procedure, compared with the pharyngeal anesthesia group.

Another trial showed that performing endoscopy without sedation was moderately less well tolerated by patients but did not require a long time for the procedure, the risks were not higher and the patients' reserves to undergo a subsequent procedure did not increase (Bonta *et al*, 2003). In this study, however, there was no control group, only blinded (both patients and endoscopists), sedation and placebo groups. More recently, it was found that male patients, patients with previous bowel resection, those with a high body mass index (BMI) and those without gynecological surgery didn't need sedation to complete colonoscopy (Tsai *et al*, 2008).

Hypnosis has also been used to facilitate endoscopy (Conlong *et al*, 1999). Compared with intravenous Midazolam, its use was associated with greater patient discomfort (assessment made by the patient), and the lack of amnesia for the procedure. A higher technical difficulty of the endoscopist was also reported. However, using hypnosis led to less patient agitation, according to assessments made by independent observers compared with patients receiving throat spray and no intravenous sedation and those receiving midazolam.

3.2 Topical anesthesia

The use of throat sprays with various local anesthetics (lidocaine, tetracaine and benzocaine) as preparation for endoscopy is widespread, although few studies have evaluated their effectiveness.

A recent meta-analysis (Evans *et al*, 2006) of five randomized controlled trials on 500 patients showed that the use of local anesthetic sprays reduced throat discomfort and technical difficulties evaluated by the endoscopist. The main adverse effects are inhibition of gag reflex and the risk of pulmonary aspiration. There have also been reported systemic adverse effects such as arrhythmias and convulsions due to absorption of topical pharmacological agent, however extremely rare.

There is a small risk of methaemoglobinemia (Kane *et al*, 2007) especially for benzocaine, and some evidence that aspiration may occur after local anesthetic with throat spray (Ertekin *et al*, 2000).

3.3 Sedation and analgesia agent used for endoscopy

A key principle of medical sedation in GI endoscopy, especially in ambulatory units where narcotic and benzodiazepines administration have a long tradition, is that drugs should be administered in incremental dosages in order to achieve the desired sedative effect. Although certain patient characteristics (such as patient age, comorbidities, body mass, race, previous responses to sedation and routine use of oral narcotics or benzodiazepines) may help pre-establish the drug dose required to achieve adequate sedation, the exact dose that will be needed for a particular patient is impossible to be accurately predicted. This is because the pharmacological response of the patient is variable and individual to specific sedative agents. Therefore, the anesthesiologist is trying to achieve moderate sedation by administering an initial bolus selected through a process of clinical estimation and then to titrate the increased doses to achieve the desired sedative effect. The general principle is to start with a low dose, followed by an assessment of patient responsiveness, sedation lever and ventilatory and cardiovascular function and status, and then gradually continue with increasing doses. The knowledge of the pharmacokinetic properties of pharmacological agents used is critical. However, it is possible that a variable number of individual responses might exist for any sedative or analgesic used (Gourlay, 1988; Levy, 1989; Wood, 1989).

Sedation agent	Pharmacokinetics			
	Onset of action (min)	Duration of action	Elimination half-life	Excretion metabolism
Meperidine	5	2–4 h	2–7 h	Hepatic; excreted in urine
Midazolam	1.0–2.5	2–6 h	1.8–6.4 h	Hepatic and intestinal; excreted in urine
Droperidol	5-10	2-4 h	2.3 h	Hepatic; Excreted in urine
Fentanyl	≤1.5	1–2 h	2–7 h	Hepatic; excreted in urine
Propofol	<1	3–10 min	Triphasic: 2.2 min, 20 min, 8 h	Hepatic; excreted in urine
Diphenhydramine	1-10	2-6 h	2.4-9.3 h	Hepatic; excreted in urine

Table 3. Pharmacological properties of sedative agents for endoscopy (Roseveare *et al*, 1998; Rudner *et al*, 2003)

For this reason, the determination of any pharmacological schemes for moderate endoscopic sedation should include an observation period supervised by an anesthesiologist, followed by a supervised drug administration period in which the anesthesiologist selects and distribute that medicine (Rex, 2006).

Reversal agents	Initial IV dose	Onset of action	Duration of action
Naloxone (for opioids)	0.2–0.4 mg (also IM)	1–2 min	45 min
Flumazenil (for benzodiazepines)	0.1–0.2 mg	30–60 s	30–60 min

Table 4. Commonly used reversal agents

Another important principle for moderate sedation in endoscopy is that combinations of drugs from different classes have synergistic effects, without being additive. Thus, even a small amount of narcotic can substantially reduce the required amount of benzodiazepines (Arrowsmith *et al*, 1991, Bailey *et al*, 1990) or propofol (Clarke *et al*, 2001, Cohen *et al*, 2004, Kern *et al*, 2004, Roseveare *et al*, 1998, Rudner *et al*, 1998) necessary to perform the endoscopy. Similarly, benzodiazepines have a synergistic effect with narcotics (Arrowsmith *et al*, 1991, Bailey *et al*, 1990) and propofol (Clarke *et al*, 2001, Cohen *et al*, 2004; Paspatis *et al*, 2002; Seifert *et al*, 2000, Reimann *et al*2000). The understanding and knowledge of the clinical impact of synergistic effects determine the appropriate selection of drug doses needed to achieve moderate sedation.

A final general principle for endoscopic moderate sedation is that each sedative agent has unique properties in terms of time period between intravenous injection and onset of sedative action and maximum drug effect (Huang&Eisen, 2004, Horn&Nesbit, 2004). If additional drug boluses are administered before reaching previous boluses plasmatic peak, the sedative effects may rapidly accumulate and may cause unwanted deeper levels of sedation. Therefore, for each pharmacological agent used, the clinician must wait an appropriate time to reach its maximum effect before injecting additional boluses of medication during the initial titration and during the maintenance phase of sedation. For example, midazolam has a longer period for achieving the maximum effect (8-12min) than diazepam (2-5 min) (Buhren *et al*, 1995). Propofol has a very short time to onset of action (45-60 seconds) and undergoes a rapid metabolism. These features have led to the necessity of quite frequent propofol administration (especially when it is used as single agent) to maintain sedation levels. For this reason, propofol administration requires more specialized attention and supervision compared to narcotics and benzodiazepines. There is the possibility that non-anesthesiologists to administer propofol for endoscopy, but the pharmacological properties of the drug are quite different from those of currently used narcotics and benzodiazepines and therefore higher risks. The use of narcotics and benzodiazepines to produce moderate sedation is already familiar to most of the endoscopists.

Key points and practical issues concerning the use of pharmacological agents for sedation and analgesia in GI endoscopy (Thomson *et al*, 2010):

- Endoscopy with intravenous sedation is a routine practice in many countries and therefore is very important that the selection of sedative drugs to be made for a maximum patient and endoscopist comfort and with minimal side effects. One option is to spray the throat with local anesthetic that could be associated with soothing music, reducing the necessary amounts of intravenous sedative drugs.

- The pre-procedural assessment of patients undergoing sedation endoscopy is very important. Cardiovascular, respiratory and neurological comorbidities should be rigorously evaluated. Allergies and adverse reactions to sedative drugs, smoking, alcohol consumption, routinely sedatives use should also be known. The person who used pharmacological agents and monitors the effects of sedative should evaluate the nature of the proposed procedure, its likely duration and the potential for complications. This person should ideally be a physician anesthesiologist.
- Intravenous sedation for GI endoscopy should be administered only if there is sufficient space to allow easy personnel movement and require specialized monitoring equipment readily available: oximeter, frequent measurement of blood pressure, the insertion of intravenous cannula for the fluids administration.
- Propofol and its pro-drug, fospropofol can be safely administered in quality moderate sedation without patient safety compromising with low doses of narcotics and/or benzodiazepines and ideally by a physician anesthesiologist.
- Due to their pharmacological profiles, Midazolam, Fentanyl, Propofol and newer Fospropofol remain the most commonly used drugs for intravenous sedation in GI endoscopy. If sedatives are administered by the endoscopist, total dose of Midazolam and Fentanyl should not exceed 5 mg and 100 micrograms, respectively.

3.4 Anesthesia and sedation in pediatric gastrointestinal procedures

In children there are some particular morphological characteristics: the tongue fills the upper airways more than in adults, while the tonsils and adenoids may compromise the airway freedom. In addition, relatively high oxygen consumption in children and larger surface may lead to clinically significant hypoxemia, dehydration and hypothermia if not provided adequate strategies to prevent them. Endoscopy performed especially in children under 10 years of age almost always requires deep sedation with endotracheal intubation. In order to reduce the anxiety caused by the separation from parents and to improve the implementing of an intravenous catheter the physician can orally administer low doses of midazolam (0.5 mg/kg) (Liacouras *et al* 1998) before the procedure, together with special counseling for children (Mahajan *et al* 1998).

In performing GI endoscopy in children, two types of sedation are being used: minimal sedation and deep anesthesia. In deep sedation, combinations of midazolam, fentanyl and ketamine are useful; however they must be used with caution (Balsells *et al*, 1997; Bahal-O'Mara *et al*, 1994; Bouchut *et al*, 1997, Green *et al*, 2001). Even with the extensive experience of the anesthetist, there is a risk of laryngo-spasm (Green *et al*, 2001) and hypoxia (Cote *et al*, 2000). Usually the recovery is prolonged and Naloxone and Flumazenil antagonists are often required (Balsells *et al*, 1997; Lamireau *et al*, 1998). General anesthesia performed by an anesthesiologist offers safe conditions to perform endoscopic procedures in children, however, is perceived by the endoscopists as being expensive and requiring specialized personnel. However, short-term action of certain drugs such as propofol (Khoshoo *et al*, 2003) and sevoflurane (Montes & Bohn, 2000) can reduce costs because the post-anesthesia recovery time is shorter. Colonoscopy performed in pediatric patients causes pain due to bowel distension, which may alert the endoscopist about a possible perforation of the colon. General anesthesia reduces colonic tone and, therefore, deep sedation may be safer in this

respect. Conscious sedation can be used successfully in cooperating children, using combinations of opioids with benzodiazepines or nitrous oxide alone (Michaud, 2005; Annequin *et al*, 2000).
Minimum anesthesia for upper endoscopy in children does not require tracheal intubation as diagnostic procedures may take no longer than 10 minutes and cause no significant unpleasant effects afterwards. Two key points for the safety of the procedure should be highlighted: the endoscope can compress and obstruct the trachea (especially in infants) (Barbi *et al*, 2006; Casfeel *et al*, 1992) and achalasia is very dangerous (esophageal residue should be drained before any sedation or anesthesia in children). Tracheal intubation is much safer in these two situations. The anesthesia for endoscopy lasting 15-30 min, can be more easily done with a device for airway intubation, such as masks (Rauch&Brener, 2003) or laryngeal mask with a special port for the endoscope (Lopez-Gil *et al*, 2006).
Minimum anesthesia with an initial bolus of propofol (2-3 mg/kg) will suppress the gag reflex enough to allow easy introduction of the endoscope, and smaller doses as boluses or continuous infusion are also effective later on (Barbi *et al*, 2006; Khoshoo *et al*, 2003; Kaddu *et al*, 2002, Walker *et al*, 2003, Perera *et al*, 2006). Usually, no additional opioids are needed.
In children sedated endoscopy, two aspects are important: the safety of a technique in which gastric contents are not aspirated and the endoscopist's training and skill in using propofol. Barbi *et al* reported their experience in propofol use in a study involving 811 children who received upper endoscopies (Barbi *et al*, 2006). Desaturation (SpO_2 <90%) occurred in 16% of cases, but this was reduced to only 3% when supplemental oxygen was administered. Major desaturation occurred in six cases, three of them being infants (12% of all children). They required assisted ventilation by face mask and endoscopy was abandoned in three cases. None of them aspirated the gastric content in their lungs and did not require tracheal intubation. The anesthesia was made by non- anesthetists in all cases. In a study with a smaller group of 57 children, Perera *et al* (pediatric anesthesiologists) have successfully used Propofol, only a child was given suxamethonium to remove the occurring laryngospasm (Perera *et al*, 2006). Tracheal intubation was not necessary.

3.5 Anesthesia and sedation in pregnant and lactating women

Some small retrospective trials regarding intravenous sedation during upper and lower gastrointestinal endoscopy in pregnant women showed that there were no maternal or fetal adverse effects, nor did it associate congenital malformations (Capella *et al*, 1996a, 1996b). Notwithstanding this goal, endoscopy should be avoided during pregnancy, and if possible, especially during the first trimester of pregnancy to avoid potential teratogenic effects during embryogenesis. However there should be some therapeutic safety guidelines or protocols which include a minimum set of safety procedures in case of use of anesthetic care especially in emergency situations. In pregnant patients with higher gestational age, a lying position should be avoided because the uterus could compress the aorta and inferior vena cava.
Frequently administered benzodiazepines (midazolam and diazepam), fentanyl and propofol are all classified by the Australian Drug Evaluation Committee (Australian Drug Evaluation Committees [ADECE], 1999) as part of category "C", as their pharmaceutical effects may cause potential harmful effects on the human fetus or neonate without causing malformations.

In regard to women who are breastfeeding and want sedation for endoscopic procedures, data are limited. It is recommended that patients who received Midazolam should not breastfeed for at least 4 hours after its administration. Breastfeeding restriction time after propofol administration is not well documented, although it is likely to be higher because the maximum concentration in breast milk occurs in 4 to 5 hours after administration. Hence, it is indicated to collect breast milk in a container and subsequently throw it a few hours before resuming breastfeeding. Fentanyl administration is not considered a contraindication for breastfeeding (Qureshi *et al*, 2005).

4. Conclusion

Sedation practices are extremely varied, having individual particularities throughout different regions of the world. Cultural, religious, ethical and procedural aspects come into play, dictating the use of a particular type of sedation, exclusion of different classes of agents, or even banning sedation altogether. Even though no or minimum sedation do provide higher safety and shorter follow-up periods, there is an increased tendency, especially in Western patients, to expect some level of sedation. As well as different levels of sedation, different levels of qualification of the individual providing the sedation are expected, depending on the location and the type of the medical unit and the complexity of the investigation.

In current practice, a various number of sedative agents are used, each with their respective indications and strengths, balanced by a series of unwelcome side-effects and inerrant short-comings. Particularities such as age, gender, associated conditions, even weight and height, should be taken into consideration when choosing a particular type of sedation level or determining the use of a specific agent. Pediatric gastrointestinal endoscopies present particularities when considering sedation, given the distinctive morphological features of the young, developing body. Particular conditions, such as pregnancy or lactation, should come into play as well, restricting the use of particular agents with proven or suspected effects on the fetus or infant.

5. References

Annequin, D.; Carbajal, R.; Chauvin, P.; Gall, O.; Tourniaire, B. & Murat, I. (2000). Fixed 50% nitrous oxide oxygen mixture for painful procedures: a French survey. Pediatrics, Vol.105, No.4, (April 2000), E 47, ISSN 1098-4275

American Society of Anesthesiologists (2002). Task force on sedation and analgesia by non-anesthesiologists. Practice guidelines for sedation and analgesia by non-anesthesiologists. Anesthesiology, Vol.96, No.4 (April 2002), pp. 1004-1017, ISSN 0003-3022

Amorós A, Aparicio JR, Garmendia M, Casellas JA, Martínez J, Jover R. Deep sedation with propofol does not precipitate hepatic encephalopathy during elective upper endoscopy. Gastrointest. Endosc. 2009; 70: 262–8.

Arrowsmith, J.; Gerstman, B.; Fleischer, D. & Benjamin S.B. (1991). Results from the American Society for Gastrointestinal Endoscopy/U.S. Food and Drug Administration collaborative study on complication rates and drug use during gastrointestinal endoscopy. Gastrointestinal Endoscopy, Vol.37, No.4, (July-August 1991), pp. 421-427, ISSN 1097-6779

Australian Drug Evaluation Committee. (1999). Prescribing Medicines in Pregnancy. In An Australian Categorisation of Risk of Drug Use in Pregnancy, 4th edn. 1999. Available from URL: http://www.tga.gov.au/docs/pdf/medpreg.pdf

Bahal-O'Mara, N.; Nahata, M.C.; Murray, R.D.; Linscheid, T.R.; Fishbein, M.; Heitlinger, L.A.; Li, B.U.; McClung H.J.; Potter, C. & Lininger, B. (1994). Sedation with meperidine and midazolam in pediatric patients undergoing endoscopy. European Journal of Clinical Pharmacoogy, Vol. 47, No.4, pp. 319–323, ISSN 1432-1041

Bailey, P.; Pace, N.; Ashburn, M.; Moll J. W.; East K.A. & Stanley T.H. (1990). Frequent hypoxemia and apnea after sedation with midazolam and fentanyl. Anesthesiology, Vol.73, No.5 (November 1990), pp. 826-830, ISSN 0003-3022

Balsells, F.; Wyllie, R.; Kay, M. & Steffern R. (1997).Use of conscious sedation for lower and upper gastrointestinal endoscopic examinations in children, adolescents, and young adults: a twelve-year review. Gastrointestinal Endoscopy, Vol. 45, No.5, (May 1997), pp. 375-380, ISSN 1097-6779

Barbi, E.; Petaros, P.; Badina, L.; Pahor, T.; Giuseppin, I.; Biasotto, E.; Martelossi, S.; Di Leo, G.; Sarti, A. & Ventura A. (2006). Deep sedation with propofol for upper gastrointestinal endoscopy in children, administered by specially trained pediatricians: a prospective case series with emphasis on side effects. Endoscopy, Vol. 38, No.4, (April 2006), pp. 368–375, ISSN 1438-8812

Bell, G. D. (2004). Preparation, premedication, and surveillance. Endoscopy, Vol.36, No.1, (January 2004), pp. 23–31, ISSN 1438-8812

Bonta PI, Kok MF, Bergman JJ *et al.* Conscious sedation for EUS of the esophagus and stomach: a double-blind, randomized, controlled trial comparing midazolam with placebo. Gastrointest. Endosc. 2003; 57: 842–7.

Bouchut, J.C.; Godard, J.; Lachaux, A. & Diot, N. (2001). Deep sedation for upper gastrointestinal endoscopy in children. Journal of Pediatric Gastroenterology and Nutrition, Vol. 30, No.5, (May 2000), pp. 477-485, ISSN 1536-4801

Brill JV. Endoscopic sedation: legislative update and implications for reimbursement. Gastrointest. Endosc. Clin. North Am. 2008; 18: 665–78.

Buhren, M.; Maitre, P.O.; Crevoisier, C. & Stanski D.R.(1995).Pharmacodynamic modeling of the electroencephalographic effects of midazolam and diazepam. Clinical Pharmacology & Therapeutics, Vol.48, No.5, pp. 555–567, ISSN 1532-6535

Bytzer, P. & Lindeberg, B. (2007). Impact of an information video before colonoscopy on patient satisfaction and anxiety—a randomized trial. Endoscopy, Vol. 39, No.8, (August 2007), pp. 710–714, ISSN 1438-8812

Cappell, M.S.; Colon, V.J. & Sidhom, O.A. (1996). A study at 10 medical centers of the safety and efficacy of 48 flexible sigmoidoscopies and 8 colonoscopies during pregnancy with follow-up of fetal outcome and with comparison to control groups. Digestive Diseases Sciences, Vol.41, pp. 2353–2361, ISSN 1573-2568

Cappell, M.S.; Colon, V.J.; & Sidhom, O.A. (1996). A study of eight medical centers of the safety and clinical efficacy of esophagogastroduodenoscopy in 83 pregnant females with follow-up of fetal outcome with comparison control groups. The American Journal of Gastroenterology, Vol.91, pp. 1963–1967, ISSN 1572-0241

Casfeel, H.B.; Fiedorek, S.C. & Kiel, E.A (1992). Arterial blood oxygen desaturation in infants and children during upper gastrointestinal endoscopy. Gastrointestinal Endoscopy, Vol. 36, No.5, (September 1990), pp. 448-449, ISSN 1097-6779

Clarke AC, Chiragakis L, Hillman LC, Kaye GL. Sedation for endoscopy: the safe use of propofol by general practitioner sedationists. Med. J. Aust. 2002; 176: 158–61.

Clarke, A.C. (2007). Consent for direct access endoscopy. Journal of Gastroenterology and Hepatology, Vol.22, No.12, (December 2007), pp. 2051-2052, ISSN 1440-1746

Cohen, L.B.; Hightower, C.D.; Wood, D.A.; Miller, K.M. & Aisenberg, J.(2004) Moderate level sedation during endoscopy: a prospective study using low-dose propofol, meperidine/fentanyl, and midazolam. Gastrointestinal Endoscopy, Vol.59, No.7, (June 2004), pp. 795-803, ISSN 1097-6779

Coté, C.J.; Karl, H.W.; Notterman, D.A.; Weinberg, J.A. & McCloskey, C.(2000). Adverse sedation events in pediatrics: analysis of medications used for sedation. Pediatrics, Vol.106, No.4, pp. 633–644, ISSN 1098-4275

Conlong P, Rees W. The use of hypnosis in gastroscopy: a comparison with intravenous sedation. Postgrad. Med. J. 1999; 75: 223–5.

Evans LT, Saberi S, Kim HM, Elta GH, Schoenfeld P. Pharyngeal anesthesia during sedated EGDs: is "the spray" beneficial? A meta-analysis and systematic review. Gastrointest. Endosc. 2006; 63: 761–6.

Ertekin C, Kiylioglu N, Tarlaci S, Keskin A, Aydogdu I. Effect of mucosal anaesthesia on oropharyngeal swallowing. Neurogastroenterol. Motil. 2000; 12: 567–72.

Faigel, D.O.; Baron, T.H.; Goldstein, J.L.; Hirota, W.K.; Jacobson, B.C.; Johanson, J.F.; Leighton, J.A.; Mallery, J.S.; Peterson, K.A.; Waring, J.P.; Fanelli, R.D. & Wheeler-Harbaugh, J. (2002). Guidelines for the use of deep sedation and anesthesia for GI endoscopy. Gastrointestinal Endoscopy, Vol.56, No.5, (November 2002), pp. 613–617, ISSN 1097-6779

Faulx AL, Vela S, Das A *et al*. The changing landscape of practice patterns regarding unsedated endoscopy and propofol use: a national Web survey. Gastrointest. Endosc. 2005; 62: 9–15.

Fechner J, Ihmsen H, Hatterscheid D, *et al*. Comparative pharmacokinetics and pharmacodynamics of the new propofol prodrug GPI 15715 and propofol emulsion. Anesthesiology 2004; 101: 626–39

Gibiansky E, Struys MM, Gibiansky L, *et al*. AQUAVAN injection, a water-soluble prodrug of propofol, as a bolus injection: a phase I dose-escalation comparison with DIPRIVAN (part 1): pharmacokinetics. Anesthesiology 2005; 103: 718–29.

Gourlay, G.K.; Kowalski, S.R.; Plummer, J.L.; Cousins, M.J. & Armstrong, P.J. (1988). Fentanyl blood concentration–analgesic response relationship in the treatment of postoperative pain. Anesthesia & Analgesia, Vol.67, No.4, (April 1988), pp. 329-337, ISSN 1526-7598

Green, S.M.; Klooster, M.; Harris, T.; Lynch, E.L. & Rothrock, S.G. (2001). Ketamine sedation for pediatric gastroenterology procedures. Journal of Pediatric Gastroenterology and Nutrition, Vol. 32, No.1, (January 2001), pp. 26-33, ISSN 1536-4801

Hayee B, Dunn J, Loganayagam A *et al*. Midazolam with meperidine or fentanyl for colonoscopy: results of a randomized trial. Gastrointest. Endosc. 2009; 69 (Suppl. 3): 681–7.

Huang, R. & Eisen, G.M. (2004). Efficacy, safety, and limitations in current practice of sedation and analgesia, Gastrointestinal Endoscopy Clinics of North America, Vol.14, No.2 (April 2004), pp. 269-288

Holm C, Christensen M, Schulze S, Rosenberg J. Effect of oxygen on tachycardia and arterial oxygen saturation during colonoscopy. Eur. J. Surg. 1999; 165: 755–8.

Horn, E. & Nesbit, S.A. (2004). Pharmacology and pharmacokinetics of sedatives and analgesics. Gastrointestinal Endoscopy Clinics of North America, Vol.14, No.2 (April 2004), pp. 247-268

Ionescu, D. (2005). Intravenous anesthetics, In: Clinical anesthesia, I. Acalovschi, (Ed.), 209-210, Clusium, ISBN 973-555-443-7, Cluj-Napoca, Romania

Kaddu, R.; Bhattacharya, D.; Metriyakool, K.; Thomas, R. & Tolia, V. (2002). Propofol compared with general anesthesia for pediatric GI endoscopy: is propofol better? Gastrointestinal Endoscopy, Vol.55, No.1, (January 2002), pp. 27-32, ISSN 1097-6779

Kane GC, Hoehn SM, Behrenbeck TR, Mulvagh SL. Benzocaine-induced methemoglobinemia based on the Mayo Clinic experience from 28 478 transesophageal echocardiograms: incidence, outcomes, and predisposing factors. Arch. Int. Med. 2007; 167: 1977–82.

Kanto J, Gepts E. Pharmacokinetic implications for the clinical use of propofol. Clin. Pharmacokinet. 1989; 17: 308–26.

Kulling D, Orlandi M, Inauen W. Propofol sedation during endoscopic procedures: how much staff and monitoring are necessary? Gastrointest. Endosc. 2007; 66: 443–9.

Kern, S.E.; Xie, G.; White, J.L. & Egan, T.D. (2004). A response surface analysis of propofol–remifentanil pharmacodynamic interaction in volunteers. Anesthesiology, Vol.100, No.6 (June 2004), pp. 1373-1381, ISSN 0003-3022

Khoshoo, V.; Thoppil, D.; Landry, L.; Brown, S. & Ross, G. (2003). Propofol versus midazolam plus meperidine for sedation during ambulatory esophagogastroduodenoscopy. Journal of Pediatric Gastroenterology and Nutrition, Vol. 37, No.2, (August 2003), pp. 146-149, ISSN 1536-4801

Lamireau, T.; Dubreuil, M. & Daconceicao, M. (1998). Oxygen saturation during esophagogastroduodenoscopy in children: general anesthesia versus intravenous sedation. Journal of Pediatric Gastroenterology and Nutrition, Vol. 27, No.2, (August 1998), pp. 172-175, ISSN 1536-4801

Lazzaroni M, Bianchi Porro G. Preparation, premedication, and surveillance. Endoscopy 2001; 33: 103–8

Levy, G. (1989). Impact of pharmacodynamic variability on drug delivery. Advanced Drug Delivery Reviews, Vol.33, No.3, (September 1998), pp. 201-206

Liacouras, C.A.; Mascarenhas, M.; Poon, C. & Wenner, W.J. (1998). Placebo-controlled trial assessing the use of oral midazolam as a premedication to conscious sedation for pediatric endoscopy. Gastrointestinal Endoscopy, Vol.47, No.6, (June 1998), pp. 455-460, ISSN 1097-6779

Lopez-Gil, M.; Brimacombe, J. & Diaz-Reganon, G. (2006). Anesthesia for pediatric gastroscopy: a study comparing the ProSeal laryngeal mask airway with nasal cannulae. Pediatric Anesthesia, Vol 16, No.10, (October 2006), pp. 1032–103, ISSN 1460-9592

Louis S, Bassett M, Clarke A, Thomson A. Anaesthetic support for endoscopic retrograde cholangio pancreatograms in Australian teaching hospitals. Int. Med. J. 2004; 34: 368–9.

Lytle, J. (2005). Anesthesia in ambulatory surgery, In: Clinical anesthesia, I. Acalovschi, (Ed.), 842-843, Clusium, ISBN 973-555-443-7, Cluj-Napoca, Romania

Mahajan, L.; Wyllie, R.; Steffen, R.; Kay, M.; Kitaoka, G.; Dettorre, J.; Sarigol, S. & McCue, K. (1998). The effects of a psychological preparation program on anxiety in children and adolescents undergoing gastrointestinal endoscopy. Journal of Pediatric Gastroenterology & Nutrition, Vol.27, No.2, pp.161-165, ISSN 0277-2116

Michaud L. (2005). Sedation for diagnostic upper gastrointestinal endoscopy: a survey of the Francophone Pediatric Hepatology, Gastroenterology, and Nutrition Group. Endoscopy, Vol.37, No.2, pp. 167–170, ISSN 1438-8812

Montes, R.G. & Bohn, R.A. (2000). Deep sedation with inhaled sevoflurane for pediatric outpatient gastrointestinal endoscopy. Journal of Pediatric Gastroenterology and Nutrition, Vol. 31, No.1, (May 2000), pp. 41-46, ISSN 1536-4801

Morrow JB, Zuccaro G Jr, Conwell DL, *et al*. Sedation for colonoscopy using a single bolus is safe, effective, and efficient: a prospective, randomized, double-blind trial. Am J Gastroenterol 2000; 95: 2242–7.

Padmanabhan U, Leslie K. Australian anaesthetists' practice of sedation for gastrointestinal endoscopy in adult patients. Anaesth. Intensive Care 2008; 36: 436–41.

Paspatis, G.; Manolaraki, M.; Xirouchakis, G. Papanikolaou, N.; Chlouverakis, G. & Gritzali,A. (2002). Synergistic sedation with midazolam and propofol versus midazolam and pethidine in colonoscopies: a prospective, randomized study. The American Journal of Gastroenterology, Vol.24, No.8, (August 2002), pp. 1963–1967, ISSN 1572-0241

Pena LR, Mardini HE, Nickl NJ. Development of an instrument to assess and predict satisfaction and poor tolerance among patients undergoing endoscopic procedures. Dig. Dis. Sci. 2005; 50: 1860–71.

Perera, C.; Strandvik, G.F.; Malik, M. & Sen, S. (2006). Propofol anesthesia is an effective and safe strategy for pediatric endoscopy. Pediatric Anesthesia, Vol.16, No.2, (February 2006), pp. 220–221, ISSN 1460-9592

Pruitt R, Cohen LB, Gibiansky E, *et al*. A randomized, open-label, multicenter, dose-ranging study of sedation with Aquavan injection (GPI 15714) during colonoscopy. Gastrointest Endosc 2005; 61: AB111.

Qadeer MA, Rocio Lopez A, Dumot JA, Vargo JJ. Risk factors for hypoxemia during ambulatory gastrointestinal endoscopy in ASA I-II patients. Dig. Dis. Sci. 2009; 54: 1035–40.

Qureshi, W.A.; Rajan, E. & Adler, D.G. (2005). American Society for Gastrointestinal Endoscopy. ASGE Guideline: guidelines for endoscopy in pregnant and lactating women. Gastrointestinal Endoscopy, Vol.61, No.3, (March 2005), pp. 357-362, ISSN 1097-6779

Rauch, R.Y. & Brener, C.E. (2003). Airway management for pediatric esophagogastroduodenoscopy using an endoscopy mask. Anesthesia & Analgesia, Vol. 96, No.1, (January 2003), pp. 303–304, ISSN 1526-7598

Reimann, F., Samson, U., Derad, I.; Fuchs, M.; Schiefer, B. & Stange, E.F. (2000) Synergistic sedation with low-dose midazolam and propofol for colonoscopies Endoscopy, Vol. 32, No.3, (March 2000), pp. 239-244, ISSN 1438-8812

Ristikankare M, Hartikainen J, Heikkinen M, Julkunen R. Is routine sedation or topical pharyngeal anesthesia beneficial during upper endoscopy? Gastrointest. Endosc. 2004; 60: 686–94.

Rex, D.K. (2006). Moderate sedation for endoscopy: sedation regimens for non-anaesthesiologists. Alimentary Pharmacology & Therapeutics, Vol.24, No.2, (July 2006), pp.163-171, ISSN 1365-2036

Rex DK, Deenadayalu VP, Eid E *et al.* Endoscopist-directed administration of propofol: a worldwide safety experience. Gastroenterology 2009 137: 1229–37.

Rex, D.K.; Heuss, L.T.; Walker, J.A. & Qi, R. (2005). Trained registered nurses/endoscopy teams can administer propofol safely for endoscopy. Gastroenterology, Vol.129, No.5, (November 2005), pp.1384–139, ISSN 1528-0012

Roseveare, C.; Seavell, C.; Patel, P.; Criswell, J.; Kimble, J.; Jones, C. & Shepherd H. (1998). Patient-controlled sedation and analgesia, using propofol and alfentanil, during colonoscopy: a prospective randomized controlled trial. Endoscopy, Vol. 30, No.9, (November 1998), pp. 768-773, ISSN 1438-8812

Rudner, R.; Jalowiecki, P.; Kawecki, P.; Gonciarz, M.; Mularczyk, A. & Petelenz, M. (2003). Conscious analgesia/sedation with remifentanil and propofol versus total intravenous anesthesia with fentanyl, midazolam, and propofol for outpatient colonoscopy. Gastrointestinal Endoscopy, Vol.57, No.6, (May 2003), pp. 657-663, ISSN 1097-6779

Seifert, H.; Schmitt, T.; Gultekin, T.; Caspary, L. & Wehrmann, S. (2000). Sedation with propofol plus midazolam versus propofol alone for interventional endoscopic procedures: a prospective, randomized study. Alimentary Pharmacology & Therapeutics, Vol.14, No.9, (September 2000), pp.1207-1214, ISSN 1365-2036

Sitcai, N. (2004). Outside hospital anesthesiology practice. Guide for private medicine, Callisto, ISBN 973-87261-0-7

Snyder SH, Enna SJ, Young AB. Brain mechanisms associated with therapeutic actions of benzodiazepines: focus on neurotransmitters. Am. J. Psychiatry 1977; 134: 662–5

Stark RD, Binks SM, Dutka VN, O'Connor KM, Arnstein MJ, Glen JB. A review of the safety and tolerance of propofol ('Diprivan'). Postgrad. Med. J. 1985; 61 (Suppl. 3): 152–6.

Thomson, A.; Andrew, G. & Jones, D.B. (2010). Optimal sedation for gastrointestinal endoscopy: Review and recommendations. Journal of Gastroenterology and Hepatology, Vol.25, No.3, (March 2010), pp. 469-478, ISSN 1440-1746

Tsai MS, Su YH, Liang JT, Lai HS, Lee PH. Patient factors predicting the completion of sedation-free colonoscopy. Hepatogastroenterology 2008; 55: 1606–8.

Trapani G, Altomare C, Liso G, Sanna E, Biggio G. Propofol in anesthesia. Mechanism of action, structure-activity relationships, and drug delivery. Curr. Med. Chem. 2000; 7: 249–71.

Tu RH, Grewall P, Leung JW, *et al.* Diphenhydramine as an adjunct to sedation for colonoscopy: a double-blind randomized, placebo-controlled study. Gastrointest Endosc 2006; 63: 87–94.

VanNatta ME, Rex DK. Propofol alone titrated to deep sedation versus propofol in combination with opioids and/or benzodiazepines and titrated to moderate sedation for colonoscopy. Am. J. Gastroenterol. 2006; 101: 2209–17.

Yi SY, Shin JE. Midazolam for patients undergoing upper gastrointestinal endoscopy: a prospective, single-blind and randomized study to determine the appropriate amount and time of initiation of endoscopy. J. Gastroenterol. Hepatol. 2005; 20: 1873–9.

Zuccaro G Jr. Sedation and analgesia for GI endoscopy. Gastrointest Endosc 2006; 63: 95–96.

Walker, J.A.; McIntyre, R.D.; Schleinitz, P.F.; Jacobson, K.N.; Haulk, A.A.; Adesman, P.; Tolleson, S.; Parent, R.; Donnelly, R. & Rex, D.K. (2003). Nurse-administered propofol sedation without anesthesia specialists in 9152 endoscopic cases in an ambulatory surgery center. American Journal of Gastroenterology, Vol. 98, No.8, (August 2003), pp. 1744–1750, ISSN 1572-0241

Wang, T.H. & Lin, J.T. (1999). Worldwide use of sedation and analgesia for upper intestinal endoscopy. Gastrointestinal Endoscopy Vol.50, No.6, (December 1999), pp. 888-889, ISSN 1097-6779

Wood, M. (1989). Variability of human drug response. Anesthesiology, Vol.71, No.5 (November 1989), pp. 631-634, ISSN 0003-3022

4

Sedation for Pediatric Endoscopies

Vidyut Bhatia[1] and Narendra Kumar Arora[2]
[1]*Apollo Centre for Advanced Pediatrics, Indraprastha Apollo Hospital, New Delhi*
[2]*The INCLEN (International Clinical Epidemiology Network) Trust International India*

1. Introduction

Endoscopy can be a very traumatic event for a child and it is essential that the procedure be smooth, painless and anxiety-free. Hence, endoscopy in children normally requires the simultaneous administration of sedation to warrant the patient's well-being, comfort, and cooperation throughout the procedure. The endoscopist has to balance the benefits with the possible adverse events because sedation related complications are reported to be much more than procedure related events like perforation and bleeding (Thakkar, Elserag et al. 2007). Although there is little agreement amongst pediatric endoscopists on best sedation practices everyone does agree that ensuring the child's safety is paramount (Lightdale, Mahoney et al. 2007).

2. Goals

The goal is always to optimize patient safety and minimize complications. The goals of sedation can be divided into two main categories. These are patient specific and physician/ endoscopist specific. The patient specific goals are anxiolysis, analgesia and amnesia for the procedure. From an endoscopists' perspective, the goals of sedation are cooperation from the patient, completion of the procedure, and no complications.

3. Patient assessment and risk stratification

Patient assessment and risk stratification is the most important initial step in planning for endoscopy in a child. This should be done at two stages. The first time is when the decision to perform an endoscopy has been made (i.e. in the outpatient clinic etc.) and once just before commencing the procedure. It is just like doing a pre-anesthetic check-up before any surgery.

4. ASA classification for pre anesthetic status

The ASA classification is used to identify at risk patients and plan sedation accordingly (Table. 1). This classification system although in vogue for nearly 5 decades does not specifically address issues related to children. Healthy neonates and infants do not tolerate similar anesthetics well in comparison to older children and young adults. For these reasons, in further discussions, sedation for endoscopy infants and neonates has been taken up separately.

ASA class	Status
1	A normal healthy patient
2	A patient with mild systemic disease
3	A patient with severe systemic disease
4	A patient with severe systemic disease that is a constant threat to life
5	A moribund patient who is not expected to survive without the operation
6	A declared brain-dead patient whose organs are being removed for donor purposes

Table 1. ASA (American Society of Anesthesiologist) classification of physical status

5. Sedation levels

Depending on the type of endoscopic procedure, children may require no sedation (e.g., flexible sigmoidoscopy in an infant), intravenous sedation, or general anesthesia. Levels of sedation range from a continuum of mild sedation to deep sedation (Mahoney and Lightdale 2007). Therefore it is important to keep in mind that the child can pass on from light sedation to a deep sedation easily with the same combination of drugs and dosage. The endoscopist has to remain prepared for such eventualities.

5.1 No sedation

Unsedated upper endoscopy has been routinely performed in very young and adolescent patients at several institutions without any difference in outcomes (Bishop, Nowicki et al. 2002). In particular, flexible sigmoidoscopy, changes or removals of percutaneous endoscopically placed gastrostomy tubes and placement of pH or impedance probes can be performed without sedation (Mahoney and Lightdale 2007). The advantages of not getting sedation include minimal complications, earlier recovery and lower cost of the procedure.

5.2 Light to moderate sedation

This is an another name for conscious sedation and defined as a medically controlled state of depressed consciousness that allows protected reflexes to be maintained, retains the ability to maintain a patent airway independently and continuously, and permits appropriate responses by the patient to physical stimulation or verbal commands; for example, "open your eyes."

5.3 Deep sedation/analgesia

Deep sedation is defined as a medically controlled state of depressed consciousness or unconsciousness from which the patient is not easily aroused. It may be accompanied by a partial or complete loss of protective reflexes, and includes the inability to maintain a patent airway independently and respond purposefully to physical stimulation or verbal command.

5.4 General anesthesia

General anesthesia is defined as a medically controlled state of unconsciousness accompanied by a loss of protective reflexes, including the inability to maintain an airway independently and no purposeful response to physical stimulation or verbal command.

Children with the American Society of Anesthesiologists (ASA) physical status 3 and 4 and patients who are going to have procedures such as achalasia dilation, foreign body removal, and percutaneous endoscopic gastrostomy placement are typically selected for general anesthesia and should be assessed by an anesthesiologist.

6. Method of sedation

Sedatives should not be administered in a facility unsupervised by medically trained personnel or where appropriate monitoring equipment and manpower are not available, since unrecognized complications may lead to disaster. The method of sedation is determined by the endoscopist and the needs of the patient. Many factors must be considered, including the patient's condition, ASA classification, patients age, the type of procedure (i.e., diagnostic versus therapeutic), the anticipated level of cooperation from the patient, the parents' and patient's preference after being provided these choices and explanation of their risks, as well as the endoscopist's experiences.

There is a wide variation in the method of practice of sedation. Within city of Delhi, India five pediatric gastroenterology setups practice different approaches ranging from no sedation at all to moderate sedation and a mix of deep sedation and general anaesthesia. From other published literature as well, the message is not consistent (Lightdale, Mahoney, et al. 2007). This probably reflects an uncertainty in the optimal method of sedation and the lack of proper guidelines according to the authors. Comfort of pediatric endoscopist for particular types of sedation is equally important.

A conscious sedation protocol is followed at the pediatric gastroenterology division of All India Institute of Medical Sciences, New Delhi, India. For infants below 6 months no sedation is given, while all other children including those under going procedures receive moderate IV sedation.

All children are given the following drugs according to the following protocol prior to endoscopy (Table 2).

Drug	Concentration (mg/ml)	Preparation	Concentration after dilution (mg/ml)	Dose (mg/kg)	Dose after dilution (ml/kg)
Atropine	0.6	Dilute 1 ampoule in 5ml of saline	0.1	0.1	0.15
Diazepam	5.0	2ml diazepam + 2ml 2% lignocaine* + 6ml saline	1.0	0.1	0.1
Ketamine	5.0	2ml of drug + 8 ml of saline	10.0	2.0	0.2

* Lignocaine is added for its cardiac stability

Table 2. Concentration, method of preparation and dosage of drugs used for pediatric sedation at the Pediatric Gastroenterology division, Department of Pediatrics, All India Institute of Medical Sciences, New Delhi, India

7. Preparation for the procedure

7.1 Fasting

Conventionally, fasting for solids for 6 hours and liquids for 2 to 4 hours is recommended (Tolia, Peters et al. 2000). Longer periods of fasting may be required for conditions such as achalasia and gastric outlet obstruction, because retained food in the esophagus or stomach may increase the risk of aspiration. Infants and neonates are not fasted for long and often require to be put on IV fluids during fasting.

7.2 Antibiotic prophylaxis

Children with congenital heart diseases or a compromised immune system are candidates for endocarditis prophylaxis. We administer single injection of amoxicillin and gentamicin just before start of the procedure. In children sensitive to amoxicillin, vancomicin is given. For ERCP, a flouroquinolone is also added.

7.3 Time out

"Time-out" is an important component before any procedure on the patient. It is done immediately prior to starting the procedure and is performed to prevent any medical error by conducting a final verification of correct patient, procedure, and site. The timeout should also ensure that correct equipment, drugs and personnel to perform sedation are available. It is an active communication among all procedural team members that should be consistently performed prior to all procedures.

On-site equipment of appropriate sizes should be available prior to the procedure and include the following: (i) pulse oximetry (ii) suction and catheters; (iii) noninvasive blood pressure measurement equipment (iv) positive pressure O_2 delivery system (v) emergency kit with age and size appropriate drugs and resuscitation equipment.

7.4 Documentation before sedation

Although endoscopy has a relatively low risk as compared to other surgical procedures, it is important that all pediatric endoscopists be prepared for complications associated with either the procedure or the sedation. In turn, all patients and their families must be well informed prior to the endoscopy and the initiation of sedation about the possible risks of the procedure and of the sedation. It is extremely important to find a delicate balance between the full disclosure of the invasive nature of the procedure and related complications and anticipated parental and patient responses to the disclosed information.

Documentation before sedation must include the following:

1. Informed consent: Informed consent must involve disclosure by the endoscopist and deliberation by the parents or legal guardians. If the patient is an adolescent, it is appropriate to obtain informed assent. A separate consent form for sedation may be required.
2. Verbal instructions
3. Dietary precautions
4. Health evaluation

7.5 Topical anesthetic spray and premedication

For upper gastrointestinal endoscopy, pre-medication with topical sprays and oral sedatives prior to IV line insertion are used at many centers. Topical lidocaine applications (gel, sprays, inhalers or lollipops) have been used as an addition to sedation with varying results. Some formulations are associated with nausea, vomiting and gagging and might increase the need for sedation. Ayoub et al. performed a single-blind, randomized, prospective study (Ayoub, Skoury et al. 2007) to compare topical lidocaine application by means of a lollipop with the spray group and found that, gag reflexes in the lollipop group were significantly weaker and patients were better able to tolerate scope introduction and manipulation during the procedure. Sedation was needed by 96% of patients given spray, but by only 32% of patients in the lollipop group (P <0.001). All these were adults and its extrapolation to pediatric population may be difficult.

Topical application is only effective when the anesthetic is delivered to the posterior pharynx. This system requires depression of the tongue and elicitation of a gag reflex with a tongue blade during spraying, which may be highly unpleasant for children. Opponents of the pharyngeal anesthesia postulate that this increases the distress in children (Ament, Berquist et al. 1988), whereas the proponents have propagated the more generally held view that it is the pharyngeal stimulation from the endoscope that causes more patient agitation (Evans, Saberi et al. 2006). We have in our setup never used topical anesthetics prior to endoscopy and after giving IV sedation, children of all ages tolerate endoscope well.

8. Post procedure instructions

After the procedure, children are retained in the hospital for 2 hours (conscious sedation) - 8 hours (general anaesthesia) depending upon the types of anaesthesia and the procedures. If any intervention has been done, child is advised to stay longer till they are stable. Approximately 2 hours after the procedure, if the child is conscious and awake, he / she can be offered something to drink. Most children sleep after leaving the hospital. When child wakes, he or she may be drowsy. Some children are sleepy for the remainder of the day. After child wakes up, do not allow him or her to walk alone for at least 4 hours. Child may feel suddenly dizzy and fall without warning. The sedative can affect the child's coordination ability and balance. For the first 12 hours after waking up the child should not do anything that requires alertness, coordination, or balance. The care providers are told that the sedative sometimes causes the child to behave in unexpected ways. However, by the next day child's behavior should return to normal. For infants it is okay to give "clear liquids" (water, apple juice, tea) after getting home. Wait approximately 30 minutes to make sure child does not choke or vomit. Then milk, formula or other foods may be given. If child can drink without vomiting or choking, he or she can have the foods he or she usually eats. The patient is instructed to return/seek medical help for recurrent vomiting and if any of the common effects listed above last more than 12 hours, or if child's pain increases. We also advise the patient not to travel if he/she has had sclerotherapy in the past 24 hours.

9. Sedation related complications and their management

There are no good published studies that have documented adverse events following pediatric sedation. Cote et al reported on the adverse sedation events in children in a study published in 2000 (Cote, Notterman et al. 2000). This study was a critical incident analysis of contributory factors. The primary event in both the hospital-based and non-hospital-based patients was respiratory, the secondary event was cardiac arrest, and the third was inadequate resuscitation. Drug-drug interactions, inadequate monitoring, inadequate medical evaluation, lack of an independent observer, and inadequate management of resuscitation were also some of the other causes of adverse sedation events. Successful outcome was related to the use of pulse oximetry in patients compared to those without any monitoring. At pediatric gastroenterology division of All India Institute of Medical Sciences, New Delhi, India, 4874 endoscopies were done over the past two and a half years. Following adverse events were observed amongst them (Table 3). Most complications from sedation are avoidable. Children below one year are at the highest risk and need special attention. Desaturation and apnea are the most frequently encountered adverse effects which can be quickly reversed with administration of 0_2/ increasing flow. Uniform guidelines for both in hospital and out of hospital sedation must include appropriate personnel skilled in airway management and resuscitation. Health care personnel who sedate children for procedures must have advanced airway and resuscitation skills.

Adverse event	N=4874
Ineffective sedation	351 (7.2%)
Respiratory depression (Hypoxemia)	975 (20%)
Bronchospasm/ laryngospasm	101 (0.21%)
Combativeness/delirium	238 (0.49%)
Allergic reaction to drugs	118 (0.24%)

Table 3. Incidence of various adverse events observed over a period of two and a half years following endoscopies at the pediatric gastroenterology division of All India Institute of Medical Sciences, New Delhi, India

10. Pharmacological options

The main classes of drugs used for sedation analgesia for diagnostic and therapeutic procedures are narcotics, benzodiazepines, systemic anesthetics and reversal agents. They are described briefly in the following paragraphs.

10.1 Narcotics

10.1.1 Fentanyl

Fentanyl is a fat-soluble drug that rapidly enters the blood–brain barrier. It is more potent and fast acting than both morphine and meperidine. Fentanyl should be administered to children as a slow IV push since rapid administration has been associated with chest wall and glottic rigidity. Fentanyl's onset of action is approximately 30 seconds, and its opioid effects last approximately 30 to 45 minutes. Fentanyl should be administered in small doses to slowly titrate to effect, with several minutes allowed between each dose. Because its termination of action occurs with redistribution rather than from metabolism, the respiratory depressive effects of fentanyl outlast its analgesic effects.

10.1.2 Meperidine and the lytic cocktail

Until recently, meperidine was a favorite in longer procedures since its clinical duration of action is 2–4 hours. It may be given intravenously in dosage of 0.5–1.0 mg/kg, with maximum being 4 mg/kg. The time of peak effect for meperidine is 1–3 minutes after intravenous administration. In addition to respiratory depression, the active metabolite meperidine (nor-meperidine) may cause seizures. Meperidine should not be used long-term or in patients with poor renal clearance. Special consideration includes avoidance in patients taking monoamine oxidase inhibitors and in patients with cardiovascular instability. The other adverse reactions following meperidine include delirium, nausea, vomiting, urinary retention, pruritis, smooth muscle spasm, and hypotension. Central nervous system toxicity may occur in patients taking tricyclic antidepressants and phenothiazines. Meperidine in the past was commonly used as a cocktail mixed with promethazine and chlorpromazine. The cocktail is still, on occasion, used by some but it has very long sedation duration, anywhere from 7 to 19 hours. It can also be associated with hypotension seizures, extra pyramidal reactions, and severe prolonged life-threatening respiratory depression.

10.2 Benzodiazepines

10.2.1 Midazolam

Midazolam has now become the preferred drug in many pediatric endoscopy suites. It is a benzodiazepine with three to six times greater potency than diazepam. It is given in the dose of 0.1-0.3 mg/kg/dose intravenously. Midazolam provides three advantages over diazepam. It provides patients better anterograde and retrograde amnesia for the procedure. It has a shorter half life and there appears to be no resedation as seen with diazepam. The onset of action for a dose of midazolam is within 1 to 5 minutes, and it achieves its peak effect in approximately 30 minutes to 1 hour. Unlike other benzodiazepines, the clearance of midazolam is dose related (i.e., increased clearance with increased dosage).

10.3 Systemic anesthetics

10.3.1 Ketamine

Ketamine in low doses can cause intense analgesia with minimal respiratory and cardiovascular depression. Typical doses are 1–2 mg/kg intravenous. The onset occurs in less than 1 minute, with a peak effect in several minutes and duration of action in approximately 15 minutes. Higher doses (2mg/kg) or supplementation with other sedatives or narcotics may produce deep sedation or general anesthesia. Ketamine should always be administered with an atropine (0.1 mg/kg) or glycopyrrolate (0.01 mg/kg) since profuse secretions from ketamine alone may induce laryngospasm.

Cardiovascular stability and blood pressure are usually maintained. Typically, ketamine has been associated with hallucinations during emergence in up to 12% of patients. It may be reduced by administration of benzodiazepam. It is contraindicated in patients with head injury, open globe injury, hypertension, and psychosis. It is recognized that ketamine can induce apnea in neonates as well as a decrease response to hypocarbia, laryngospasm, and coughing. There is no antagonist available.

10.3.2 Propofol

Propofol is a short-acting sedative hypnotic. It is available in an Intralipid formulation. It has no analgesic properties, but it does have antiemetic and antipruritic properties. Although small doses of propofol (25–50 μg/(kg min) can provide "conscious sedation" in adults with deep sedation, airway obstruction quickly occurs in pediatric patients. It is titrated with an infusion pump and should be administered by individuals with advanced airway skills. There has been a lot of enthusiasm in using this agent in pediatric intensive care units and in Endoscopy suites. Cases of fatal metabolic acidosis, mild cardiac failure, and lipemic serum have been reported in children which limits its use for prolonged periods of time. Short-term sedation with propofol has been associated with no such problems. Propofol should be administered in large veins since it can cause pain on injection. Respiratory depression/apnea and hypotension are related to the dose, rate and co-adminstration with other CNS depressants. Hypotension occurs from using the medication, especially when it is given rapidly. Anaphylactic reactions and bacterial contaminations have been described and have been attributed to the lipid formulation in which it is dispensed. Strict aseptic technique must be used when one uses propofol because it may support the growth of microorganisms. The dosage of this drug should be lowered if the patients are hemodynamically unstable. There is no antagonist available for this drug.

10.4 Antagonists/reversal agents

Flumazenil is a specific benzodiazepam antagonist and will rapidly reverse the sedative and respiratory effects of benzodiazepines. In patients who are taking benzodiazepines for seizures or drug dependency, seizures may recur if flumazenil is given. The recommended dose of flumazenil is 10 µg/kg up to 1 mg intravenously. Antagonism begins within 1–2 minutes and lasts approximately 1 hour. Since resedation after 1 hour is known to occur with diazepam, the patient must be carefully monitored for at least 2 hours. Flumazenil should not be administered for the routine reversal of the sedative effects of benzodiazepam, but reserved for reversal of respiratory depression only.

Naloxone reversal of meperidine due to respiratory depression may precipitate seizures caused by normeperidine. The initial dose for respiratory depression is 1–2 µg/kg titrated to affect every 2–3 minutes. A dose of 10–100 µg/kg up to 2 mg may be required for respiratory arrest.

11. Conclusions

Sedation for pediatric endoscopy is generally given to have a smooth and comfortable procedure. With proper safety precautions and adopting uniform guidelines, adverse events can be reduced to very low levels. However, pediatric endoscopy team must always be prepared for severe respiratory adverse events.

12. References

Ament, M. E., W. E. Berquist, et al. (1988). "Fiberoptic upper intestinal endoscopy in infants and children." Pediatr Clin North Am 35(1): 141-155.

Ammar and M. (2003). "Complications after outpatient upper GI endoscopy in children: 30-day follow-up." The American Journal of Gastroenterology 98(7): 1508-1511.

Ayoub, C., A. Skoury, et al. (2007). "Lidocaine lollipop as single-agent anesthesia in upper GI endoscopy." Gastrointest Endosc 66(4): 786-793.

Bishop, P. R., M. J. Nowicki, et al. (2002). "Unsedated upper endoscopy in children." Gastrointestinal endoscopy 55(6): 624-630.

Cote, C. J., D. A. Notterman, et al. (2000). "Adverse sedation events in pediatrics: a critical incident analysis of contributing factors." Pediatrics 105(4 Pt 1): 805-814.

Evans, L. T., S. Saberi, et al. (2006). "Pharyngeal anesthesia during sedated EGDs: is "the spray" beneficial? A meta-analysis and systematic review." Gastrointest Endosc 63(6): 761-766.

Lightdale, J. R., L. B. Mahoney, et al. (2007). "Methods of sedation in pediatric endoscopy: a survey of NASPGHAN members." J Pediatr Gastroenterol Nutr 45(4): 500-502.

Mahoney, L. B. and J. R. Lightdale (2007). "Sedation of the Pediatric and Adolescent Patient for GI Procedures." Curr Treat Options Gastroenterol 10(5): 412-421.

Thakkar, K., H. Elserag, et al. (2007). "Complications of pediatric EGD: a 4-year experience in PEDS-CORI." Gastrointestinal Endoscopy 65(2): 213-221.

Tolia, V., J. M. Peters, et al. (2000). "Sedation for pediatric endoscopic procedures." J Pediatr Gastroenterol Nutr 30(5): 477-485.

5

Intravenous Sedation for Pediatric Gastrointestinal Endoscopy in a Developing Country

Somchai Amornyotin
Department of Anesthesiology and Siriraj GI Endoscopy Center, Faculty of Medicine, Siriraj Hospital, Mahidol University, Bangkok, Thailand

1. Introduction

The field of pediatric sedation and analgesia has evolved over the past two decades. The growing number of pediatric gastrointestinal endoscopy procedures requiring sedation and analgesia are recognized even in developing countries. It is well accepted that children undergoing diagnostic and therapeutic gastrointestinal endoscopic procedures should receive sedation and/or anesthesia. Nevertheless, considerable practice variation prevails. The ability to provide safe and effective sedation and analgesia is an important skill for physicians involved in pediatric patients. Children are more prone to anxiety in the acute setting. Procedural sedation and analgesia is the use of sedative, analgesic and dissociate drugs to provide anxiolysis, analgesia, sedation and motor control during painful and unpleasant procedures.

Intravenous sedation for pediatric gastrointestinal endoscopic procedure is ubiquitous in any hospital that cares for children and depending on the institution and country. The developing countries have no their practice guidelines. The guidelines established by the American Academy of Pediatrics (AAP) (Cote et al., 2006), the American Society of Anesthesiologists (ASA, 2002) and the Joint Commission on Accreditation of Healthcare Organizations (JCAHO) serve as the standard for institutional policy development in the area of pediatric intravenous sedation.

The guideline defines terms throughout and in particular:

Minimal sedation: a drug-induced state which patients respond normally to verbal commands.

Moderate sedation (conscious sedation): a drug-induced depression of consciousness which patients respond purposefully to verbal commands. Spontaneous ventilation is adequate. Cardiovascular function is usually maintained.

Deep sedation: a drug-induced depression of consciousness which patients can not be easily aroused but respond purposefully after repeated verbal or painful stimulation. Spontaneous ventilation may be inadequate. Cardiovascular function is usually maintained.

General anesthesia: a drug-induced loss of consciousness which patients are not arousable, even by painful stimulation. Patients often require assistance in maintaining a patent airway. Cardiovascular function may be impaired.

In this report, the author will seek to examine the role of anesthesiologists in determining the field of pediatric intravenous sedation, and the current status of intravenous sedation for pediatric gastrointestinal endoscopic procedures in Siriraj GI Endoscopy Center, Siriraj Hospital, Thailand. Additionally, this review is divided into three parts: 1. the pre-pediatric gastrointestinal endoscopic assessment period, 2. the intra-pediatric gastrointestinal endoscopic management period, and 3. the post-pediatric gastrointestinal endoscopy period.

2. Pre-pediatric gastrointestinal endoscopic assessment period

The general health status of each patient undergoing pediatric procedural intravenous sedation must be evaluated. A physical examination should focus primarily on the upper airway, lungs, cardiovascular system, and baseline neurological status. To aid in assessment risk, the American Society of Anesthesiologists (ASA) has developed a classification system for patients, which categorizes individuals on a general health basis. Several studies have documented the fact that sedation risk in children rises with increasing ASA physical status (Cote et al., 2006; Krauss & Green, 2006; Vespasiano et al., 2007). ASA physical status 1 and 2 are considered low risk patient populations. ASA physical status 3 and 4 are high risk patient populations. The specific high risk patient populations in which anesthesia consultation may be warranted including known respiratory or hemodynamic instability, obstructive sleep apnea, high risk airway management, ASA physical status ≥4, infants born <37 weeks and <60 weeks post conception, history of sedation related adverse events, and patients with neuromuscular disease affecting respiratory or brain stem function.

In this pre-assessment period, there are no differences in a routine practice between the developed countries and the developing countries. Additionally, the majority of intravenous sedation practices for pediatric gastrointestinal endoscopic procedures in the developing countries were sedated by anesthesiologists and/or anesthetic personnel in the operating room.

3. Intra-pediatric gastrointestinal endoscopic management period

Any time sedative and analgesic medications are to be given to a pediatric patient, a clearly worded informed consent should be obtained. This consent should include a listing of the possible consequences of adverse drug reactions, allergic reactions and airway difficulties. Prior to undertaking intravenous sedation, there are some key pieces of equipment that must be in place. These equipments that should be in place before starting a sedation are suction, oxygen, airway, pharmacy, monitors, and extra equipment such as defibrillator (SOAPME) (Cote et al., 2006). In general, intravenous sedation for pediatric gastrointestinal endoscopic procedures is done by anesthesiologists or anesthetic personnel directly supervised by the anesthesiologist or anesthetic personnel.

In a developing country where pediatric endoscopy is performed at increasing rates, the majority of cases (as noted by anecdotal observation) are treated under general anesthesia in the operating room. At Siriraj Hospital, there is a dedicated endoscopy unit with dedicated anesthesia service. Over the last four years, 2006–2010, we performed most pediatric gastrointestinal endoscopic procedures with intravenous sedation technique. We followed the guidelines provided by the American Academy of Pediatrics (Cote et al., 2006) and American Society of Anesthesiologists standards (ASA, 2002). Our review of intravenous sedation practice in pediatric population showed that intravenous sedation can be done safely with various sedative combinations with proper monitoring and anesthesiology service supervision.

Patient monitoring during the procedure should be included continuous monitoring of heart rate and oxygen saturation, and intermittent recording of respiratory rate and blood pressure. Additionally, capnography detects increasing levels of carbon dioxide before desaturation occurs and can detect early inadequately ventilation (Krauss & Green, 2000). However, the cost of capnometer is relatively high. The developing countries like Thailand have none or few capnometers, though this monitor is not routinely used. A sedative drug can only be considered safe after experience in hundreds or thousands of cases. Good protocols are important for the safety and success of the intravenous sedation technique. Depending on the procedure, pediatric intravenous sedation can involve monotherapy or combination therapy. Each regimen and administration of intravenous sedation must be carefully personalized for each patient. When administered, the drugs should be given as an appropriate initial dose with subsequent doses until titrated to effect. However, the most important factor is the judgement of the physician (ASA, 2002; Sury, 2004; Cote et al., 2006; Krauss & Green, 2006; Vespasiano et al., 2007; Meredith et al., 2008).

Common drug-receptor systems used by anesthesiologists in Thailand include the following:

1. Opioid receptors: fentanyl, meperidine
2. Gamma-aminobytyric acid (GABA) receptors: propofol
3. Benzodiazepine receptors: midazolam
4. N-methyl-D-aspartate (NMDA) receptors: ketamine

Sedation should be administered based on the patient's weight and titrated by response. Dosing requirements for individual patients may vary significantly based on the patient's psychosocial development and attention to the surrounding environment by the endoscopy team. Adequate time should be allowed between doses to assess sedation effects and determine the need for additional medication. For example, midazolam should be titrated to the effect with at least three minutes between doses, while fentanyl should have five minutes between doses. Higher doses of sedative/analgesic agents are frequently needed in preschool, school aged and preteen patients compared with those used in teenage children. The most common intravenous sedation regimen for pediatric gastrointestinal endoscopic procedure is the use of an opioid and a benzodiazepine combination to achieve analgesia and amnesia (Dar & Shah, 2010). Many safe regimens were reported. Consequently, anesthesiologist or the anesthetic personnel must exercise extreme caution while administering the intravenous sedation for pediatric gastrointestinal endoscopic procedure. The use of intravenous sedation drugs is reliability, efficacy and easy titration to achieve the end point. However, monitoring during the procedure is essential.

3.1 Analgesic drugs

3.1.1 Fentanyl

Fentanyl is a potent synthetic opioid with no intrinsic anxiolytic or amnestic properties. It has high lipid solubility allows for quick penetration of the blood-brain barrier, resulting in a very rapid onset of action (<1 minute) and short duration of action (30-45 minutes) (Nowicki & Vaughn, 2002; Dar & Shah, 2010). Fentanyl lacks of direct of myocardial depressant effects, and absence of histamine release, making it an excellent choice for intravenous sedation. Intravenous fentanyl can be easily and rapidly titrated for painful procedures (Kennedy et al., 1998; Pitetti et al., 2003). The combination of fentanyl and midazolam is a popular intravenous sedation regimen, with a safety profile when both drugs are carefully titrated (Kennedy et al., 1998; Pena & Krauss, 1999; Pitetti et al., 2003). Fentanyl can cause respiratory depression and apnea, especially when combined with other sedatives or in infants less than 3 months of age (C.L. Algren & C.T. Algren, 1997). Fentanyl-induced bradycardia may need treatment with a vagolytic drug such as atropine. Chest wall and glottic rigidity has been observed with rapid administration of fentanyl. Safe intravenous administration therefore requires slow titration of 0.5-1.0 mcg/kg boluses, and may repeat every 3 minutes, but the maximum cumulative dose is 4 to 5 mcg/kg in one hour (Tolia et al., 2000).

3.1.2 Meperidine (Pethidine)

Meperidine is a synthetic opioid and has grown out of favor in past years. The metabolites of meperidine are toxic to the central nervous system at high doses and in patients with renal impairment. Meperidine has a long and favorable experience in intravenous sedation for pediatric gastrointestinal endoscopic procedure (Bahal-O'Mara et al., 1993). Meperidine 0.5-1.0 mg/kg i.v. combined with midazolam 0.05-0.1 mg/kg i.v. provides effective sedation for gastrointestinal endoscopy. However, meperidine is not recommended for intravenous sedation in the emergency department (Lewis & Stanley, 1999; Mace, 2004). Side effects of meperidine are respiratory depression, nausea, vomiting, and dysphoria (Goad & Webster, 1997). It causes less histamine release and urticaria than morphine (C.L. Algren & C.T. Algren, 1997). Fatal reactions have also occurred in patients taking monoamine oxidase inhibitors.

3.2 Sedative drugs

3.2.1 Propofol

Propofol is a phenol derivative with sedative, hypnotic and anesthetic properties. It has a rapid onset (< 1 minute), shorter duration of action, and rapid recovery. Its clinical effects are dose dependent. Propofol has antiemetic, anxiolytic, hypnotic, amnestic and anesthetic properties. However, it does not have analgesic effects. Propofol can be given to children in the settings of gastroenterology (Barbi et al., 2003; Amornyotin et al., 2009, 2010), emergency department (Bassett et al., 2003; Green & Krauss, 2003), and critical care series (Lowrie et al., 1998) with good efficacy, rapid recovery, and apparent safety. The most serious adverse effect of propofol is potent respiratory depression and apnea can occur suddenly. The respiratory depression rates vary extensively by the study (Green & Krauss, 2003). Propofol can also produce hypotension, although this effect is typically transient and of little clinical importance in healthy patients (Green & Krauss, 2003). Propofol is well known to be painful upon injection, the addition of lidocaine has been shown to decrease the incidence of pain during injection (Bassett et al., 2003).

Currently, most centers utilize an anesthesiologist or nurse anesthetist to administer propofol (Sury & Smith, 2008), although recently nurse administered and patient controlled dosing has been reported in adult patients. In our endoscopy center, propofol is also administered by an anesthesiologist or nurse anesthetist. Propofol provides equal or better control and more rapid recovery when compared with midazolam for sedation (O'Hare et al., 2001). Initial intravenous bolus dose of propofol is 1.0 mg/kg and is followed by 0.5 mg/kg, and the repeated dose is needed. In my experience, I use the initial bolus dose of propofol and follow by the continuous intravenous technique. The continuous intravenous infusion of propofol dose is 100-150 mcg/kg/min. Majority of our patients received propofol in combination with other sedatives. Over the last decade, the use of propofol for endoscopic sedation has increased. It has gained wide acceptance among adult gastroenterologist. The use of propofol in pediatric population has been shown to be safe, effective, and reliable (Balsells et al., 1997; Kaddu et al., 2002). The drug, now commonly used outside the operating room, has demonstrated an excellent safety profile, despite a narrow therapeutic window. Desirable properties of propofol for endoscopic procedures include ease of use, quick onset of action, and rapid metabolization leading to shorter recovery time (Aouad M.T. et al., 2008).

3.2.2 Midazolam

Midazolam is the drug most commonly used for sedation in children during procedures (Kennedy et al., 1998; Pena & Krauss, 1999). It is a shorting, water soluble benzodiazepine with anxiolytic, amnestic, sedative, muscle relaxant, and anticonvulsant properties. It is very widely used because of its more rapid onset of action and shorter duration of effect compared with diazepam (Tolia et al., 2000). Disadvantages of midazolam include transient hypotension and vomiting. Midazolam is approved for many routes, including intravenous, oral and nasal and is most useful for intravenous sedation. Because of greater clearance of midazolam in children, larger weight-adjusted dosages may be required in pediatric patients than in adult to achieve similar levels and duration of sedation (Gilger, 1993 & Tolia et al., 2000). The shorter clinical half-life of the drug necessitates additional boluses for longer or complicated procedures. Less midazolam is needed when fentanyl is administered than when meperidine is given with midazolam. Initial intravenous dose of midazolam is 0.025-0.1 mg/kg and may repeat another dose, but the maximum recommended dose is 0.4-0.6 mg/kg. In our endoscopy center, we commonly use midazolam combined with low dose propofol and/or low dose fentanyl.

3.2.3 Ketamine

Ketamine is a phencyclidine derivative with dissociative sedative, analgesic and amnestic properties (Green & Krauss, 2000). It is one of the most sedative-analgesic agents and results in a number of desired clinical effects that are dose dependent (Krystal et al., 1994). Typically spontaneous respiration and airway reflexes are maintained although may not be totally normal. Neuropsychiatric effects of ketamine include visual hallucinations that may be accompanied by emergence phenomena and agitation. Ketamine generally causes an increase in heart rate, blood pressure, cardiac output, intracranial pressure, and intraocular pressure. Ketamine can induce salivation, and cholinergics have traditionally been coadministered. The single most severe adverse effect with ketamine sedation is laryngospasm. Ketamine is clinically effective by a number of different routes. Intravenous dose of ketamine is 1-1.5 mg/kg, and may repeat dose every 10 minutes as needed. In Thailand, we commonly used low dose of ketamine, and combined with low dose of midazolam, opioid drug, and/or low dose of propofol (Amornyotin et al., 2009). This combination technique produces stable hemodynamic effects, and can reduce the sedation related adverse effects.

The ideal combination of sedative drugs for intravenous sedation in pediatric patients undergoing gastrointestinal endoscopic procedure is unknown. The drug combination provides synergistic action while lowering the doses of each agent. The combination regimen may be a superior sedation technique (Cohen et al., 2004; Van Natta & Rex, 2006). Our practice reflects this technique where many different combination regimens were used. Midazolam and fentanyl are the most common agents used in combination with propofol in this study. The next most common combination includes midazolam, fentanyl, ketamine, and propofol.

Cardiopulmonary complications account for more than half of the major complications during endoscopy (Lamireau et al., 1998) and are often related to hypoxia, especially in children less than 1-year old (Lamireau et al., 1998 & Lightdale et al., 2008). In a study by Barbi et al., using propofol in 811 children undergoing upper endoscopy, desaturation on supplemental oxygen is 3%, and major desaturation was noted in 0.7% of all the children. Additionally, a study by Yldzdas et al. demonstrated that the use propofol and midazolam/ fentanyl in 126 children who were randomly assigned to different sedation regimens had a 16.6% incidence of respiratory depression as shown by high end-tidal carbon dioxide (>50 mmHg). The higher incidence of respiratory depression reflected the better detection of respiratory depression by the use of end-tidal carbon dioxide. The adverse events in our clinical practice are comparable to those in the studies that did not use end-tidal carbon dioxide monitoring (Balsells et al., 1997; Malviya et al., 1997 & Barbi et al., 2006).

4. Post-pediatric gastrointestinal endoscopic period (Recovery and discharge)

Following sedation it is important that patient monitoring continue until the children are fully awake and ready for discharge. The recovery area should be equipped with oxygen, suction, and equipment for tracheal intubation. Monitoring equipment including non-invasive blood pressure, pulse oximetry, electrocardiography, and ventilation monitoring should be available as well. Patients should be discharged only when they have met specific criteria.
The criteria for discharge should include:

1. stable vital signs
2. a return to the level of consciousness that is similar to the baseline for that patient
3. pain under control
4. adequate muscle strength to maintain a patent airway
5. speech and ambulation appropriate for age should return to pre-sedation level
6. nausea and/or vomiting should be controlled.

Patients who received reversal drugs such as naloxone or flumazenil may require longer periods of observation, because the half-life of the offending agent may exceed that of the reversal medication and lead to resedation. At the time of discharge, specific written and verbal instruction and information as well as the status of the child should be given to a parent, legal guardian or other responsible adult. Specific instructions should be given to the child's family instructing them what to do if the child should appear sedated or have any other medical problems. In the western countries, most of GIE procedures for children can be safely done with ambulatory setting. However, the majority of pediatric GIE procedures in eastern countries like Thailand are done with inpatient setting.

In summary, no method of intravenous sedation can be universally applied to all children requiring gastrointestinal endoscopic procedures. However, in a tertiary care teaching hospital in a developing country, intravenous sedation for pediatric gastrointestinal endoscopic procedures can be safely and effectively performed outside the operating room with a multi-drug sedation regimen utilizing anesthesiologists and anesthetic personnel with appropriate basic monitoring.

5. References

Algren, C.L. & Algren, C.T. (1997). Pediatric sedation: essentials for the perioperative nurse. *Nursing Clinics of North America*, Vol. 32, No. 1, pp. 17-30

American Society of Anesthesiologists. (2002). Practice guidelines for sedation and analgesia by non-anesthesiologists. *Anesthesiology*, Vol. 96, No. 4, pp. 1004-1017

Amornyotin S. et al. (2009). Experience of intravenous sedation for pediatric gastrointestinal endoscopy in a large tertiary referral center in a developing country. *Pediatric Anesthesia*, Vol. 19, No. 8, pp. 784-791

Amornyotin, S. & Aanpreung, P. (2010). Clinical effectiveness of an anesthesiologist-administered intravenous sedation outside of the main operating room for pediatric upper gastrointestinal endoscopy in Thailand. *International Journal of Pediatrics*, Vol. 2010, Article. ID 748564, 6 pages, doi:10.1155/2010/748564

Aouad M.T. et al. (2008). Addition of ketamine to propofol for initiation of procedural anesthesia in children reduces propofol consumption and preserves hemodynamic stability. *Acta Anaesthesiologica Scandinavica*, Vol. 52, No. 4, pp. 561–565

Barbi E. et al. (2006). Deep sedation with propofol for upper gastrointestinal endoscopy in children, administered by specially trained pediatricians: a prospective case series with emphasis on side effects. *Endoscopy*, Vol. 38, No. 4, pp. 368–375

Bahal-O'Mara N. et al. (1993). Efficacy of diazepam and meperidine in ambulatory pediatric patients undergoing endoscopy: a randomized, double-blind trial. *Journal of Pediatric Gastroenterology and Nutrition*, Vol. 16, No. 4, pp. 387-392

Balsells F. et al. (1997). Use of conscious sedation for lower and upper gastrointestinal endoscopic examinations in children, adolescents, and young adults: a twelve-year review. *Gastrointestinal Endoscopy*, Vol. 45, No. 5, pp. 375–380

Barbi E. et al. (2003). Deep sedation with propofol by nonanesthesiologists: a prospective pediatric experience. *Archieves of Pediatric and Adolescent Medicine*, Vol. 157, No. 11, pp. 1097-1103

Bassett K.E. et al. (2003). Propofol for procedural sedation in children in the emergency department. *Annals of Emergency Medicine*, Vol. 42, No. 6, pp. 773-782

Cohen L.B. et al. (2004). Moderate level sedation during endoscopy: a prospective study using lowdose propofol, meperidine / fentanyl, and midazolam. *Gastrointestinal Endoscopy*, Vol. 59, No. 7, pp. 795–803

Cote C.J. et al. (2006). Guidelines for monitoring and management of pediatric patients during and after sedation for diagnostic and therapeutic procedures: an update. *Pediatrics*, Vol. 118, No. 6, pp. 2587-2602

Dar, A.Q. & Shah, Z.A. (2010). Anesthesia and sedation in pediatric gastrointestinal endoscopic procedures: a review. *World Journal of Gastrointestinal Endoscopy*, Vol. 2, No. 7, pp. 257-262

Gilger M.A. (1993). Conscious sedation for endoscopy in the pediatric patient. *Gastroenterology Nursing*, Vol. 16, No. 2, pp. 75-79

Green, S.M. & Krauss, B. (2000). The semantics of ketamine. *Annals of Emergency Medicine*, Vol. 36, No. 5, pp. 480-482

Green, S.M. & Krauss, B. (2003). Propofol in emergency medicine: pushing the sedation frontier," *Annals of Emergency Medicine*, Vol. 42, No. 6, pp. 792-797

Joint Commission on Accreditation of Healthcare Organizations. (2005). Comprehensive accreditation manual for hospitals. Oakbrook Terrace, IL: Joint Commission on Accreditation of Healthcare Organizations

Kaddu R. et al. (2002). Propofol compared with general anesthesia for pediatric GI endoscopy: is propofol better? *Gastrointestinal Endoscopy*, Vol. 55, No. 1, pp. 27–32

Kennedy R.M. et al. (1998). Comparison of fentanyl/midazolam with ketamine/midazolam for pediatric orthropedic emergencies. *Pediatrics*, Vol. 102, No. 4, pp. 956-963

Krauss, B. & Green, S.M. (2000). Sedation and analgesia for procedures in children. *New England Journal of Medicine,* Vol. 342, No. 13, pp. 938-945

Krauss, B. & Green, S.M. (2006). Procedural sedation and analgesia in children. *Lancet,* Vol. 367, No. 9512, pp. 766-780

Krystal J.H. et al. (1994). Subanesthetic effects of the noncompetitive NMDA antagonist, ketamine, in humans. Psychomimetic, perceptual, cognitive and neuroendocrine responses. *Archieves of General Psychiatry,* Vol. 51, No. 3, pp. 199-214

Lamireau, T.; Dubreuil, M. & Daconceicao, M. (1998). Oxygen saturation during esophagogastroduodenoscopy in children: general anesthesia versus intravenous sedation. *Journal of Pediatric Gastroenterology Nutrition,* Vol. 27, No. 2, pp. 172–175

Lewis, K.P. & Stanley, G.D. (1999). Pharmacology. *International Anesthsiology Clinics,* Vol. 37, No. 1, pp. 73-86

Lightdale J.R. et al. (2008). Efficiency of propofol versus midazolam and fentanyl sedation at a pediatric teaching hospital: a prospective study. *Gastrointestinal Endoscopy,* Vol. 67, No. 7, pp. 1067–1075

Lowrie L. et al. (1998). The pediatric sedation unit: a mechanism for pediatric sedation. *Pediatrics,* Vol. 102, No. 3, pp. e 30

Mace S.E. et al. (2004). Clinical policy: Evidence-based approach to pharmacological agents used in pediatric sedation and analgesia in the emergency department. *Journal of Pediatric Surgery,* Vol. 39, No. 10, pp. 1472-1484

Malviya, S.; Voepel-Lewis, T. & Tait, A.R. (1997). Adverse events and risk factors associated with the sedation of children by nonanesthesiologists. *Anesthesia and Analgesia,* Vol. 85, No. 6, pp. 1207–1213

Meredith J.R. et al. (2008). Pediatric procedural sedation and analgesia. *Journal of Emergencies, Trauma and Shock,* Vol. 1, No. 2, pp. 88-96

Nowicki, M.J. & Vaughn, C.A. (2002). Sedation and anesthesia in children for endoscopy. *Techniques in Gastrointestinal Endoscopy,* Vol. 4, No. 4, pp. 225-130

O'Hare R.A. et al. (2001). Recovery from propofol anesthesia supplemented with remifentanil. British Journal of Anaesthesia, Vol. 86, No. 3, pp. 361-365.

Pena, B.M.G. & Krauss, B. (1999). Adverse events of procedural sedation and analgesia in a pediatric emergency department. *Annals of Emergency Medicine,* Vol.34, No. 4, pp. 483-490

Pitetti R.D. et al. (2003). Safe and efficacious use of procedural sedation and analgesia by nonanesthesiogists in a pedatric emergency department. *Archieves Pediatric and Adolescent Medicine,* Vol. 157, No. 11, pp. 1090-1096

Sury M.R.J. (2004). Paediatric sedation. *Continuing Education in Anaesthesia, Critical Care and Pain,* Vol. 4, No. 4, pp. 118-122

Sury, M.R.J. & Smith, J.H. (2008). Deep sedation and minimal anesthesia. *Pediatric Anesthesia,* Vol. 18, No. 1, pp. 18–24

Tolia, V.; Peters, J.M. & Gilger, M.A. (2000). Sedation for pediatric endoscopic procedures. *Journal of Pediatric Gastroenterology and Nutrition,* Vol. 30, No. 5, pp. 477-485

Van Natta, M.E. & Rex, D.K. (2006). Propofol alone titrated to deep sedation versus propofol in combination with opioids and / or benzodiazepines and titrated to moderate sedation for colonoscopy. *American Journal of Gastroenterology,* Vol. 101, No. 10, pp. 2209–2217

Vespasiano, M; Finkelstein, M & Kurachek, S. (2007). Propofol sedation: intensivists' experience with 7304 cases in a children's hospital. *Pediatrics,* Vol. 120, No. 6, pp. e 1411-1417

Yldzdas, D.; Yapcoglu, H. & Ylmaz H.L. (2004). The value of capnography during sedation or sedation /analgesia in pediatric minor procedures. *Pediatric Emergency Care,* Vol. 20, No. 3, pp. 162–165.

Part 2

The Esophagus

6

Endoscopic Aspects of Eosinophilic Esophagitis: From Diagnosis to Therapy

Alfredo J. Lucendo[1] and Susana Jiménez-Contreras[2]
[1]*Department of Gastroenterology, Hospital General de Tomelloso*
[2]*Department of Gastroenterology, Hospital Virgen de Altagracia*
Spain

1. Introduction

Eosinophilic esophagitis (EoE) represents a chronic, immune/antigen mediated disease characterized by esophageal dysfunction and eosinophilic inflammation (Liacouras et al., 2011). The past few years have witnessed a progressive rise in diagnosed cases of EoE, which has become the second most common chronic esophageal disease after gastroesophageal reflux (Lucendo, 2010). In spite of this, EoE remains underdiagnosed in many cases, especially because endoscopic findings are usually much harder to detect than those observed in esophageal growths (such as neoplasms) or erosive disorders. A great variety of endoscopic findings has been described in literature for EoE patient, including an apparently normal esophagus, which suggests that changes in this organ's appearance are not only complex, but also subtle enough to be overlooked by an endoscopist unaccustomed to diagnosing this disease.

At the same time, research efforts aimed at providing efficient therapy for this chronic illness has also intensified. Unfortunately, no treatment strategies have been commonly accepted to date, making adequate management of these patients somewhat controversial (González-Castillo et al., 2010). That being said, 3 different therapeutic approaches have been used effectively in patients with EoE. The first approach involves endoscopic dilation, a technique which is frequently able to solve alterations in the caliber of the esophagus, including a narrowing of the lumen (Schoepfer et al., 2009). From the earliest documented cases, mechanical dilation has been used as a treatment option for EoE, similar to the way it is used in other cases of fibrous esophageal stenosis, such as peptic stenosis or following caustication.

The classification of EoE as an immunoallergic disorder has led to a second approach, namely that of treating patients with drugs for bronchial asthma (Furuta & Straumann, 2006). However, because no specifically approved drugs are currently available for EoE patients, these treatment must be due out label.

From the first studies performed on children with EoE, allergies to certain dietary components have been demonstrated to contribute significantly to its pathogenesis; indeed, it is well-documented that both the symptoms of the disease and histology levels improve after eliminating certain foods from the diet (Liacouras et al., 2005). However, while early studies based exclusively on elemental diets showed enormous efficacy in reverting EoE (Kelly et al., 1995), this approach is not plausible in adults or chronic patients.

One important stumbling block to determining the most effective treatment for EoE is the lack of studies directly comparing different treatment strategies for the disease. Such studies will be necessary before the best therapeutic option for EoE can be established.
In this chapter we review the various endoscopic lesions described in EoE to date. This should help relatively inexperienced endoscopists screen for patients suspected of having EoE. We will also discuss the effects and risks of endoscopic treatment by dilation in EoE patients by reviewing the current literature.

2. Diagnosis

EoE is a clinico-pathological disease characterized by symptoms related to esophageal dysfunction. Up to now, esophageal biopsies have been essential for making a diagnosis. For optimal pathological evaluation, multiple biopsies from the proximal and distal esophagus should be obtained and evaluated for a variety of pathological features, the most characteristic being an eosinophil-predominant inflammation with a minimum threshold of 15 eosinophils/high power field (hpf). However other accompanying findings reinforce the diagnosis and should also be noted by the pathologist. These include: eosinophilic microabscesses, surface layering of eosinophils, extracellular eosinophilic deposits, basal cell hyperplasia, intercellular edema, and lamina propria fibrosis (Furuta et al., 2007).
The effects of EoE are isolated to the esophagus; therefore, eosinophilic inflammation should be absent from both gastric and duodenal biopsy samples (Lucendo, 2010). Furthermore, other causes of esophageal eosinophilia should be excluded, specifically gastroesophageal reflux disease (GERD). This can effectively be excluded if there is a normal pH-metry or if eosinophils persist after treatment with full doses of proton pump inhibitors (PPI). However, the prevalence of patients suffering from both EoE and GERD make the PPI trial the method of choice for diagnosing EoE in these cases (Molina-Infante et al., 2009).

3. Endoscopic findings

The fact that EoE was first identified only 30 years ago is indicative of the frequently subtle and unspecific endoscopic finding present in most patients. In fact, common esophageal diseases causing dysphagia are usually characterized by evident endoscopic lesions, such us peptic erosions, ulcers, protruding masses or stenosis, all of which contrast with the relatively minor findings exhibited by the majority of patients with EoE. Successful diagnosis of the disease thus requires a high level of suspicion on the part of the clinician, who should perform a careful examination of the esophagus accompanied by mucosal biopsies, even if the mucosa appears to be normal.
Many patients diagnosed with EoE have had previous endoscopies for dysphagia or food impaction and received different diagnoses. In fact, one study reported that the average adult EoE patient underwent two endoscopic exams before being diagnosed correctly (Lucendo et al., 2007). Esophageal symptoms in these patients are frequently attributed to various causes, with some reported cases receiving referrals to mental health professionals because psychological rather than physiological disorders were suspected.
Only in past few years has EoE been extensively recognized, leaving behind its status as a broadly misdiagnosed disease (Gonsalves et al., 2005) to become the second cause of chronic esophagitis.

Endoscopy with esophageal biopsy remains the only reliable diagnostic test for EoE. Consequently, in order for clinicians to recognize the disease more easily, a better awareness of the distinct endoscopic features of EoE is essential. Retrospective re-evaluations of the endoscopic appearance of the esophagus in those patients eventually diagnosed with EoE have revealed that esophageal appearance had been described as normal in between one quarter to one third of the cases (Müller et al., 2007; Sgouros et al., 2006; Liacouras et al., 2005). It is important to note, however, that even though the endoscopic findings are subtle, remarkable abnormalities can still be detected in the majority of patients, as we describe below.

Endoscopy has helped identify a great number of esophageal abnormalities in patients with EoE. These include fixed esophageal rings that sometimes reduce the esophageal lumen (a phenomenon known as trachealization) and transient esophageal rings (also called feline folds or felinization). Diffuse nodularity/granularity of the mucosa has also been described, along with widespread exudative mucosal lesions, either in the form of whitish papulae of varying sizes clustered together (white spots) or as large, white, exudative fibrinoid lesions. These whitish lesions on the mucosa resemble a mild, superficial Candida infection, but histopathology shows micro-abscesses made up of eosinophils (Lucendo et al., 2007). Furthermore, a loss of the common vascular pattern of the mucosa has been described (Lucendo, 2007; Straumann et al., 2004). Some of the most common findings are longitudinal furrows (referred to as "corrugated esophagus," which is an architectural analogy to a grooved column) (Straumann et al., 2004), diffuse esophageal narrowing, and esophageal lacerations induced by passage of the endoscope. Mucosal fragility, also called *crêpe-paper* mucosa (Straumann et al., 2003), is an important feature of this pathology as it may cause tears during upper endoscopy or even if the patient tries to dislodge impacted food by inducing vomiting (Lucendo et al., 2011). However, because all of these endoscopic features have been described in other esophageal disorders, none can be considered pathognomonic for EoE.

To shed light on the varied endoscopic appearances of EoE, we have classified them according to two independent yet complementary aspects: alterations in the caliber of the esophagus and alterations in the appearance of the mucosa (Lucendo et al., 2007).

- Alterations in the caliber of the esophagus, which appear as a consequence of motor esophageal disturbances associated to EoE in children (Nurko et al., 2009) and adults (Moawad, 2011; Lucendo et al, 2007), or after fibrous remodeling of the organ. In this case, multiple simultaneous contraction rings may be observed; these may block the passage of the endoscope while still permitting observation of the distal lumen. Alternatively, the clinician may notice regular concentric strictures, which impede both passage of the endoscope and observation of the distal mucosa (Lucendo et al, 2007). The smaller caliber of the esophagus may go unnoticed in barium contrast radiography and endoscopy (Vasilopoulos et al., 2002). All of these changes may occur without mucosal lesions (e.g. erosions or ulcerations), unlike what happens in peptic disease. Alterations in the caliber are found predominantly in the mid and distal esophageal thirds and can be reverted with treatment; in fact, since motor disturbances can be successfully treated with topical steroid treatment, a functional rather than structural origin of caliber alterations in EoE should be considered.
- Alteration in the appearance of the mucosa. In a study analyzing different endoscopic findings associated with EoE in parallel with the intensity of histological lesions,

density of eosinophils, and cell activation as determined with the aid of immunostaining for Major Basic Protein (MBP) (Lucendo et al., 2007), it was observed that the density of eosinophils increased with the severity of histological changes. Qualitative analysis of the patient biopsies showed a correlation between the intensity of histopathological changes and the diverse patterns of findings from endoscopic exploration of the mucosa. Consequently, four endoscopic-histopathological patters were defined: 1. Granular pattern: mucosa with relatively defined papular elevations that give it an irregular shape. Histological analysis highlighted changes in eosinophilic infiltration and derived damage, with different intensities in different areas, which implies possible mucosal effects that are not uniform in intensity. 2. Corrugated pattern: linear longitudinal ridges or striae along the folds of the esophagus also affected by mucosal edema. The histology identified edema with growth in intercellular spaces between the epithelial cells, ballooned cells, and spongiosis. 3. Undulated pattern: this may denote contraction of the muscularis mucosae (not evaluable in endoscopic biopsies). It should not be mistaken for simultaneous contraction rings in the internal or circumferential layer of the esophageal muscularis propia, which in this case reduce the size of the lumen. 4. Exudative pattern: different-sized whitish lesions (from slight spotting to squamous lesions), creating epithelial clusters or microabscesses containing eosinophils. These patients had a high density of eosinophils on the surface of the esophagus, destruction and detachment of the most superficial strata, and more intense immunostaining for MBP.

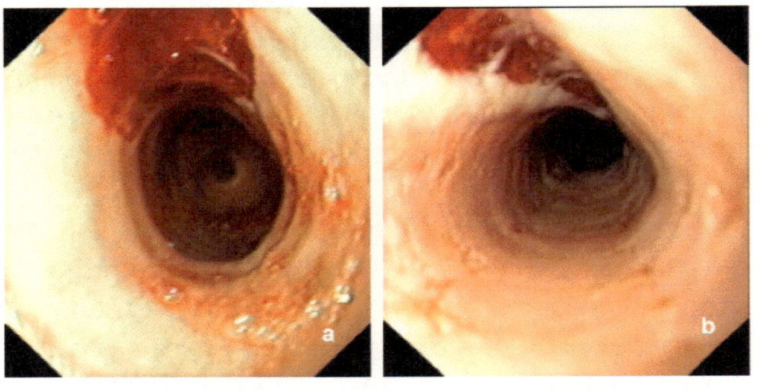

Fig. 1. Images from two patients with eosinophilic esophagitis and spontaneous esophageal tearing, withring disruption. This occurred as a result of the efforts the patients made to induce vomiting and dislodge impacted food

Several prospective studies have evaluated the utility of endoscopic findings for diagnosing EoE. In 2007, G.A. Prasad and co-workers successfully used endoscopy in conjunction with esophageal biopsies to diagnosis EoE in 15% of 222 patients who were being attended for non-obstructive dysphagia (Prasad et al., 2007). Of the 21 patients who exhibited endoscopic results characteristic of EoE, the diagnosis was confirmed in only 8 cases (38%). However, 10 of the 102 patients (9,8%) with an apparently normal endoscopic examination presented histological evidence of EoE. In 2008, S.H. Mackenzie et al. reported similar findings (Mackenzie et al., 2008). Thus, while 12% of the 261 patients suffering from dysphagia who underwent endoscopy were initially diagnosed with EoE, only 12 of 35 patients (34%) who showed esophageal rings in their endoscopic exams were confirmed to have EoE after esophageal biopsy.

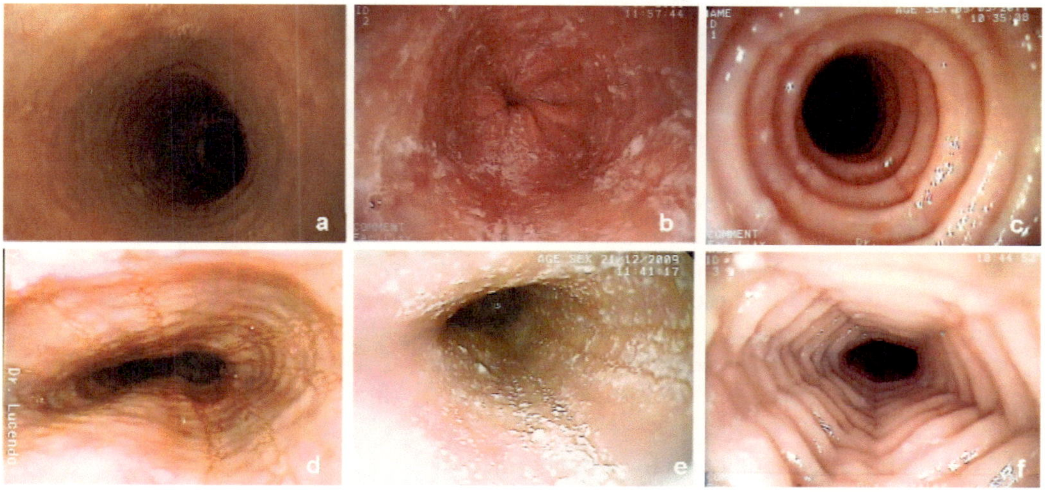

Fig. 2. Several endoscopic aspects of eosinophilic esophagitis: a: Normal- caliber esophagus with a normal appearance mucosal surface; b: Fragile-looking mucosa, with irregular surface and whitish exudates; c: Reduced-caliber, trachealized esophagus with regular mucosal surface, which allows the passage of the endoscope; d: Longitudinal linear furrows and irregular mucosa; e: The esophageal mucosal surface may be covered in cotton-like exudates mimicking candiadiasis, but biopsy finds them to be multiple eosinophil-containing micro-abscesses; f: Ringed esophagus with stenosis blocking the passage of the endoscope

In any case, EoE seems to be a very common cause of dysphagia, with a prevalence of up to 22% in patients with the non-obstructive version of this condition (Ricker, 2001). In addition, its incidence rates are significantly higher in men than in women and also in those of European descent than for other ethnicities. These findings underscore the importance of performing routine biopsies to screen for EoE in these patients (Ricker, 2011).

Because the reliability of endoscopic findings alone for diagnosing EoE does not appear to exceed 40%, few studies deal with finding ways to improve the diagnostic efficiency of endoscopy. Indeed, only one published study has examined the ability of narrow-band imaging (NBI) endoscopy to improve reliability. While this technique proved helpful in detecting mucosal details that go unnoticed in a routine white-light examination, it only managed to identify rings and furrows with fair to good reliability; no other findings were noted. Moreover, there was also great interobserver variability. The researchers thus concluded that endoscopic findings alone were not sufficiently reliable for supporting a diagnosis of EoE or for making treatment decisions (Peery, 2011).

As we have seen, none of the endoscopic features described above is pathognomonic for EoE; however, the presence of more than one of them in a given patient bolsters the case for a diagnosis of EoE. It is our hope that a greater awareness of these subtle characteristics will help clinicians avoid overlooking them to more accurately diagnose patients. Of course, any preliminary diagnosis must then be confirmed through biopsies. Indeed, as we emphasized above, biopsy sampling should also be performed in cases of non-obstructive dysphagia, even when the esophagus appears normal.

4. Endoscopic treatment for Eosinophilic Esophagitis (EoE)

Since the first descriptions of EoE appeared in the literature, the disease has been associated with alterations in the caliber of the esophagus, which specialists have sought to correct by means of endoscopic dilation. In this sense, endoscopic therapy has always been recognized as one of the main treatment modalities in EoE patients, together with systemic and topical steroids and changes in diet.

The efficacy of endoscopic treatment in EoE patients is clear in emergency situations, in which it is needed to resolve food impactions that block the esophageal lumen, and also in scheduled explorations of patients with esophageal symptoms, especially if these are accompanied by a reduced esophageal caliber. The characteristic fragility of the esophageal wall in these patients initially led several authors to consider endoscopic techniques to be a risky treatment option (Lucendo, 2007). We will discuss this assertion in greater depth after reviewing new evidence from the latest studies.

4.1 Emergency endoscopy and food desimpaction

The impaction of food in the esophagus is common in EoE patients and is, together with dysphagia, the clinical hallmark of the disease. Additionally, food impaction is the clinical manifestation which most frequently leads to diagnosis of EoE in adult patients, constituting a complication that must be urgently remedied. In this manner, 43.3% of the 30 adult patients studied in a Spanish series underwent endoscopy as an emergency treatment to resolve food impaction before being diagnosed with EoE (Lucendo et al., 2007). Furthermore, an analysis of 251 Swiss patients with EoE showed that 34.7% required extraction of the impacted bolus with the aid of flexible or rigid esophagoscopy, with the latter causing a 20% rate of transmural perforations (Straumann et al., 2008). Bolus removal by means of rigid endoscopy thus constitutes a high-risk procedure and should be avoided in EoE patients. Food impaction in pediatric forms of EoE seems to be uncommon, with no definitive explanation for this difference.

4.2 Dilation treatment for EoE

From the earliest documented cases, mechanical dilation with through-the-scope hydropneumatic balloons or Savary bougies has been employed as a treatment option for EoE, similar to the way it is used in other cases of rigid or fibrous esophageal stenosis resulting from the cicatrization of prolonged esophageal inflammatory processes such as GERD or after the ingestion of caustic substances. The chronic inflammatory phenomena which characterize EoE seem to cause subepithelial collagen deposition and fibrous remodeling, as recently shown in both childhood (Chehade et al., 2007; Aceves et al., 2007) and adult (Straumann et al., 2010, 2011) forms of the disease as well as in animal models (Mishra et al., 2008). Also, in recent years, various studies have addressed the relationship between EoE and GERD (Spechler et al., 2007), proving that both diseases can coexist in the same patient, causing dysmotility of the distal third of the esophagus, poor acid clearance, and the possibility of lesions – particularly Schatzki rings (Nurko et al., 2004) – from reflux.

Several aspects should be considered before defining the real role of endoscopic treatment through dilation in EoE patients:

- There are no universally accepted therapeutic goals for EoE to date. Currently, treatment objectives range from merely controlling the symptoms to resolving the epithelial inflammatory infiltrate. A group of EoE experts have recommended treating asymptomatic cases of EoE to avoid the potential consequences of fibrous remodeling of the organ (Liacouras et al., 2011), although the long-term consequences are not really known. The experience of each center and the availability of techniques and studies also limit the treatment options and the objectives established in each case. However, we should keep in mind that if left untreated, EoE is a chronic disease involving persistent histological inflammation over time, with detrimental effects on a patient's quality-of-life (Straumann, 2008).

- With regard to what constitutes the best therapeutic option for EoE patients, no studies comparing different therapeutic modalities have been carried out. Moreover, several published EoE case studies involve dilation with concomitant drug therapy (either with steroids or montelukast), which makes it difficult to clearly establish the effect of the individual treatment modalities.
- Additionally, esophageal symptoms are frequently intermittent in EoE patients, who can experience prolonged asymptomatic periods despite the persistence of eosinophilic inflammation. This raises doubts about the convenience of restricting therapy to symptomatic periods only or whether to prescribe a maintenance treatment.
- Narrowing of the esophageal lumen can originate in two ways: by muscle contractions due to motor disturbances secondary to eosinophilic infiltration of deep esophageal wall structures, or by fibrous structures derived from fibrous remodeling and collagen deposits in the subepithelial strata. A combination of both mechanisms may also be possible. In addition, it is difficult to make routine distinctions between patients who have a definite stricture and those in whom it can be reversed through drug or diet therapy.
- A relevant difficulty in assessing the efficacy of individual therapeutic modalities in EoE patients comes from the lack of a validated, commonly accepted score for symptoms in this disease. This makes it difficult not only to extrapolate results from one study to another, but also to objectively evaluate the effect of treatment on clinical manifestations. In this scenario, and with regard to endoscopic treatment, the most valuable criterion for response is the need for repeated dilations.

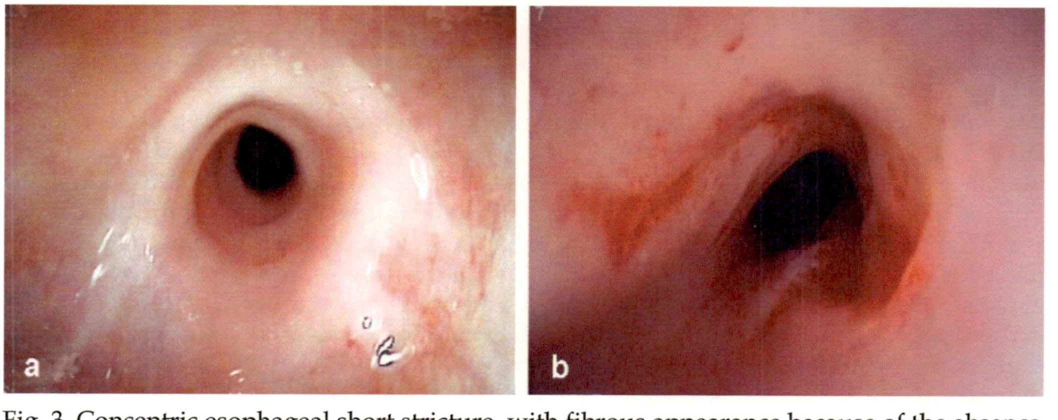

Fig. 3. Concentric esophageal short stricture, with fibrous appearance because of the absence of vascular pattern, before (a) and after (b) endoscopic dilation using a trough-the-scope balloon. A deep mucosal tear can be observed

In this context, endoscopic dilation can be restricted to two well-established subgroups of EoE patients: those unresponsive to medical therapy and those with a persistent or definitive stricture (Schoepfer et al., 2008). The identification of such patients should be made prior to endoscopic therapy, which in clinical practice implies not using endoscopic dilation as an initial treatment.

4.3 Safety of esophageal dilation in EoE patients

A review of the literature indicates that esophageal dilation is an efficient treatment for EoE, providing immediate relief of symptoms (Zuber-Jerger et al., 2006; Roberts-Thomson, 2009), which is why many authors regard it as a front-line treatment (Vasilopoulos et al., 2002; Straumann, 2010). However, initial reports on the use of esophageal dilation in EoE patients also found a high rate of complications ranging from chest pain to esophageal perforation, which appeared in 7% and 5% of all reported cases, respectively (Furuta et al., 2007; Hirano, 2010). These rates are substantially higher than those for esophageal dilation for other benign strictures. Most described cases of esophageal perforation (spontaneous or after endoscopic procedures) only led to pneumomediastinum (Eisenbach et al., 2006; Rajagopalan & Triadafilopoulos, 2009), but in some cases, an emergency esophagectomy by means of thoracotomy or esophagogastroplasty was required (Lucendo et al., 2011; Riou et al., 1996; Liguori et al., 2008). Although no patient fatalities have been reported to date, the seriousness of these complications has led some researchers to warn that endoscopic dilation poses a higher risk of complications in patients with EoE. That, along with the efficacy and proved safety of dietary modification and topical steroids for this disease, has caused several authors to recommend that dilations not be performed until the presence of an eosinophilic infiltrate has been ruled out (Lucendo & De Rezende, 2007). A trial with corticosteroids before dilation has been also proposed in order to reduce active inflammation and the risk for complications (Sgouros et al., 2006).

The exact cause of the extreme fragility described for esophageal mucosa in EoE has not been clearly established, but it seems to be directly related to the inflammatory infiltrate and the cytotoxic effect of eosinophils. These eosinophils contain several cytotoxic proteins in their cytoplasmic granules capable of damaging tissues (Rothenberg et al., 2001), the risk of which is likely to be higher in patients with a high density of eosinophils and long-term symptoms (Straumann et al., 2008). Multiple evidence obtained from patients (Landres et al., 1978) and from animal models of EoE (Mishra et al., 2001) has shown that the inflammatory infiltrate penetrates deeply into the esophageal wall, reaching the muscle layers. Indeed, fibrous remodeling of the esophageal wall, which reduces the elastic properties of its components, has also been described in EoE patients (Aceves et al., 2004; Straumann et al., 2011). In this sense, esophageal distensibility, which alters the mechanical properties of the esophageal wall (Kwiatek et al., 2011), has been shown to be significantly reduced in adult EoE patients in comparison to controls. Accordingly, both the resistance and distension of the organ may be impaired in EoE, leading to increased fragility during endoscopic dilation procedures (Lucendo & De Rezende, 2007) and in traction movements around the gastroesophageal junction in cases of nausea and vomiting. Thus, a simple brush of the endoscope may give rise to mucosal rents, with cases of spontaneous esophageal perforation (Prasad & Arora, 2005) and Boerhaave's syndrome (Lucendo et al, 2011) having been reported in EoE patients after the mere passage of the endoscope (Kaplan et al., 2003). For these patients especially, then, the various endoscopic procedures must be performed gently.

Two recent retrospective, uncontrolled studies developed in adult EoE patients and published in 2010 and 2011 attempted to assess the safety of esophageal dilation with bougies or through-the-scope balloons in a total of 363 dilation procedures (Dellon et al., 2010; Jung et al., 2011). In the first study, Dellon and coworkers observed an overall symptom improvement of 83% with a concomitant increase in esophageal caliber. The authors also observed a 7% complication rate, with 2 deep mucosal rents and 3 episodes of chest pain, but no transmural perforations. In the second study, Jung's group found that 9.2% of patients suffered deep mucosal tears while major bleeding and immediate perforation occurred in 0.3% and 1.0% of the patients, respectively. Complication rates from these two studies contrast with the high rates of perforation reported in earlier EoE literature. Moreover, none of the perforations reported in these two studies required surgical intervention (Table 1).

Several predictive factors for complications during dilation have been identified, including a long evolution of dysphagia, the existence of esophageal stenosis, and a high density of eosinophils (Cohen et al., 2007). Complications were also significantly associated with younger age and repeated procedures (Dellon et al., 2010), along with luminal narrowing in the upper and middle esophageal thirds, a luminal stricture incapable of being traversed with a standard upper endoscope, and the use of Savary bougies (Jung et al., 2011).

4.4 Sustained efficacy of endoscopic dilation in EoE patients

In spite of these data, it should be noted that because endoscopic dilation is a mechanical procedure with no effect on the underlying inflammatory process (Schoepfer et al., 2010), its efficacy is probably limited over time. In the case studies published to date, the duration of the effect cannot be appropriately estimated owing to the short monitoring period, although it usually ranges from 3 to 12 months. Still, it is common for patients to undergo repeated dilations, in some cases up to 9 times, to control their symptoms (Schoepfer et al., 2008; Dellon et al., 2010; Pasha et al., 2007). Also noteworthy is the fact that a proportion of patients undergoing endoscopic dilation also receive concomitant drug therapy, which may mask the clinical effect of endoscopic therapy in and of itself (Dellon et al., 2010).

Taking all this into account, endoscopic dilation should be considered as an alternative treatment for patients with EoE and esophageal stenosis when other measures (especially topical steroid treatment) have failed. It is also advisable that the procedure be used together with other therapy modalities in order to avoid complications derived from active eosinophilic inflammation of the organ. Further studies should be carried out to determine which patients are the best candidates for this kind of treatment due to their better clinical results and/or lower complication rates. This will probably require the definition of different patient subgroups or phenotypes according to several variables which are as yet unidentified.

4.5 How endoscopic dilations should be done in EoE?

As noted above, endoscopic dilation constitutes an effective treatment for EoE and should therefore be considered in those patients exhibiting a reduced esophageal caliber and persisting esophageal symptoms despite topical steroid treatment and/or dietary modifications. Dilation should preferably be done when the active inflammatory infiltrate has been banned or significantly reduced (Sgouros et al., 2006). Endoscopic dilation should be carried out by experienced endoscopists and under sedation to avoid provoking Boherhaave's syndrome if the technique is tolerated badly (Nantes et al., 2009). In order to minimize complications, the procedure should be carried out gently with medium-sized bougies, gradually increasing the caliber and never dilating fully to the larger calibers used in the treatment of other forms of stenosis.

Author and year	Patients dilated	Efficiency	Repeated sessions	Perfora-tion	Other complications
Riou PJ. et al., 1996	1 patient	Stenotic esophagus despite dilation	No	Yes	Pneumomediastinum and early mediastinitis, requiring subtotal esophagectomy.
Morrow JB. et al., 2001	16 adults	16 clinically improved	1 required repeated dilation	No	Deep mucosal tears Increased post endoscopy analgesia. Difficulty in inserting the endoscope.
Vasilopoulos S. et al., 2002	5 adults	5/5 clinically improved	Yes (4 of them)	No	2 extensive esophageal tearing, chest pain and overnight hospitalization.
Straumann A. et al., 2003	11 adults	A single dilation of 7 patients 50% reduction in symptoms 1 patient did not show improvement of symptoms	Yes (in 4 patients)	No	Severe mucosal tearing.
Croese J. et al., 2003	17 adults	16/17 improved clinically	Mean 3.4 dilations per patient, range 1-13)	No	Tears were recorded in 13 (87%).
Straumann A. et al., 2003	5 adults	5 asymptomatic for 3 to 24 months	No	No	Development of disquieting lesions in response to the procedure.
Nurko S. et al., 2004	7 children	5 total symptomatic relief 2 partial response	Not specified	No	No.
Potter JW. et al., 2004	13 adults	7/13 showed transient (<3 months) improvement	Repeated in 6 patients at least twice over the following year	No	Extensive esophageal trauma. Moderate chest pain. Overnight hospitalization.
Langdom DE. 2005	11 (not specified)	Not specified	Not specified	Yes	2–3 day hospitalization, severe chest pain and odynophagia.
Zimmerman SL. et al., 2005	8 adults	8 temporary relief of dysphagia.	Four patients with recurrent dysphagia (mean number of procedures, 2.5; range, 2–4) over an average period of 4.5 years (range 1–10 years).	No	No.

Author and year	Patients dilated	Efficiency	Repeated sessions	Perfora-tion	Other complications
Cantù P. et al., 2005	2 adults	Both cases	No	No	No.
Eisenbach C. et al., 2006	1 adult	Asymptomatic	Repeated esophageal dilation	Yes	No.
Zuber-Jerger I. et al., 2006	1 adult	Clinical improvement for 3 years	Yes, after dysphagia recurred.	No	No.
Pasha SF. et al., 2007	13 adults	11/13 clinically improved	Mean number of dilations was 2 (range, 1-5)	No	Superficial mucosal tears occurred in 31% of dilations.
Schoepfer AM. et al., 2008	10 adults	10/10 clinically improved over an average 6-month period	Mean number of dilations was 2.7 (range, 1-5)	No	Transient postprocedural odynophagia for 1-3 days.
Rajagopalan J. et al., 2009	1 adult	Symptoms improved for 6 months	Two dilations in a 6-week period	No	Severe pain during the subsequent 24-48-hour period.
Dellon ES. et al., 2010	36 patients	Overall clinical response in 20 (83%)	Mean no. of dilations per patient 1.9 (range 1-9).	No	5 complications reported: 2 deep mucosal rents and 3 episodes of chest pain, on of them needing hospitalization.
Jung KW. et al., 2011	161 patients	Not specified	Mean no. of dilations per patient 1.8±1.4	Yes	Deep mucosal tear in 9,2% of dilations and major bleeding in 0,3% of dilations.
Swan MP. et al., 2011	29 patients	Not specified	Mean of 2.07 dilations per patient	No	2 cases admitted with postdilatation pain.

Table 1. Summary of published cases of dilations, their results and complications

No definitive data exist with regard to which dilation technique(s) should be used. Some clinicians prefer using through-the-scope balloons to dilate EoE patients since this method allows the endoscopist a direct visualization of the mucosa during the procedure (Dellon et al., 2010), but the use of Savary bougies has also been reported to be a safe method (Swan et al., 2011).

Multiple strictures are also possible in patients with EoE, but a common strategy in such cases has likewise yet to be established. Inflating a balloon segmentally in multiple areas can dilate the entire esophagus quickly if necessary while maintaining direct visualization at all times (Dellon et al., 2010), but the final method employed should preferably depend on the endoscopist's experience.

5. Conclusion

Eosinophilic esophagitis is a rapidly emerging disease which has become a common pathology in clinical practice. A wide range of endoscopic findings typical of EoE has been described in the literature, but none of them is pathognomonic for the disease. If a patient presents more than one typical finding, a diagnosis of EoE can be proposed with a certain amount of confidence, but the definitive diagnosis must be confirmed through biopsies, which should also be performed on patients with compatible clinical data, even if their esophagus appears to be normal.

Endoscopic dilation should only be considered in cases in which symptoms and/or a reduced esophageal caliber persist despite topical steroid or dietary therapies. The procedure should be carried out gently under sedation with medium-sized hydropneumatic balloons or bougies, and only up to smaller calibers than those used in other forms of strictures.

6. References

Aceves, SS., Newbury, RO., & Dohil, R. (2007). J Allergy Clin Immunol. *Esophageal remodeling in paediatric eosinophilic esophagitis*, Vol.119, No.1, (January 2007), pp. 206-212, ISSN 0091-6749

Chehade, M., Sampson, HA., & Morotti, RA. (2007). J Pediatr Gastroenterol Nutr. *Esophageal subepithelial fibrosis in children with eosinophilic esophagitis*, Vol.45, No.3, (September 2007), pp. 319-328, ISSN 1536-4801

Cheung, KM., Oliver, MR., & Cameron, DJS. (2003). J Pediatr Gastroenterol Nutr. *Esophageal eosinophilia in children with dysphagia*, Vol.37, No.4, (October 2003), pp. 498-503, ISSN 1536-4801

Cohen, MS., Kaufman, AB., & Palazzo, JP. (2007). Clin Gastroenterol Hepatol. *An audit of endoscopic complications in adult eosinophilic esophagitis*, Vol.5, No.10, (October 2007), pp. 1149-1153, ISSN 1198-1206

Dellon, ES., Gibbs, WB., & Rubinas, TC. (2010). Gastrointest Endosc. *Esophageal dilation in eosinophilic esophagitis: safety and predictors of clinical response and complications*, Vol.71, No.4, (April 2010), pp. 706-712, ISSN 0016-5107

Eisenbach, C., Merle, U., & Schirmacher, P. (2006). Endoscopy. *Perforation of the esophagus after dilation treatment for dysphagia in a patient with eosinophilic esophagitis*, Vol.38, Suppl.2, (November 2006), pp. E43-E44, ISSN 1068-9249

Furuta, GT., & Straumann, A. (2006). Aliment Pharmacol Ther. *Review article: the pathogenesis and management of eosinophilic esophagitis*, Vol.24, No.2, (July 2006) , pp. 173-182, ISSN 1365-2036

Furuta, GT., Liacouras, CA., & Collins, MH. (2007). Gastroenterology. *Eosinophilic esophagitis in children and adults: a systematic review and consensus recommendations for diagnosis and treatment*, Vol.133, No.4, (October 2007), pp. 1342-1363, ISSN 0016-5085

González-Castillo, S., Arias, Á., & Lucendo, AJ. (2010). J Clin Gastroenterol. *Treatment of eosinophilic esophagitis: how should we manage the disease?*, Vol.44, No.10, (December 2010), pp. 663-671, ISSN 1539-2031

Hirano, I. (2010). Gastrointest Endosc. *Dilation in eosinophilic esophagitis: to do or not to do?*, Vol.71, No.4, (April 2010), pp. 713-714, ISSN 0016-5107

Jung, KW., Gundersen, N., & Kopacova, J. (2011). Gastrointest Endosc. *Occurrence of and risk factors for complications after endoscopic dilation in eosinophilic esophagitis*, Vol.73, No.1, (January 2011), pp. 15-21, ISSN 0016-5107

Kaplan, M., Mutlu, EA., & Jakate, S. (2003). Clin Gastroenterol Hepatol. *Endoscopy in eosinophilic esophagitis: 'feline' esophagus and perforation risk*, Vol.1, No.6, (November 2003), pp. 433-437, ISSN 1198-1206

Kelly, KJ., Lazenby, AJ., & Rowe, PC. (1995). Gastroenterology. *Eosinophilic esophagitis attributed to gastroesophageal reflux: improvement with an amino acid-based formula.* Vol.109, No.5, (November 1995), pp. 1503-1512, ISSN 0016-5085

Kwiatek, MA., Hirano, I., & Kahrilas, PJ. (2011). Gastroenterology. *Mechanical properties of the esophagus in eosinophilic esophagitis*, Vol.140, No.1, (January 2011), pp. 82-90, ISSN 0016-5085

Korsapati, H., Babaei, A., & Bhargava, V. (2009). Gut. *Dysfunction of the longitudinal muscles of the oesophagus in eosinophilic oesophagitis*, Vol.58, No.8, (August 2009), pp. 1056-1062, ISSN 1468-3288

Kwiatek, MA., Hirano, I., & Kahrilas, PJ. (2011). Gastroenterology. *Mechanical properties of the esophagus in eosinophilic esophagitis*, Vol.140, No.1, (January 2011), pp. 82-90, ISSN 0016-5085

Landres, RT., Kuster, GGR., & Strum, WB. (1978). Gastroenterology. *Eosinophilic esophagitis in a patient with vigorous achalasia*, Vol.74, No.6, (June 1978), pp. 1298-1301, ISSN 0016-5085

Liacouras, CA., Spergel, JM., & Ruchelli, E. (2005). Clin Gastroenterol Hepatol. *Eosinophilic esophagitis: a 10-year experience in 381 children*, Vol.3, No.12, (December 2005), pp. 1198-1206

Liacouras, CA., Furuta, GT., & Hirano, I. (2011). J Allergy Clin Immunol. *Eosinophilic esophagitis: Updated consensus recommendation for children and adults,* Vol.6, (April 2011), Epub ahead of print, ISSN 0091-6749

Liguori, G., Cortale, M., & Cimino, F. (2008). World J Gastroenterol. *Circumferential mucosal dissection and esophageal perforation in a patient with eosinophilic esophagitis*, Vol.14; No.5, (February 2008), pp. 803-804, ISSN 1007-9327

Lucendo, AJ. (2007). Med Clin (Barc). *Eosinophilic esophagitis*. Vol.128, No.5, (April 2007), pp. 590-597, ISSN 0025 -7753

Lucendo, AJ., & De Rezende, L. (2007). Endoscopy. *Endoscopic dilation in eosinophilic esophagitis: a treatment strategy associated with a high risk of perforation*, Vol.39, No.4, (April 2007), pp. 376, ISSN 1068-9249

Lucendo, AJ., Castillo, P., & Martín-Chávarri, S. (2007). Eur J Gastroenterol Hepatol. *Manometric findings in adult eosinophilic oesophagitis: A study of 12 cases*, Vol.19, No.5, (May 2007), pp. 417-424, ISSN 1473-5687

Lucendo, AJ., Pascual-Turrión, JM., & Navarro, M. (2007). Endoscopy. *Endoscopic, bioptic and manometric findings in eosinophilic esophagitis before and after steroid therapy: a case series*, Vol.39, No.9, (September 2007), pp. 765-771, ISSN 1068-9249

Lucendo, AJ. (2010). Scand J Gastroeneterol. *Eosinophilis diseases of the gastrointestinal tract*, 2010, Vol.45, No.9, (September 2010), pp. 1013-1021, ISSN 1502-7708

Lucendo, AJ., Friginal-Ruiz, AB., & Rodríguez, B. (2011). Dis Esophagus. *Boerhaave's syndrome as the primary manifestation of adult eosinophilic esophagitis. Two case reports and a review of the literature*, Vol.24, No.2, (February 2011), pp. E11-E15, ISSN 1442-2050

Mackenzie, SH., Go, M., & Chadwick, B. (2008). Aliment Pharmacol Ther. *Eosinophilic oesophagitis in patients presenting with dysphagia--a prospective analysis*, Vol.28, No.9, (November 2008), pp. 1140-1146, ISSN 1365-2036

Mishra, A., Hogan, SP., & Brandt, EB. (2001). . J Clin Invest. *An etiological role for aeroallergens and eosinophils in experimental esophagitis*, Vol.107, No.1, (January 2001), pp. 83-90, ISSN 0021-9738

Mishra, A., Wang, M., & Pemmaraju, VR. (2008). Gastroenterology. *Esophageal remodeling develops as a consequence of tissue specific IL-5-induced eosinophilia*, Vol.134, No.1, (January 2008), pp. 204-214, ISSN 0016-5085

Moawad, FJ. (2011). Dig Dis Sci. *Esophageal Motor Disorders in Adults with Eosinophilic Esophagitis*, Vol.18, Epub ahead of print, (March 2011), ISSN 1573-2568

Molina-Infante, J., Ferrando-Lamana, L., & Fernandez-Bermejo, M. Am J Gastroenterol. *Eosinophilic esophagitis in GERD patients: a clinicopathological diagnosis using proton pump inhibitors*, Vol.104, No.11, (November 2009), pp. 2856-2857, ISSN 1572-0241

Müller, S., Pühl, S., & Vieth, M. (2007). Endoscopy. *Analysis of symptoms and endoscopic findings in 117 patients with histological diagnoses of esinophilic esophagitis*, Vol.39, No.4, (April 2007), pp. 339-344, ISSN 1068-9249

Nantes, Ó., Jiménez, FJ., & Zozaya, JM. (2009). Endoscopy. *Increased risk of esophageal perforation in eosinophilic esophagitis*, Vol.41, Suppl.2, (July 2009), pp. E177-E178, ISSN 1068-9249

Nurko, S., Teitelbaum, J., & Husain, K. (2004). J Pediatr Gastroenterol Nutr. *Association of Schatzki ring with eosinophilic esophagitis in children*, Vol.38, No.4, (April 2004), pp. 431-441, ISSN 1536-4801

Nurko, S., Rosen, R., & Furuta, GT. (2009). Am J Gastroenterol. *Esophageal dysmotility in children with eosinophilic esophagitis: a study using prolonged esophageal manometry*, Vol.104, No.12, (December 2009), pp. 3050-3057, ISSN 1572-0241

Pasha, SF., DiBaise, JK., & Kim, HJ. (2007). Dis Esophagus. *Patient characteristics, clinical, endoscopic, and histologic findings in adult eosinophilic esophagitis: a case series and systematic review of the medical literature*, Vol.20, No.4 (2007), pp. 311-319, ISSN 1442-2050

Peery, AF., Cao, H., & Dominik, R. (2011). Clin Gastroenterol Hepatol. *Variable Reliability of Endoscopic Findings with White-Light and Narrow-Band Imaging for Patients with Suspected Eosinophilic Esophagitis*, Vol.4, Epub ahead of print, (March 2011), ISSN 1542-7714

Prasad, GA., & Arora, AS. (2005). Dis Esophagus. *Spontaneous perforation in the ringed esophagus*, Vol. 18, No.6 (June 2005), pp. 406-409, ISSN 1442-2050

Prasad, GA., Talley, NJ., & Romero, Y. (2007). Am J Gastroenterol. *Prevalence and predictive factors of eosinophilic esophagitis in patients presenting with dysphagia: a prospective study*, Vol.102, No.12, (December 2007), pp. 2627-2632, ISSN 1572-0241

Rajagopalan, J., & Triadafilopoulos, G. (2009). Dis Esophagus. *Ring(s)-related esophageal meat bolus impaction: biopsy first, dilate later*, Vol.22, No.5 (November 2009), pp. E14-E16, ISSN 1442-2050

Ricker, J., McNear, S., & Cassidy, T. (2011). Therap Adv Gastroenterol. *Routine screening for eosinophilic esophagitis in patients presenting with dysphagia*, Vol.4, No.1, (January 2011), pp. 27-35, ISSN 1756-2848

Riou, PJ., Nicholson, AG., & Pastorino, U. (1996). Ann Thorac Surg. *Esophageal rupture in a patient with idiopathic eosinophilic esophagitis*, Vol.62, No.6 (December 1996), pp. 1854-1856, ISSN 1552-6259

Roberts-Thomson, IC. (2005). J Gastroenterol Hepatol. *Images of interest. Gastrointestinal: Eosinophilic esophagitis*, Vol.20, No.8, (August 2005), pp. 1299, ISSN 1440-1746

Roman, S., Hirano, I., & Kwiatek, MA. (2011). Neurogastroenterol Motil. *Manometric features of eosinophilic esophagitis in esophageal pressure topography*, Vol.23, No.3, (March 2011), pp. 208-214, ISSN 1365-2982

Schoepfer, AM., Gschossmann, J., & Scheurer, U. (2008). Endoscopy. *Esophageal strictures in adult eosinophilic esophagitis: dilation is an effective and safe alternative after failure of topical corticosteroids*, Vol.40, No.2, (February 2008), pp. 161-164, ISSN 1068-9249

Schoepfer, AM., Gonsalves, N., & Bussmann, C. (2009). Am J Gastroenterol. *Esophageal Dilation in Eosinophilic Esophagitis: Effectiveness, Safety, and Impact on the Underlying Inflammation*, Vol. 105, No.5, (May 2009), pp. 1062-1070, ISSN 1572-0241

Sgouros, SN., Bergele, C., & Mantides, A. (2006). Eur J Gastroenterol Hepatol. *Eosinophilic esophagitis in adults: a systematic review*, Vol.18, No.2, (February 2006), pp. 211-217, ISSN 1473-5687

Sgouros, SN., Bergele, C., & Mantides, A. (2006). Endoscopy. *Eosinophilic esophagitis in adults: what is the clinical significance?*, Vol.38, No. 5, (May 2006), pp. 515-520, ISSN 1068-9249

Spechler, SJ., Genta, RM., & Souza, RF. (2007). Am J Gastroenterol. *Thoughts on the complex relationship between gastroesophageal reflux disease and eosinophilic esophagitis*, Vol.102, No.6, (June 2007), pp. 1301-1306, ISSN 1572-0241

Straumann, A., Rossi, L., & Simon, HU. (2003). Gastrointest Endosc. *Fragility of the esophageal mucosa: a pathognomonic endoscopic sign of primary eosinophilic esophagitis?*, Vol.57, No.3, (March 2003), pp. 407-412, ISSN 0016-5107

Straumann, A., Spichtin, HP., & Grize, L. (2004). Digestion. *Eosinophilic esophagitis: red on microscopy, white on endoscopy*, Vol.70, No.2 (September 2004), pp. 109-116, ISSN 1421-9867

Straumann, A. (2008). Gastrointestinal Endosc Clin North Am. *The natural history and complications of eosinophilic esophagitis*, Vol.18, No.1, (January 2008), pp. 99-118, ISSN 1052-5157

Straumann, A., Bussmann, C., & Zuber, M. (2008). Clin Gastroenterol Hepatol. *Eosinophilic Esophagitis: Analysis of Food Impaction and Perforation in 251 Adolescent and Adult Patients*, Vol.6, No.5, (May 2008), pp. 598-600, ISSN 1542-7714

Straumann, A. (2010). Gastrointest Endosc Clin N Am. *The natural history and complications of eosinophilic esophagitis*, Vol.18, No.1, (January 2010), pp. 99-118, ISSN 1052-5157

Straumann, A., Conus, S., & Degen, L. (2010). Gastroenterology. *Budesonide is effective in adolescent and adult patients with active eosinophilic esophagitis*, Vol.139, No.5, (November 2010), pp. 1526-1537, ISSN 0016-5085

Straumann, A., Conus, S., & Degen, L. (2011). Clin Gastroenterol Hepatol. *Long-term budesonide maintenance treatment is partially effective for patients with eosinophili esophagits*, Vol.28, Epub ahead of print (January 2011), ISSN 1542-7714

Swan, MP., Donnellan, F., & Kandel, G. (2011). Gastrointest Endosc. *Safe and effective dilatation in eosinophilic esophagitis: the tale of two subgroups*, Vol.72, No.2, (February 2011), pp. 408, ISSN 0016-5107

Vasilopoulos, S., Murphy, P., & Auerbach, A. (2002). Gastrointest Endosc. *The small-caliber esophagus: an unappreciated cause of dysphagia for solids in patients with eosinophilic esophagitis*, Vol.55, No.1, (January 2002), pp. 99-106, ISSN 0016-5107

Zuber-Jerger, I., Ratiu, N., & Kullman, F. (2006). J Gastrointestin Liver Dis. *Long-lasting effect of endoscopic dilation of an esophageal stenosis due to eosinophilic esophagitis*, Vol.15, No.2, (June 2006), pp. 167-170, ISSN 1842-1121

7

Expression of Reactive Oxygen Species in Reflux Disease

Emma Andreasson and Anna Casselbrant
Department of Gastrosurgical Research and Education, Institute of Clinical Sciences, Sahlgrenska Academy, University of Gothenburg, Sweden

1. Introduction

Reflux of acidic gastric contents, or bile and pancreatic enzymes into the esophagus may cause mucosal inflammation (esophagitis or red streak). This disorder is commonly called gastroesohageal reflux disease (GERD), and in signs of esophageal mucosal injuries the disorder is called 'erosive reflux disease' (ERD). If the reflux is frequent and long standing such episodes can elicit severe inflammation or damage of the esophageal squamous epithelium (1-2).

Oxygen is a requirement for life but oxygen metabolites can cause serious tissue injuries. It is normal for the immune system to respond to injury to the mucosa or pathogens by producing oxygen and nitrogen radicals. Reactive oxygen species (ROS) are an often-used term that includes true radicals that have unpaired electrons as well as chemicals that can gain or loose electrons. Oxidative stress is a general term used to describe the steady state of oxidative damage in a cell, tissue or organ, caused by ROS. If there is an unbalance between the production of ROS and the systems ability to detoxify the reactive species or easily repair the resulting damage, oxidative stress is caused and this is a reality in most living organisms. ROS are used in immune system to attack and eliminate pathogens but ROS are also involved in the development of many diseases such as atherosclerosis and cancer (3-5).

There are many different sources by which ROS are generated. Among a lot of enzymes and molecules that cause oxidative stress there are three major enzymes; myeloperoxidase (MPO), nicotinamide adenine dinucleotide phosphate oxidase (NADPH oxidase) and nitric oxide syntase (NOS) that produce the products superoxide (O_2^-), hydrogen peroxide (H_2O_2), nitric oxide (NO) and hypocloric acid (HOCl).

We have previously shown that extremely high levels of NO are formed when nitrite in swallowed saliva meets acidic refluxates in the distal esophagus (6). NO has radical-characteristics and has been suggested to initiate esophageal carcinogenesis (7). This view may be questioned because luminally formed NO appears to be quite harmless and is rapidly eliminated during normal tissue conditions. However, in inflamed tissue with production of ROS it is reasonable to assume that luminal NO will react with particularly O_2^- and form the extremely labile oxidising compound peroxynitrite ($ONOO^-$). Such oxidative species have potential roles in all steps of carcinogenesis including DNA

mutation, activation of proto-oncogenes and inactivation or loss tumor suppressor genes (5, 7).
The aim of the present study is to elucidate the presence of radical producing enzymes, represented by NADPH oxidase, MPO and iNOS and also the expression of radical formation marker for $ONOO^-$ activity as well as nitro radical end products; nitrotyrosine. The second aim is to elucidate the histological changes and number of inflammatory cells as well as the expression of inflammatory markers IL1β and IL6 in human esophageal biopsies from healthy volunteers and patients with ERD.

2. Material and methods

2.1 Subjects and tissue

Biopsies were taken from healthy controls (n=7, mean age 36, 4 female) and patients with ERD (n=13, mean age 48, 3 female). The biopsies were collected during endoscopy and specimens were immediately frozen in liquid nitrogen (for later western blot analysis) or snap frozen in RNA STAT-60 (Nordic Bio Site AB, Stockholm, Sweden) (for later rt-PCR analysis) and subsequently stored in liquid nitrogen or fixed in buffered 4% formaldehyde (for later histo-morphology evaluation). The biopsies were taken in the 3 o´clock position 2 cm proximal to the gastro esophageal junction, and in the altered area for the esophagitis (red streak)(8). Protein expressions of MPO, NADPH oxidase, iNOS and nitrotyrosine were assessed by western blot technique and immunohistochemistry. Expression of the IL1β and IL6 were assessed by both western blot and rtPCR.
The Los Angeles classification was used by the endoscopist to decide the degree of esophageal inflammation (1). All patients who contributed for this study were classified as LA-A.
Ethics. All participants had given informed consent and the study had been approved by Ethical Committee of Göteborg University and was performed in accordance with the Declaration of Helsinki.

2.2 Western blot analyses

The frozen specimens were sonicated in a PE buffer (10 mM potassium phosphate buffer, pH 6,8 and 1mM EDTA) containing 10 mM 3-[(3-cholamidopropyl) dimethylammonio]-1-propane sulphonate (CHAPS: Boehringer Mannheim, Mannheim, Germany) and protease inhibitor cocktail tablet Complete (Roche Diagnostics AB, Stockholm, Sweden). The homogenate was then centrifuged (10,000 g for 10 min at 4°C) and the supernatant was analysed for protein content by the Bradford method and stored at -80°C (9). Samples were diluted in SDS buffer and heated at 70°C for 10 min before they were loaded on a NuPage 10% Bis-Tris gel, and electrophoresis run using a MOPS buffer (Invitrogen AB, Lidingo, Sweden). One lane of each gel was loaded with prestained molecular weight standards (SeeBlue, NOVEX, San Diego, CA, USA). A positive control was loaded on each gel (Table 1). After the electrophoresis the proteins were transferred to a polyvinyldifluoride transfer membrane, Hybond, 0.45µm, RPN303F, (Amersham, Buckinghamshire, UK) using an iBlot (Invitrogen AB). Membranes were than incubated with polyclonal specific antibodies directed at the MPO, NADPH oxidase ($p47^{phox}$-subunit), iNOS, nitrotyrosine, IL-1β and IL-6 respectively (Table 1). An alkaline phosphatase conjugated goat anti-mouse or goat anti-rabbit IgG antibody (Santa Cruz) and CDP-Star (Tropix, Bedford, MA, USA) were used as a substrate to identify immunoreactive proteins by means of chemiluminescense. Images were captured by a Chemidox XRS cooled CCD camera, and analyzed with Quantity One software (BioRad laboratories, Hercules, CA, USA). Glyceraldehyde-3-phosphate dehydrogenase (GAPDH) antibody (Imgenex, San Diego, CA, USA) was used as control for equal loading, and for each tested sample the ratio of primarily antibody/GAPDH was used.

Target protein	*Primary antibody*	*Positive control*
MPO	Antimyeloperoxidase 07-496 Upstate/Millipore	Hl-60 sc-2209 Santa Cruz
Nitrotyrosine	Antinitrotyrosine 06-284 Upstate/Millipore	Nitrotyrosine 12-354 Upstate
iNOS	Transinos N 32030 TransductionLab/BioSite	RAW 264.7 sc-2212 Santa Cruz
NADPH-oxidase ($p47^{phox}$)	H-195 sc-14015 Santa Cruz	Hl-60 sc-2209 Santa Cruz
GAPDH	Glyceraldehyde-3-phosphate dehydrogenase Imgenex/BioSite	Loading control for western blot
IL-1β	Interleukin-1 Beta Sc-52012 Santa Cruz	Serum was used as positive control
IL-6	Interleukin-6 Sc-28343 Santa Cruz	Serum was used as positive control

MPO; myeloperoxidase, iNOS; inducible nitric oxide synthase, NADPH-oxidase; nicotinamide adenine dinucleotide phosphate oxidase, GAPDH; Glyceraldehyde-3-phosphate dehydrogenase, IL; interleukin

Table 1. Antibodies and controls used in Western Blot analyses and immunohistochemistry

2.3 Immunohistochemistry

The mucosal specimens were fixed in buffered 4% formaldehyde and embedded in paraffin. Sections for immunohistochemistry (3μm) were deparaffinized and then boiled for 15 min in 10mM citrate buffer (pH 6.0) for antigen retrieval. The Immunocruz TM Staining System (Santa Cruz Biotechnology, Santa Cruz, CA, USA) was used for the immunohistochemistry protocol. After inhibition of endogenous peroxidase activity, the slides were pre-incubated with serum block and then incubated with primary antibodies against MPO, NADPH oxidase iNOS and nitrotyrosine (see table 1) over night in dilutions of 1:200, 1:50, 1:1000 and

1:500 respectively. Control sections were incubated with normal rabbit or mouse IgG 0.4μg/μL instead of the primary antibody. After being washed, the slides were incubated with biotinylated secondary antibody and the complex was detected using horseradish peroxidase (HRP)-streptavidin. The colour was developed using 3,3′-diaminobenzidine.

2.4 Reverse transcriptase polymerase chain reaction

The biopsy was snap frozen in liquid nitrogen. Frozen tissue was homogenised and total RNA was extracted according to the methods suggested by the manufacturer, following phenol-chloroform extraction and ethanol precipitation. Reverse transcription from 2.5 μg of total RNA was carried out using the SUPERSCRIPT™ First-Strand Synthesis System (Invitrogen, Lidingö, Sweden) with Oligo (dT) Primers (Life Technologies, Täby, Sweden). Resulting cDNA was stored at – 20°C until use.

Lightcycler Q-PCR (Roche Diagnostics AB, Stockholm, Sweden) was performed using the FastStart DNA Master SYBR Green I (Roche Diagnostics AB, Stockholm, Sweden). PCR was performed containing 2 μl of each RT sample using the hot-start technique. MgCl2 concentration was optimised to 4 mM to obtain the highest signal intensity and lowest background. For each tested sample the copy number of the PCR products was calculated by dividing these values by the genometric mean copy number of the reference gene (GAPDH). The quantification was performed by the software supplied by Roche Diagnostics (Mannheim, Germany). The primer sequences, PCR products sizes and references are listed in Table 2.

	rtPCR Primer sequences	Size (bp)	Reference
IL-1β	F:5´- aaacagatgaagtgctccttccag-3´ R:5´- tggagaacaccacttgttgctcca-3´	388	10
IL-6	F:5´- ggtcaggggtggttattgcatc -3´ R:5´- tgtgtgaaagcagcaaagaggc-3´	276	10
GAPDH	F:5´- cccatcaccatcttccaggag-3´ R:5´- gttgtcatggatgaccttggcc-3	284	11

IL; interleukin, GAPDH; Glyceraldehyde-3-phosphate dehydrogenase

Table 2. rt-PCR-related information

2.5 Histology

The fixed biopsy were dehydrated and embedded in paraffin. A histo-pathologist evaluation of mucosal inflammation and histological changes were performed in coded three-micron sections stained with eosin-hematoxylin. Histological evaluation of inflammation (number of mucosal lymphocytes, plasma cells and eosinophilic granulocytes) and morphometric investigations concerning: basal cell layer thickness (BCL), papillary length (PL), total epithelium thickness, and dilatation of intracellular spaces (DIS), were performed on the mucosal specimens.

3. Statistics

Significant differences for multiple independent groups of observation were identified using Kruskal-Wallis and contrasted by Mann-Whitney U-test. Significant differences for dependent group of observation was identified using Wilcoxon´s signed rank test. Nonparamitric correlation analysis was performed by Spearman´s rank correlation test. A p-value ≤0.05 was considered to be of statistical significance.

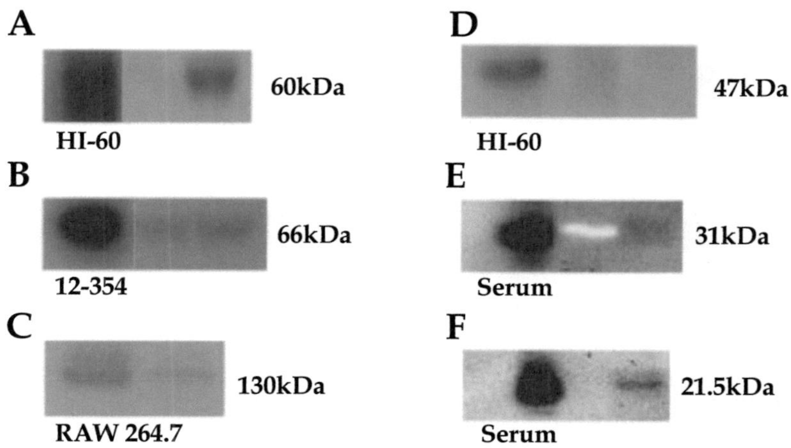

Fig. 1. Typical western blot for MPO (Panel A), NADPH oxidas (Panel B), iNOS (Panel C), nitrotyrosine (Panel D), IL-1β (Panel E) and IL-6 (Panel F) with a band at 60 kDa, 66 kDa, 130 kDa, 47 kDa, 31 kDa and 21.5 kDa respectively, in the positive control cell lysate HL-60, cell lysate 12-354, mouse macrophage cell line RAW 264.7 and serum, and in human esophageal mucosal biopsy retrieved during endoscopy

4. Results

4.1 Biochemical signs of inflammation

A typical western blot for MPO, NADPH oxidase, iNOS, nitrotyrosine, IL-1β and IL-6 are shown in figure 1A-F. A significant increase of MPO protein expression (ERD, p=0.0001, red streak, p=0.005) as well as a significant increase of nitrotyrosine expression (ERD, p=0.05, red streak, p=0.05) was detected in ERD-patients compared healthy controls using western blotting (figure 2A and D). No significant differences in expression of NADPH oxidase, iNOS (figure 2B and C), IL1β or IL6 were detected (data not shown). However at gene expression level using rt-PCR technique, IL6 was significantly increased in ERD-patients (p=0.01), whereas there was no difference in IL1β between the groups at gene level (data not shown).

Immunohistochemistry performed on endoscopically retrieved mucosal biopsies revealed a distinct staining for MPO in epithelial lymphocytes and also weak staining in the squamous epithelial cells (figure 3 A). Immunostaining for NADPH oxidase was detected in basal layer of the epithelium and papillae (figure 3B), whereas iNOS was localized mainly to the upper and mid-zone layer in the epithelium (figure 3C). Nitrotyrosin immunoreactivity was detected in the epithelium in both the basal and in the upper layer (figure 3D).

4.2 Histological signs of inflammation

No signs of active inflammation, defined as presence of lymphocytes, amount of eosinophiles granulocyts or plasmacells, were detected in the esophageal mucosa (table 3).

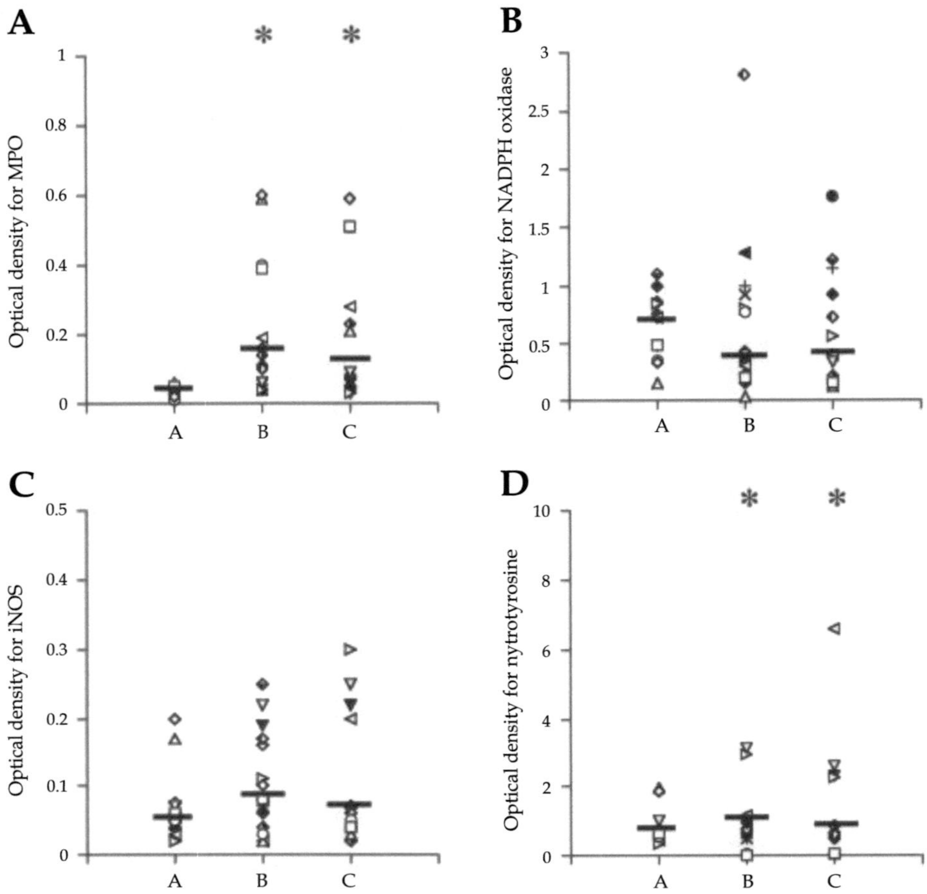

A. Control; B. ERD; C. Red streak

Fig. 2. Western blot analysis of the MPO (Panel A), NADPH oxidas (Panel B), iNOS (Panel C) and nitrotyrosine (Panel D) in human esophageal biopsies taken from macroscopically normal squamous mucosa in healthy subjects (n=7), patients with erosive reflux disease (ERD)(n=13) and from the red streak areas in ERD-patients (n=13). Tissue sample were taken in the 3 o´clock position 2 cm proximal to the gastro esophageal junction. Significant differences are indicated with asterisks (*=p≤0.01; Mann-Whitney U-test). The median value in each group is indicated

	Control	**ERD**	**Red streak**
Mucosal lymphocytes	6.29±2.0	5.8±0.9	8.9±2.1
Eosinophilic granulocytes	0	4.6±3.1	0.67±0.4
Plasma cells	0	0	0

ERD; Errosive reflux disease

Table 3. The number of inflammatory cells in human esophageal mucosa

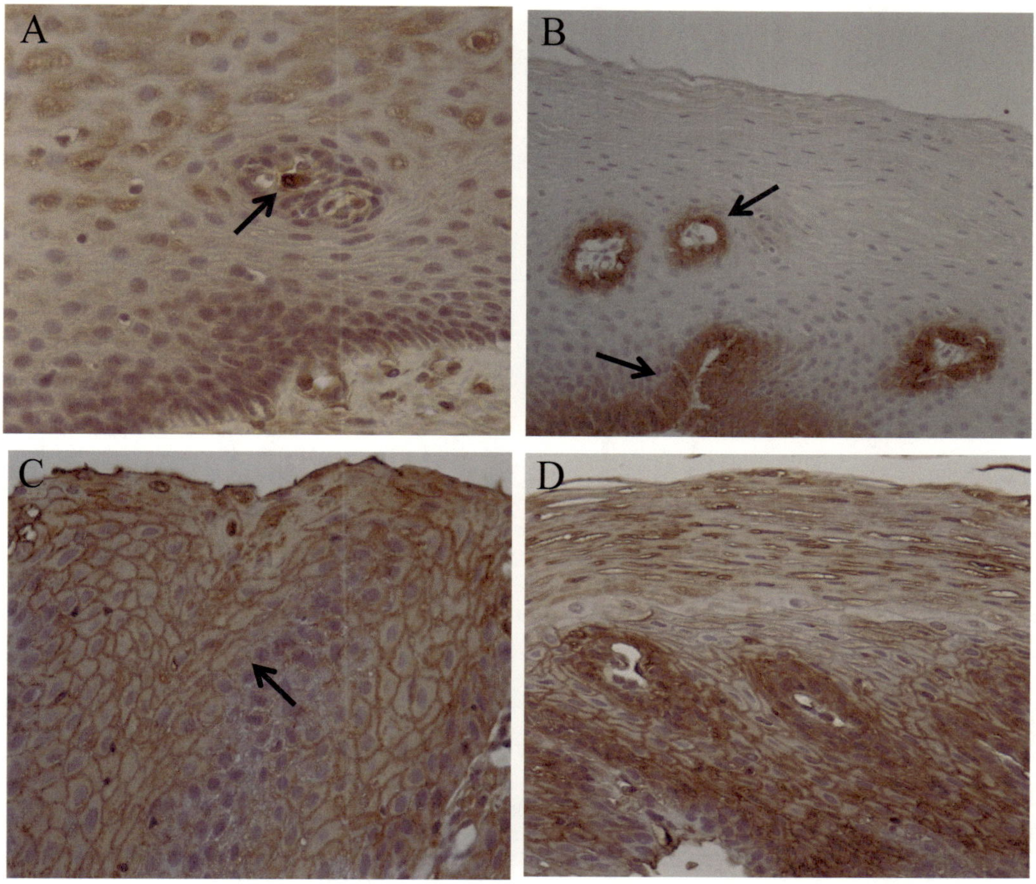

Fig. 3. Immunostaining of the human esophageal epithelium at X40 magnification with brown indicating positive immunoreactivity. (Panel A) Staining for MPO was localized in lymphocytes (arrow) as well as in upper layer epithelial cells. (Panel B) Immunostaining for NADPH oxidas is most obvious in basal epithelial cells and around the papillae (see arrows). (Panel C) Staining for iNOS was localized in stratum superficiale and spinosum (arrow). (Panel D) Immunoreactivity for nitrotyrosine is most obvious in upper layer epithelial cells and around the papillae

4.3 Histology

Histological signs of erosive mucosal disease were confirmed. In the red streak, the squamous epithelium showed a significantly thicker basal cell layer (p=0.016), longer papillae (p=0.001), thicker total epithelium thickness (p=0.016) and wider intercellular space (p=0.003) compared to biopsies taken in healthy control subjects (Figure 4A-D). Furthermore, also when compared to unaffected squamous mucosa in ERD-patients the epithelium showed a significantly thicker basal cell layer (p=0.022), longer papillae (p=0.022), and thicker total epithelium thickness (p=0.001), compared to biopsies from healthy controls (Figure 4A-D).

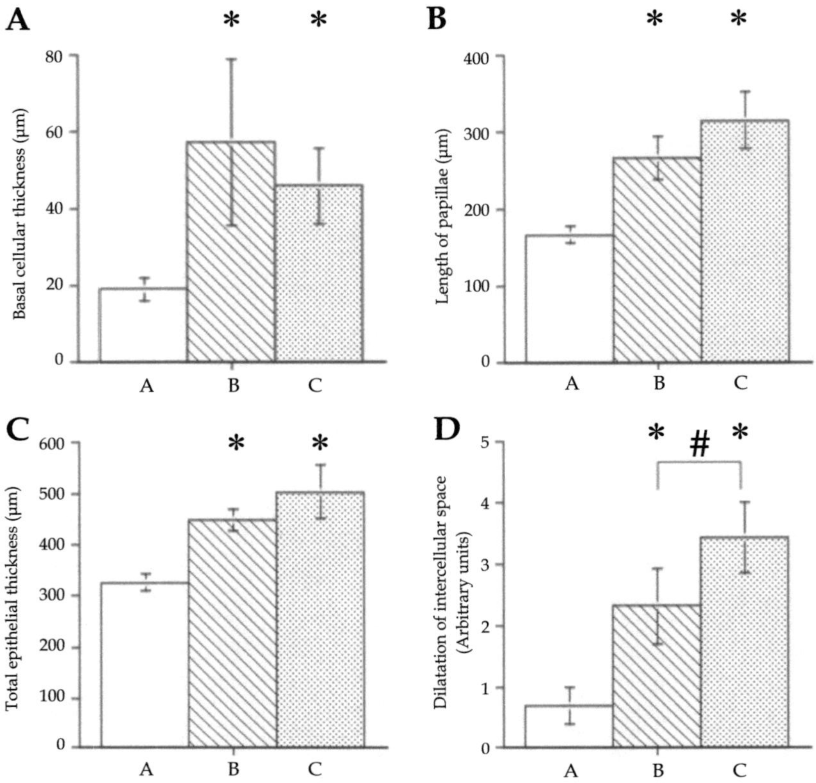

Fig. 4. Histological appearance in biopsies from macroscopically normal squamous mucosa of control subjects and patients with erosive reflux disease (ERD), and from the red streak areas in ERD-patients. Tissue sample were taken in the 3 o´clock position 2 cm proximal to the gastro esophageal junction. (Panel A) thickness of basal cellular layer, (Panel B) length of intraepithelial papillae, (Panel C) total epithelial thickness, and (Panel D) dilatation of intracellular space. Significant differences are indicated with asterisks (*=$p \le 0.01$; Mann-Whitney U-test, #=$p<0.01$; Wilcoxon´s signed rank test). Data is showed as means±SEM

4.4 ROS expression correlation analysis with histopathological alterations and immunocells

Correlation analysis revealed a positive correlation of increased expressions of nitrotyrosine with the histopathological alteration PL ($r=0.65$, $p=0.05$) and total epithelium thickness ($r=0.73$, $p=0.025$) in biopsies taken in the red streak area from ERD-patients (Figure 5A, B). No other correlation was found nor for the histopathological alterations or the number of inflammatory cells (data not shown).

5. Discussion

This study is attempted to elucidate the total generation of ROS that is produced by enzymes and molecules in the esophageal mucosa. In the present exploration of the human

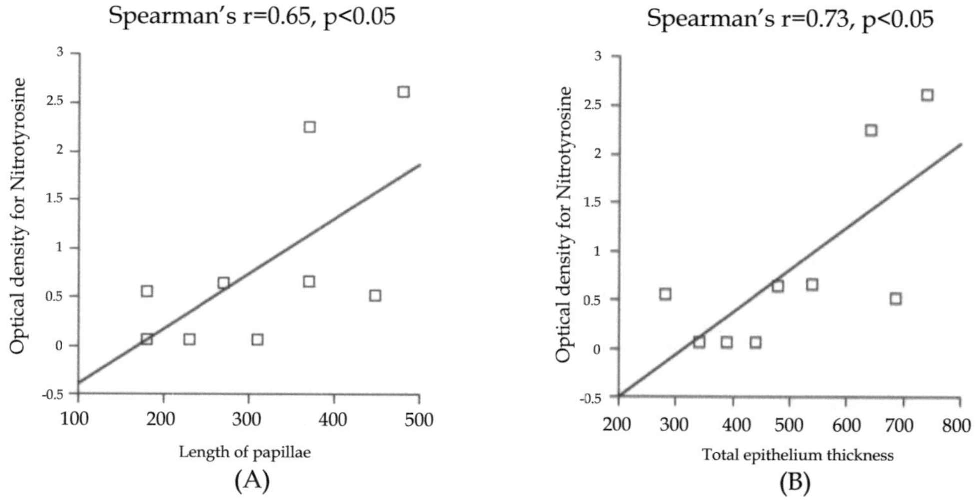

Fig. 5. Positive correlation of nitrotyrosine expression with histopathological changes papillary length (A) and total epithelium thickness (B) in biopsies taken in the red streak area from patients with erosive reflux disease

esophageal mucosa a number of reactive changes were observed. Firstly, the histological signs of erosive mucosal diseases were confirmed, also in macroscopically normal squamous epithelium from ERD-patients were changed. Secondly, there were clear signs of increased radical forming capacity in the epithelium despite absence of histological inflammation. Taken together these findings indicate that a significant change of the esophageal mucosa had occurred in association to ERD.

Nitration of tyrosine results in nitrotyrosine. The nitrate is mainly donated by peroxynitrite, however, nitrotyrosine formation is not solely generated by ONOO-. NADPH oxidase is a transmembrane electron transport chain, and the active NADPH oxidase catalyzes the production of O_2^- that serves as starting material for the production of different ROS (12). Oxidation of arginine by NOS creates the gas NO. NO reacts rapidly with O_2^- to produce the extremely reactive radical ONOO- which also can protonate and dissociate to give nitrogen (NO_2) (5). MPO reacts with H2O2 formed by the respiratory burst to generate HOCl that further can form nitryl chloride (NO_2Cl) (13). NO_2 and NO_2Cl can then nitrogenate tyrosine to form nitrotyrosine. It follows that all enzymes used in the study; MPO, NADPH oxidase, and iNOS activity may be involved in the formation of nitrotyrosine.

Nitrotyrosine is a very stable altered amino acid (an addition of a nitro group to the benzene ring of tyrosine) that can be found both as a single amino acid and belong to a complete protein in the cell. It has been found in elevated levels in a lot of inflammatory conditions like atherosclerosis, rheumatoid arthritis, influenza, pancratitis, cholecystitis, Diabetes Mellitus, ulcerative colitis and Crohn´s disease (5, 14-15) and is therefore a good indicator of the radical production. In the present study nitrotyrosine showed elevated levels in both the red streak and in the squamous epithelium taken from the ERD-patients compared to controls.

A number of studies have shown that MPO is elevated in reflux esophagitis, Barrett´s esophagus and adenocarcinoma (16-17). Eero *et al.* suggest that MPO is a key component of the pathway leading to oxidative stress and damage in the esophageal mucosa. They shown a step-by-step increase in MPO activity related to the severity of reflux disease (17). The expression of MPO was significant increased in the present study in both the red streak and in the squamous epithelium from ERD-patients, however no correlation was found between MPO and the morphological changes.

The expression of NADPH oxidase was not increased in the ERD-patients compared to the healthy individuals. This could be compared with studies made on gastritis caused by Helicobacter Pylori where NADPH oxidase was significant higher in infected patients compared to healthy volunteers (18). Our finding may perhaps suggest the possibility that the reflux of acid is not strong enough as triggering, compared to pathogens. A recent study made by Feagins LA et al. have found that different components of gastric juice, acidic media or acidic bile acid media, induce ROS production through different mechanisms (19). Moreover, no signs of active inflammation were detected in the esophageal mucosa, defined as presence of lymphocytes, amount of eosinophiles granulocyts or plasmacells. The present study is also made on patients with mild esophagitis, classified to LA-A by the endoscopist (1). Several studies have looked at pro-inflammatory cytokines expression along the inflammation- metaplasia- dysplasia- adenocarcinoma sequence in the esophagus and have also found a stepwise-elevated expression correlate to grade of severity of the disease (20-21). Such association was not made in the present study for IL-1β and IL-6 at protein level, whereas gene transcript for IL-6 was increased in ERD-patients indicating somewhat small alteration may exist beyond the detections level for protein.

We have previously shown that two sources of NO formation exist in esophagus, both dependent on the presence of acid in the esophageal lumen; enzymatic degradation of L-arginine by NO synthase and non-enzymatic NO-production their nitrite from the salvia is reduced when it meets the extremely low pH in refluxate, a mechanism related to dietary intake of nitrate (6). The sources of body nitrate are intake through drinking water and vegetables, and endogenous synthesis (22). Vegetables vary greatly in their nitrate content, and water nitrate content also varies with geographical location (22). It follows that luminal NO formations differ between individual dependent on nitrate intake during acidic reflux.

Enzymatic NO formation is constantly expressed but may be activated upon presence of acid in esophageal lumen (6). Several studies have described the expression of iNOS in esophageal squamous epithelium which have been associated with pathological condition such as cell transformation but also suggested a function related to epithelial integrity (6, 23-24). Thus, our results confirm the expression of iNOS in the surface epithelium. However, neither the biopsies taken from ERD-patients nor the red streak areas in ERD-patients were significant different in iNOS expression compared to controls.

The topographical organisation of the iNOS in the epithelium in combination with luminal non-enzymatic NO, may create particular conditions for NO gradients through the mucosa. Immunoreactivily to MPO and NADPH oxidase was also found in the surface epithelium. Therefore we could assume that during gastric acidic reflux huge level of NO is formed simultaneous with production of epithelial mucosal ROS leading to increased formation of ONOO-, which may contribute to cellular injury and DNA damage (7, 25).

MPO, NADPH oxidase and iNOS are usually found in phagocytes including neutrophils, eosinophils, monocytes and macrophages with the primary function of phagocytosis and destruction of microorganisms (26). However, except MPO that was localized in both lymphocytes and epithelial cells, immunostaining for NADPH oxidase and iNOS was *only* found in the esophageal epithelial cells. Thus, the presently increased radical forming capacity in the epithelium is independent of inflammatory cells.

In the morphological investigation of reflux signs we found that all parametric used, dilatation of intracellular spaces, papillary length, basal cell layer thickness, and total epithelium thickness were significantly increased in the distal esophagus in ERD-patients compared healthy subjects. Moreover, in this study the parametric dilatation of intracellular space was significantly increased at the "red streaks" of the distal esophagus of ERD-patients compared to biopsies from adjacent normal-locking epithelium. The above findings confirm previous observations for biopsies taken in the red streak and in 3 o´clock position 2 cm proximal to the gastro esophageal junction (27). Strong support for the involvement of nitrotyrosine in the pathogenesis of mucosal abnormalities in the red streak was obtained using correlation analysis.

In conclusion, there were clear signs of increased radical forming capacity in the epithelium despite absence of histological inflammation, in association to ERD. The histomorphological changes in ERD associating with nitrotyrosine expression, thus mirroring the foregoing radical formation, may suggest a role in the pathogenesis of esophagus. During acidified refluxes, epithelial ROS production in combination with luminal NO formation, may constitute aggravated factors in the carcinogenic process.

6. Acknowledgements

This study was supported by an unconditional scientific grant from AstraZeneca.

7. References

[1] Lundell LR, Dent J, Benett JR, Blum AL, Armstrong D, Galmiche JP, et al. Endoscopic assessment of oesophagitis: clinical and functional correlates and further validation of the Los Angeles classification. Gut 1999; 45:172-80

[2] Dent J, El-Serag HB, Wallander MA, Johansson S. Epidemiology of gastro-oesophageal reflux disease: a systematic rewiew Gut 2005; 54;710-17

[3] Pilar J, Piazuelo E, Sánchez MT, Ortego J, Soteras F, Lanas A. Free radicals and antioxidant systems in reflux esophagitis and Barrett´s esophagus. World J Gastroenterol 2005; 11:2697-2703

[4] Grisham M.B. Serial Review: Reactive oxygen species in immune responses. Free radical biology & medicine 2004; 36:1479-1480

[5] Grisham M.B Jourd´heuil D, Wink DA. Chronic inflammation and reactive oxygen and nitrogen metabolism-implications in DNA damage and mutagenesis. Aliment Pharmacol Ther 2000; 14:3-9

[6] Casselbrant A, Pettersson A, Ruth M, Bove M, Lundell L, Fändriks L. Sources of intra-oesophageal nitric oxide production following intraluminal acid exposure. Scand J Gastroenterol. 2002; 37:631-7

[7] Suzuki H, Iijima K, Scobie G, Fyfe V, McColl KE. Nitrate and nitrosative chemistry within Barrett´s oesophagus during acid reflux. Gut 2005; 54:1527-35

[8] Edebo A, Vieth M, Tam W, Bruno M, van Berkel AM, Stolte M, et al. Circumferential and axial distribution of esophagus mucosal damage in reflux disease. Dis Esophagus 2007; 20:232-8

[9] Bradford MM. A rapid and sensitive method for the quantitation of microgram quantities of protein utilizing the principle of protein-dye binding. Anal Biochem. 1976; 72:248-54

[10] Rieder F, Cheng L, Harnett KM, Chak A, Cooper GS, Isenberg G, Ray M, Katz JA, Catanzaro A, O´shea R, Post AB, Wong R, Sivak MV, Mccormick T, Phillips M, West GA, Wills JE, Biancani P, Fiocchi C. Gastroesophageal reflux disease-

associated esophagitis induces endogeneous cytokine production leading to motor abnormalities. Gastroenterology 2007; 132:154-165
[11] Okamura A, Rakugi H, Ohishi M, Yanagitani Y, Takiuchi S, Moriguchi K, Fennessy PA, Higaki J, Ogihara T. Upregulation of renin-angiotensin system during differentiation of monocytes to macrophages. J Hypertens 1999; 17:537-545
[12] Cross AR, Segal AW. The NAPDH oxidase of professional phagocytes-prototype of the NOX electron transport chain systems. Biochim Biophys Acta. 2004; 1657:1-22
[13] Klebanoff SJ. Myeloperoxidase. Proc Assoc Am Physicians. 1999; 111:383-9
[14] Mohiuddin I, Chai H, Lin PH, Lumsden AB, Yao Q, Chen C. Nitrotyrosine and chlorotyrosine: clinical significance and biological functions in the vascular system. J Surg Res 2006; 133:143-9
[15] Singer II, Kawka DW, Scott S, Weidner JR, Mumford RA, Riehl TE, Stenson WF. Expression of inducible nitric oxide synthase and nitrotyrosine in colonic epithelium in Inflammatory bowel disease. Gastroenterology 1996; 111:871-885
[16] Maley CC, Reid BJ. Natural selection in neoplastic progression of Barrett's esophagus Semin Cancer Biol 2005; 15:474-83
[17] Sihvo EI, Salminen JT, Rantanen TK, Rämö OJ, Ahotupa M, Färkkilä M, Auvinen MI, Salo JA. Oxidative stress has a role in malignant transformation in Barrett´s oesophagus Int J. Cancer 2002;102:551-5
[18] Elfvin A. Helicobacter pylori associated effects on inflammatory radical formation and angiotensin II receptors in the stomach. Thesis University of Gothenburg 2007. ISBN 978-91-628-7326-4
[19] Feagins LA, Zhang HY, Zhang X, Hormi-Carver K, Thomas T, Terada LS, Spechler SJ, Souza RF. Mechanisms of oxidant production in esophageal squamous cell and Barrett´s cell lines Am J Physiol 2008; 294:411-7
[20] O'Riordan JM, Abdel-latif MM, Ravi N, McNamara D, Byrne PJ, McDonald GS, Keeling PW, Kelleher D, Reynolds JV. Proinflammatory cytokine and nuclear factor kappa-B expression along the inflammation-metaplasia-dysplasia-adenocarcinoma sequence in the esophagus. Am J Gastroenterol 2005; 100:1257-64
[21] Fitzgerald RC,Onwuegbusi BA, Bajaj-Elliott M, Saeed IT, Burnham WR, Farthing MJ. Diversity in the oesophageal phenotypic response to gastro-oesophageal reflux: immunological determinants. Gut 2002; 50:451-9
[22] Granli T, Dahl R, Brodin P, Bockman OC. Nitrate and nitrite concentrations in human saliva: variations with salivary flow-rate. Food Chem Toxicol 1989; 27:675-80
[23] Wilson KT. Fu S, Ramanujam KS, Meltzer SJ. Increased expression of inducible nitric oxide synthase and cyclooxygenase-2 in Barrett´s esophagus and associated adenocarcinomas. Cancer Res 1998; 14:2929-34
[24] Bove M, Ruth M, Lundell L, Ny L. Epithelial barrier integrity and intraluminal nitric oxide production in response to acid perfusion of the ferret oesophagus. Acta Physiol Scand 2005; 183:211-8
[25] Lin KT, Xue JY, Nomen M, Spur B, Wong PY. Peroxynitrite-induced apoptosis in HL-60 cells. J Biol Chem 1995; 270:16487-90
[26] Babior BM. Phagocytes and oxidative stress. Am J Med. 2000; 109:33-44
[27] Vieth M, Fiocca R, Haringsma J, Delarive J, Wiesel PH, Tam W, Tytgat GN, Dent J, Edebo A, Lundell L, Stolpe M. Radial distribution of dilated intracellular spaces of the esophageal squamous epithelium in patients with reflux disease exhibiting discrete endoscopic lesions. Dig Dis 2004; 22:208-12

8

Combination Therapy After EMR/ESD for Esophageal Squamous Cell Carcinoma with Submucosal Invasion

Ota M., Nakamura T. and Yamamoto M.
Department of Surgery, Institute of Gastroenterology, Tokyo Women's Medical University, Tokyo, Japan

1. Introduction

Recently, nonoperative treatment such as chemotherapy or radiotherapy has commonly been performed for submucosal carcinoma of the esophagus. Although endoscopic mucosal resection[1)2)] (EMR) or endoscopic submucosal dissection[3)] (ESD) is usually done as curative treatment for mucosal cancer of the esophagus, the efficacy of multimodal therapy combined with EMR/ESD for esophageal squamous cell carcinoma (SCC) with submucosal invasion is controversial.

At our hospital, several patients who had SCC with submucosal invasion received multimodal therapy combined with EMR or ESD, and the results are reported here.

2. Patients and methods

From 1996 to 2005, 36 patients who had esophageal SCC with submucosal invasion underwent multimodal treatment. Esophagectomy was not performed because of associated complications in 19 cases and due to patient refusal in 17 cases.

In all patients, EMR/ESD was performed before any other treatment. Then chemotherapy, radiotherapy, or chemoradiotherapy was added, depending on the histopathological findings, which were classified according to the Guidelines for Clinical and Pathologic Studies on Carcinoma of the Esophagus[4)]. Submucosal invasion was classified into the following three grades: sm1: ≤200 μm, sm2: >200 μm, and sm2 EM (+): residual cancer cells at the resected margin.

In principle, radiotherapy or chemoradiotherapy was added if the resected margin was suspected to contain residual cancer cells, while chemotherapy was performed if lymphatic invasion was found in the resected specimen (Fig 1). Argon plasma coagulation was added without radiation if the residual tumor was limited to a small area.

2.1 Method of EMR

EMR was performed by the EEMR or EMRC method[1)2)]. EMRC was done by using a single-channel endoscope (GIF Q260; Olympus) with a cap (Olympus, Tokyo, Japan). After chromoendoscopy with iodine solution, saline was injected into the submucosal layer.

Next, a snare (SD-7P, Olympus) was opened inside the cap, the tumor was aspirated into the cap, and the snare was closed. The forced coagulation mode was used to perform resection. EMMR was done by using a single-channel endoscope (GIF Q260; Olympus) fitted with an EEMR-tube. The method was same as that for EMRC until the injection of saline. Then a snare (SD-7P, Olympus) was passed through a side channel of the tube and was opened over the tumor. The tumor was aspirated into the tube using the suction of the endoscope and the snare was tightened. Resection was done in the forced coagulation mode.

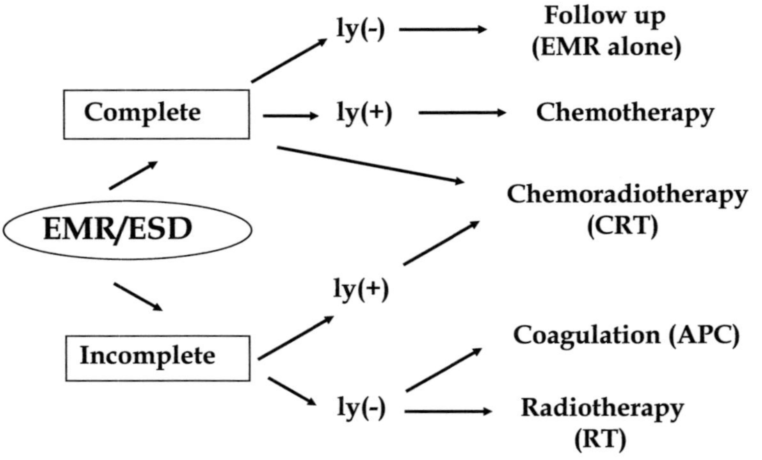

Fig. 1. Fundamental clinical course

2.2 Method of ESD

A hook knife from Olympus (Tokyo, Japan) was used for the hook knife method of ESD[3)5)] along with a single-channel endoscope (GIF Q260; Olympus) and an attachment. The electrical generator was a VIO (ERBE, Tübingen, Germany). Before marking, chromoendoscopy with iodine solution was done to identify the lateral margins of the lesion. Then marking was undertaken in the hook knife using the forced coagulation mode. After 10% glycerin was injected into the submucosal, mucosal incision was performed in the endo cut mode. Before performing submucosal dissection, hyaluronic acid solution was injected into the submucosal lesion. Then the clip with thread was attached to the oral border of the specimen and the thread was pulled in the oral direction to exert traction on the submucosal layer. Next, the submucosal lesion was dissected off the muscle layer by using the hook knife in the endo cut mode. Bleeding was controlled with hemostatic forceps (FD-411QR; Olympus) in the soft coagulation mode or with the hook knife in the spray mode. ESD was performed with the patient under sedation by intravenous administration of diazepam and pentazocine as required plus continuous infusion of propofol.

2.3 Chemotherapy and radiotherapy

Chemotherapy was performed for 2 courses if lymphatic invasion was found in the resected specimen. Patients were principally given a combination of cisplatin/5-fluorouracil or nedaplatin/5-fluorouracil (Fig. 2). Radiotherapy was given to a total dose of 50-60 Gy, with the radiation field being limited to the local tumor area (Fig. 3).

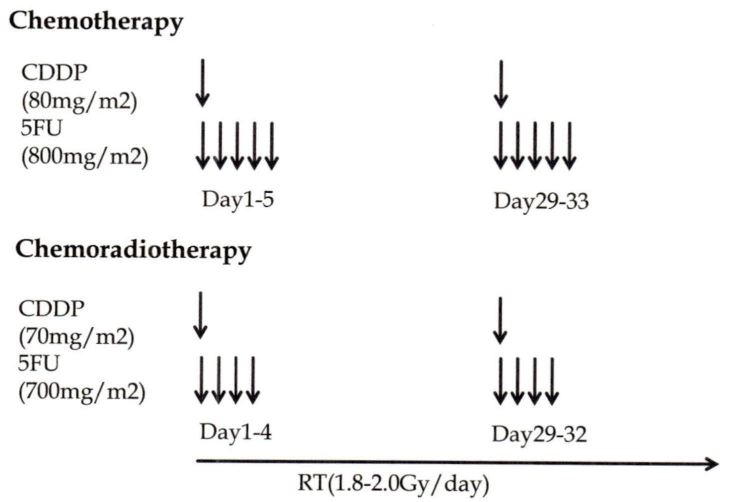

Fig. 2. Chemotherapy and chemoradiotherapy

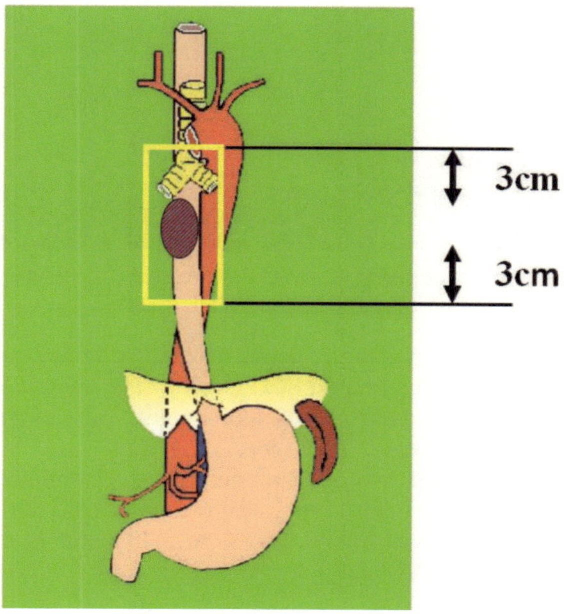

Fig. 3. The radiation field was limited to local area

3. Results

There were no complications of EMR/ESD. On histopathological examination, the depth of tumor invasion was sm1 in 22 cases, sm2 in 9, and sm2 EM (+) in 5. Lymphatic invasion (ly) was found in 18 cases (50%), and there was 1 case (3%) of vascular invasion (v).

Sixteen patients were treated with EMR alone, 8 received EMR + chemotherapy, 2 had EMR + radiotherapy, and 10 had EMR + chemoradiotherapy.

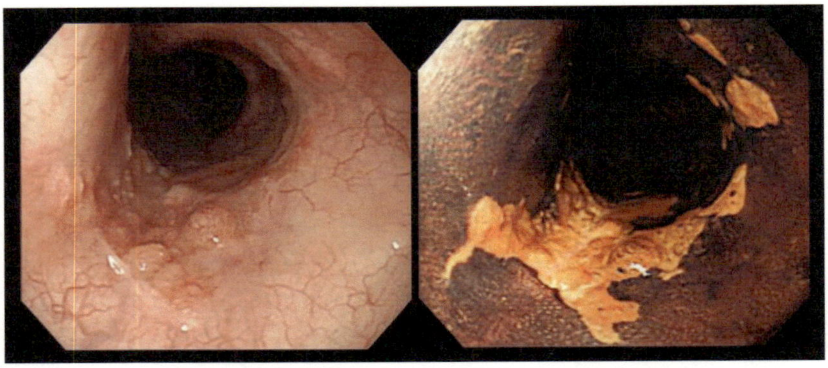

Fig. 4. 0-IIa+IIc lesion was seen in middle esophagus. EMR was performed

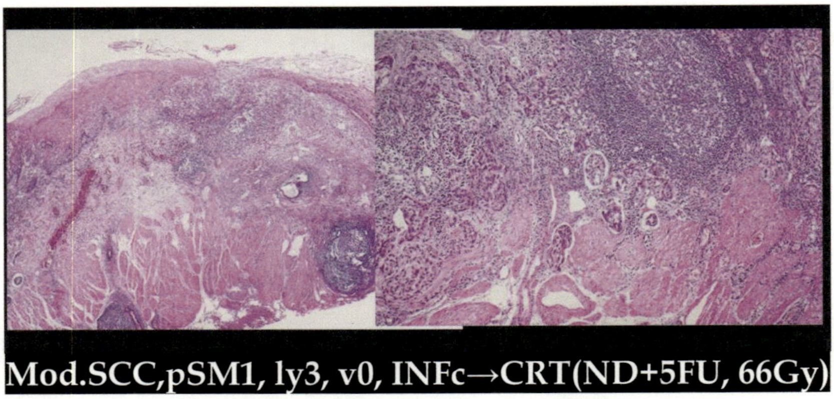

Fig. 5. Though pathological finding showed moderate. SCC, pSM1, ly3, v0, chemoradiotherapy was treated

Recurrence was diagnosed in three patients. Medistinal lymph node recurrence occurred in a man with moderately differentiated SCC (sm1, ly (-)) treated by EMR alone and cervical lymph node recurrence was detected in 1 woman with moderately differentiated SCC (sm2, ly (+)) treated by EMR alone. Both cervical lymph node recurrence and intramural metastasis were detected in 1 man with moderately differentiated SCC (sm1, ly (+)) treated by EMR + chemoradiotherapy (Fig. 4-6). Local recurrence did not occur.

There was 1 death from the primary disease and 10 patients died of other diseases. The overall survival rate was 69% (Fig. 7).

4. Discussion

Curative surgery has been considered the standard treatment for squamous cell carcinoma of the esophagus with submucosal invasion (T1b) because of the possibility of lymph node metastasis[6)7)8)]. Although chemoradiotherapy (CRT) has been performed recently for T1bN0 cancer, it is controversial whether CRT has the same therapeutic effect as surgery, and a randomized controlled trial of surgery versus CRT is still ongoing.

EMR has become widely employed for esophageal early carcinoma[1)2)] at a large number of institutions[10)]. ESD has been adopted for the treatment of early esophageal cancer as a

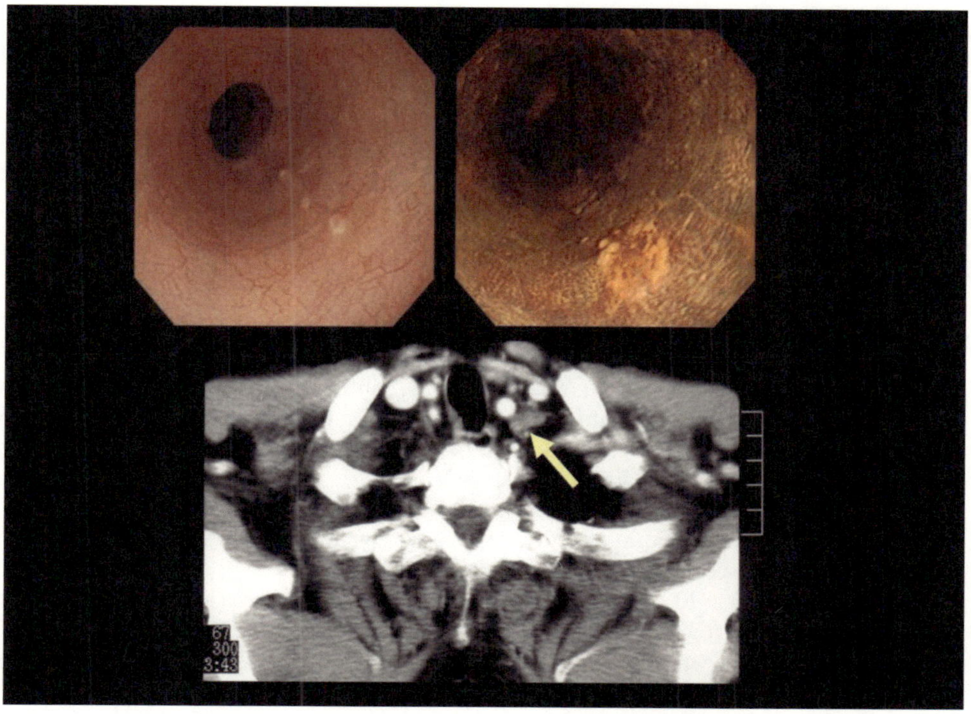

Fig. 6. After 6 month later, intrmural metastasia and cervical lymph node were detected. The patient died from the primary disease

method of excising extensive lesions en bloc. Endoscopic resection was previously considered to be curative for tumors limited to the proper mucosal layer[9]. Although the indications of EMR/ESD have been extended to tumors with invasion of the muscularis mucosae and submucosal tumors with a comparatively low rate of lymph node metastasis in recent years[11)-13)], these procedures are not indicated for tumors invading deeply into the submucosal layer.

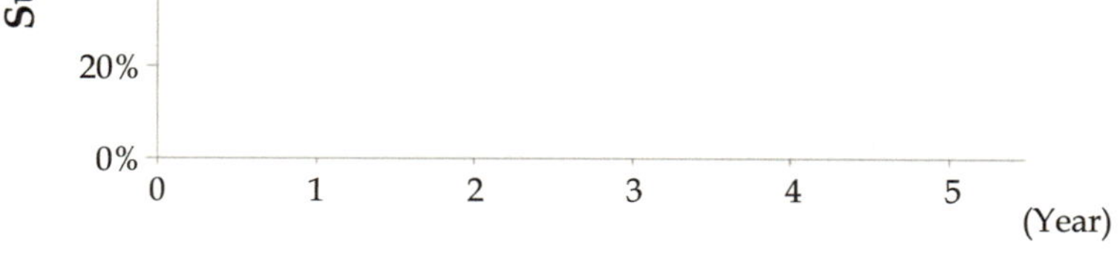

Fig. 7. Over all survival

One advantage of EMR/ESD is that histopathological examination is possible, which allows us to identify the patients who do not need chemotherapy or radiotherapy. EMR/ESD seemed to be effective because there was no local recurrence and residual tumor. There were many high risk patients in our series, so deaths from other causes were frequent. Thus, a randomized controlled trial will be needed to evaluate the correct survival rate. There were also cases of cervical and mediastinal lymph node recurrence in our series. These lymph nodes are removed by esophagectomy with 3-field dissection, so recurrences would have been avoided if esophagectomy had been performed in such patients. Accordingly, EMR/ESD needs to be selected carefully.

5. References

[1] Makuuchi H., Machimura T., Soh Y., Mizutani K., Shimada H., Sugihara T., Tokuda Y., Sasaki T., Tajima T., Mitomi T., Ohmori T., Miyoshi H. (1991) Endoscopic mucosectomy for mucosal carcinomas in the esophagus. Jpn J Surg Gastroenterol 24: 2599-2603 (Japanese, English abstract).

[2] Inoue H., Endo M., Takeshita K., Yoshino K., Muraoka Y., Yoneshima H. (1992) et al.: A new simplified technique of endoscopic esophageal mucosal resection using a cap-fitted panendoscope (EMRC). Surg Endosc 6: 264-265.

[3] Oyama T., Kikuchi Y. (2002). Aggressive endoscopic mucosal resection in the upper GI tract—Hook knife EMR method. Min Invas Ther. Allied Technol. 11: 291–5.

[4] Japanese society for esophageal disease (2007) Guidelines for clinical and pathologic studies on carcinoma of the esophagus. 10th ed., Kanehara, Tokyo.

[5] Oyama T., Tomori A., Hotta K., Morita S., Kominato, Tanaka M (2005). Endoscopic submucosal dissection of early esophageal cancer. Clin Gastroenterol Heptol 3: S67-70.

[6] Kato H., Tachimori Y., Watanabe H., Yamaguchi H., Ishikawa T., Itabashi M. (1990) Superficial esophageal carcinoma. Cancer 66: 2319-2323.

[7] Isono K., Sato H., Nakayama K. (1991) Results of nationwide study on the three-field lymph node dissection of esophageal cancer. Oncology 48: 411-420.

[8] Ide H., Kobayashi A. (1997) The choice of treatment for esophageal cancer. Ann Thorac Cardiovasc Surg 3: 87-95.

[9] Makuuchi H., Machimura T., Mizutani K., Shimada H., Sugano K., Chino O., Sugihara T., Tajima T., Mitomi T., Ohmori T., Tsuzuki T., Kumagai Y. (1993) Endoscopic mucosal resection for early esophageal cancer by the EEMR-tube method. Stomach and Intestine 28: 153-159 (Japanese, English abstract).

[10] Makuuchi H. (1996) Endoscopic mucosal resection for early esophageal cancer. Dig Endosc 8: 175-179.

[11] Nakagawa S., Watanebe H. (1994) Mucosal carcinoma of the esophagus - Their subclassification of depth of invasion, histologic risk factor and macroscopic features. Stomach and Intestine 29: 273-288 (Japanese, English abstract).

[12] Tomimatsu H., Kato Y., Yanagisawa A., Ninomiya Y., Ueda M., Matsubara T. (1999) Pathological investiganion of esophageal carcinoma with submucosal invasion: Conparison of lymph node metastasis - positive and negative cases. Endoscopia Digestiva 11: 1355-1361 (Japanese, English abstract).

[13] Makuuchi H., Shimada H., Chino O., Tanaka H., Nishi T. (1998) Possibility of endoscopic mucosal resection in patients with m3 and sm1 esophageal cancer. Stomach and Intestine 33: 993-1002 (Japanese, English abstract).

Part 3

The Stomach and Duodenum

9

Clarithromycin Resistance and *23S rRNA* Mutations in *Helicobacter pylori*

Mohammad Kargar[1], Maryam Baghernejad[1],
Abbas Doosti[2] and Sadegh Ghorbani-Dalini[3]
[1]*Department of Microbiology, Jahrom Branch, Islamic Azad University, Jahrom,*
[2]*Biotechnologe Research Center, Shahrekord Branch,*
Islamic Azad University, Shahrekord,
[3]*Department of Microbiology, Jahrom Branch, Young Researcher's Club,*
Islamic Azad University, Jahrom,
Iran

1. Introduction

Helicobacter pylori infects about 50% of the world's population and is a major cause of chronic gastritis, is strongly associated with the development of gastric and duodenal ulcers and has been linked with gastric adenocarcinoma and B-cell mucosa-associated lymphoid tissue lymphoma [1, 2].

H. pylori Infection results in a sequence of events, ultimately resulting in the development of some gastrointestinal disorders. The sequence was first suggested by Correa et al. in 1975 and has since been supported by many other studies. Colonization of the gastric mucosa by *H. pylori* first lead to the induction of an inflammatory response, predominantly by Th1 (T helper cells type 1). The initial acute gastritis is followed by active chronic gastritis, which lasts for life if the infection is not treated. Nevertheless, *H. pylori*-positive subjects are mostly unaware of this inflammation due to the lack of clinical symptoms. The Th1 response results in epithelial cell damage rather than in the removal of *H. pylori* because *H. pylori* is not an intracellular pathogen. The ongoing presence of *H. pylori* thus causes a lifelong proinflammatory response coupled to cellular damage and initiates the histological cascade. The continuous production of reactive oxygen species that results from the ongoing inflammation can result in DNA damage, thus inducing the multiple mutations thought to be required for initiation of the cancer cascade depicted in Figure 1 (3, 4).

Among the new methods of magnifying endoscopy, a prototype of endocytoscopy developed by Olympus was used for ex vivo visualization of *Helicobacter pylori* on experimentally infected gastric biopsies. Moving bacteria were observed at 1100× magnification, giving hope for a possible direct detection during endoscopy. Kim et al. also used magnifying endoscopy on 103 patients to classify the gastric surface according to four patterns: flat, irregular, papillary or nonstructured, which were then compared to the updated Sydney System for histologic gastritis. Histologic gastritis was found in 91% of the biopsy sections with a nonflat type, and among them, 96% were confirmed to harbor *H. pylori* infection. In another study, the magnified endoscopic findings in the gastric body were classified into four patterns and then correlated with histology results. Type 1 pattern corresponded to normal gastric mucosa, types 2 and 3 to *H. pylori* -infected mucosa and type 4 to atrophy. The sensitivity and specificity for these endoscopic findings were 92.7% and 100% for type 1, and 100% and 92.7% for types 2 and 3 together, respectively (5).

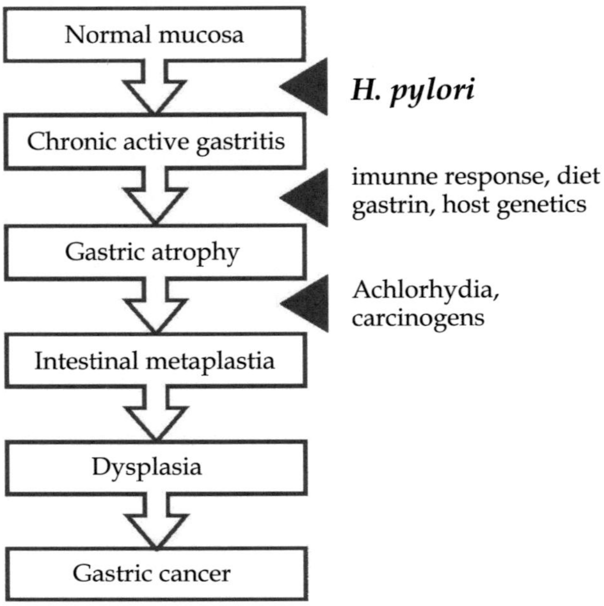

Fig. 1. Model representing the role of *H. pylori* and other factors in gastric carcinogenesis, based on the cascade proposed by Correa et al (3, 4)

2. *H. pylori* detection

Various diagnostic assays for the detection of an *H. pylori* infection are available. Histological detection and culturing of the pathogen are gold standard, which require invasive gastroduodenoscopy to obtain gastric biopsy specimens. In the last decade, noninvasive approaches, such as serological detections, the [^{13}C] and [^{14}C]urea breath test (UBT), and detection *H. pylori* antigen or DNA in feces, helped and improved the evaluation of *H. pylori* infection status in patients. Because of low sensitivities of most serological assays for younger than 12 years of age patients, they are not suitable for pediatric. The UBT is a well-established noninvasive diagnostic assay and gives excellent performance for both adults and children, but its specificity decreases for infants and young children and need. In addition, the performance of UBT with infants and young children requires trained staff for air sampling with a face mask, and the test also requires expensive instruments, such as an isotope ratio mass spectrometer or an infrared isotope ratio spectrometer. Enzyme immunoassays (EIAs) for the identification of *H. pylori* antigens in fecal specimens circumvent these difficulties. EIAs based on monoclonal antibodies have shown consistent excellent results, with very high sensitivities and specificities for both adults and children. A major disadvantage of all the noninvasive tests described above is their inability to provide information on the susceptibility or resistance of *H. pylori* to antibiotics [2].

Methods		Sensitivity and Specificity	Typical application
Invasive methods	Histology	>95%	Gold standard in routin hospital diagnostics
	Biopsy culture	>95%	Alternative gold standard
	RUT	>90%	Cost-effective and rapid test
Noninvasive methods	UBT	>95%	Alternative gold standard
	Fecal antigen	>90%	Not widely used yet
	Serology	80-90%	Mainly used for epidemiological studies

Table 1. Non-PCR base diagnosis of *H. pylori* infection (3)

3. Macrolide resistance

H. pylori infection can be cured by antibiotics, however the ideal anti-*H. pylori* treatment has yet to be found. Many factors have been implicated in treatment failure, including ineffective penetration of antibiotics into the gastric mucosa, antibiotic inactivation by low gastric pH, lack of compliance, and emergence of acquired antibiotic resistance by *H. pylori*. Despite the success of the current anti-*Helicobacter* therapies, it is suggested that eradication rates among patients with gastritis are lower than among patients with peptic ulcer disease, with the causes of this phenomenon still being the subject of speculation [6].

The macrolide class of antimicrobial agents is over 30 years old and is still at the forefront of antimicrobial therapy as well as drug discovery and development. Clarithromycin is a recently approved 14-membered macrolide with increased stability in acid and improved pharmacokinetics, including the appearance of a microbiologically active metabolite in humans. Clarithromycin possesses broad-spectrum antimicrobial activity, inhibiting a range of gram-positive and gram-negative organisms, some anaerobes, and atypical pathogens, in many cases with greater in vitro activity than erythromycin [7].

Clarithromycin is a semi-synthetic macrolide antibiotic. Chemically, it is 6-*0*-methylerythromycin. The molecular formula is $C_{38}H_{69}NO_{13}$, and the molecular weight is 747.96 (Figure 2). Clarithromycin is a white to off-white crystalline powder. It is soluble in acetone, slightly soluble in methanol, ethanol, and acetonitrile, and practically insoluble in water.

Currently, a seven-day, triple-drug regimen has been recommended as one of the first-line therapies for *H. pylori* management. This treatment includes omeprazole (a proton-pump inhibitor), clarithromycin, and amoxicillin or metronidazole [2, 8]. However, this therapy is being investigated because of increased eradication failures due to the prevalence of clarithromycin resistant *H. pylori* infections. Many studies have shown that between 0–50% of *H. pylori* isolates were clarithromycin resistant, which leads to a need for long term

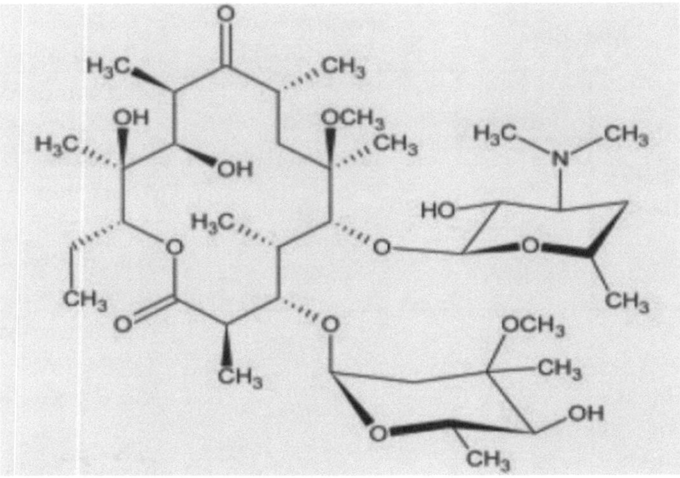

Fig. 2. The structural formula of clarithromycin

assessment of the efficacy of clarithromycin in the triple-drug regimen. It is well known that the abuse of macrolide antibiotics including clarithromycin might lead to clarithromycin resistant forms of *H. pylori* [8]. Clarithromycin is a bacteriostatic antibiotic, which belongs to a group of macrolides bound to peptidyltransferase loop of domain V and VI of the 23S rRNA molecule (Figure 3 and 4). This binding interferes with protein elongation, and thus effectively blocks bacterial protein synthesis.

The antibacterial activity of clarithromycin is similar to that of other macrolides, but clarithromycin is better absorbed in the gastric mucus layer, more acid-stable, and therefore more effective against *H. pylori*. Resistance to clarithromycin is thought to develop when substitutions in one nucleic acid at or near this binding site on the ribosome prevent the drug from binding, thereby making it ineffective [9]. Mutations A2144G, A2143G, A2142G and A2143C are the most often observed and reported by investigators, other mutations such as A2142C, A2115G, G2141A, A2142T and T2717C have been described but appear to be rare in peptidyltransferase [10, 11].

4. Detection of clarithromycin resistance

Many diagnostic assays have been developed for *Helicobacter pylori*: culture, histology, rapid urease test, urea breath test, serology, stool antigen test, and molecular-based tests [2, 5, 10, 11, 15]. Culture has the great advantage of permitting subsequent determination of the antimicrobial susceptibility of the strain isolated, in particular to macrolides. However, disadvantages of culture include special conditions for specimen transportation, the use of complicated media with special conditions for maintenance, the need for special incubation conditions, and the length of time necessary to obtain a result [10]. In routine practice the detection of clarithromycin resistance is mainly based on phenotypic methods performed after culture: agar diffusion for the E-test or the agar dilution method, which is considered the reference; however, these methods are time-consuming [16].

The association between point mutations in the *23S rRNA* gene and macrolide resistance in *H. pylori* potentially provides a new approach for diagnosing macrolide resistant *H. pylori* strains [9]. Numerous molecular-based methods are now available to assess clarithromycin

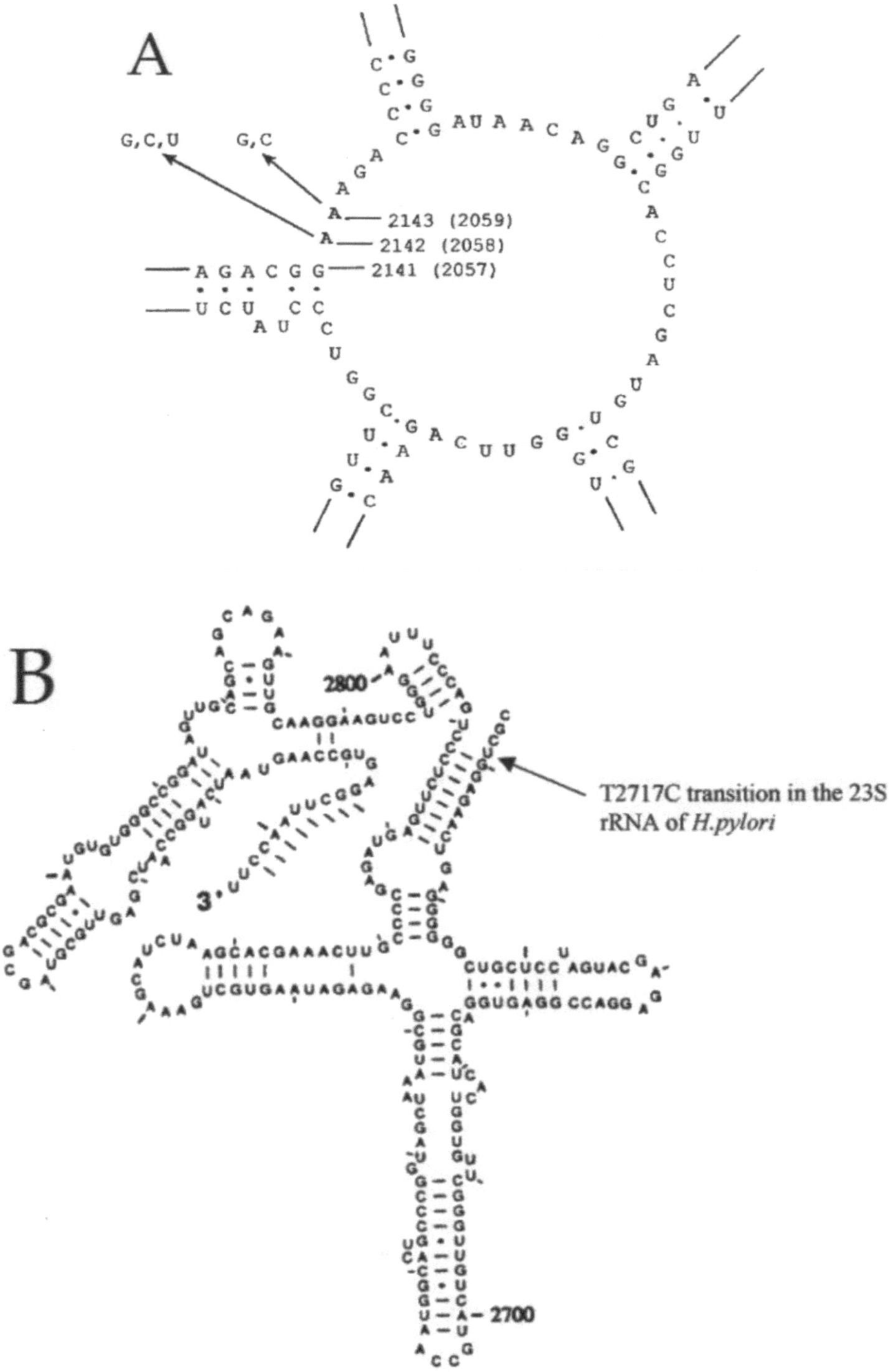

Fig. 3. Model of domain V and VI of 23S rRNA from *E. coli*, (12 , 13)

in *H. pylori*, such as PCR-RFLP, PCR-OLA, PCR-DEIA, PCR- LiPA, PCR-PHFA, 3M-PCR, real-time PCR, FISH, FRET, DNA sequencing by conventional and real-time (pyrosequencing) techniques [2, 9-11]. Most assays are polymerase chain reaction (PCR)-based using different methods to study the amplicons. The PCR-based molecular techniques are quicker than microbiological susceptibility testing, and more importantly, they can be performed directly on gastric biopsies and gastric juice [9].

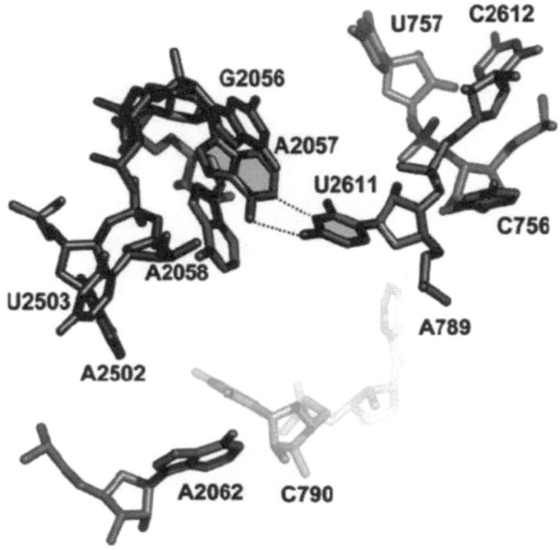

Fig. 4. A view into the macrolide-binding pocket in *E. coli* highlighting the specific geometry of the 2611–2057 base pair. H bonds are shown as dotted lines. The macrolide-binding pocket is located at the upper part of the ribosomal peptide exit tunnel, at a distance from the peptidyl transferase center that allows the accommodation of polypeptides of 5–6 residues. It is formed mainly by 23S rRNA domain V nucleotides, among which A2058 and A2059 play a prominent role in binding, selectivity, and resistance. (14)

A PCR-based approach to diagnostic testing has the advantage over existing non-culture-based tests in that it is simple to perform and can provide additional genotypic information about the infecting strain, including markers associated with antibiotic susceptibilities. In addition, although the initial cost of equipment is high, the cost of reagents and consumables for each test is extremely low in comparison with corresponding costs for other methods such as the urea breath test and stool antigen test [17]. Great advantage of PCR is that it does not require viable bacteria. The transport conditions are thus not as critical as they are for culture, and shipment costs are cheaper. The cost of the reagents necessary for our technique is reasonable: $6.20 for *H. pylori* detection only and $8.60 for detection and clarithromycin susceptibility testing. By microbiological techniques, detection is cheaper, $1.70, but the price of detection with clarithromycin susceptibility testing by E-test, $6.90, is comparable to that of PCR [10]. Nested PCR generally increases sensitivity but also has a high risk of contamination. Real-time PCR has several advantages over conventional PCR, such as short working time, high specificity, and low risk of contamination. Thus far, some studies used real-time PCR targeting either *ureC* or *16S rRNA* and *23S rRNA* for the quantitative detection of *H. pylori* in gastric biopsies [11]. FISH allowed simultaneous detection of *H pylori* and the point mutations. Also, FISH could be directly applied to formalin fixed tissue sections without extensive preparation of nucleic acid. Another advantage of this technique compared with PCR based systems became obvious when mixed strains and tissue sections harboring more than one *H. pylori* strain were examined. A mixed culture cannot be unequivocally differentiated from a strain carrying two different rRNA operons by restriction enzyme analysis or filter hybridization; this can be done easily by whole cell hybridization technology [18]. PCR-RFLP has some disadvantage than other PCR base techniques including: i: when multiple strains are present in one sample, PCR-RFLP technique can not able to identify genotypes that has low concentration, ii: PCR-RFLP technique can not able to detect two mutations A2144G and A2143C, iii: Mixed populations containing a resistant strain associated with a susceptible strain are difficult to detect by PCR-RFLP. The resistant strain is often well detected because the mutation conferring resistance produces a restriction site that results in a new band on the electrophoresis profile. However, the uncut fragment corresponding to the susceptible clone is usually not taken into consideration. The uncut fragment is indeed more often attributed to an incomplete restriction than to a mixed population. Even for pure resistant strains, a band corresponding to the uncut fragment of DNA is sometimes still present on the electrophoresis profile due to partial restriction. Thus, a mixed population containing a susceptible strain associated with a resistant strain is detected as a single resistant strain [19].

A TaqMan probe is a short oligonucleotide (DNA) that contains a 5' fluorescent dye and 3' quenching dye. To generate a light signal (i.e., remove the effects of the quenching dye on the fluorescent dye), two events must occur. First, the probe must bind to a complementary strand of DNA. Second, *Taq* polymerase, the same enzyme used for the PCR, must cleave the 5' end of the TaqMan probe (5' nuclease activity), separating the fluorescent dye from the quenching dye (Figure 5) (20).

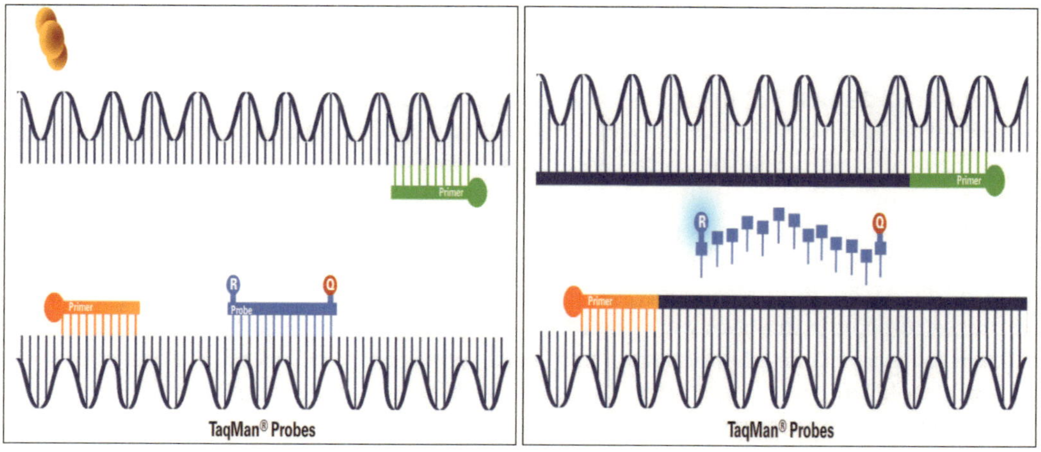

Fig. 5. Schematic model for TaqMan probe technology

Culture has the great advantage of permitting subsequent determination of the antimicrobial susceptibility of the strain isolated, in particular to macrolides. However, disadvantages of culture include special conditions for specimen transportation, the use of complicated media with special conditions for maintenance, the need for special incubation conditions, and the length of time necessary to obtain a result [10]. Low bacterial density and a patchy distribution of the pathogen may have been the reasons for the negative culture and histology results. This may also be true for the patient determined to be negative by the rapid urease test, histology, and culture but positive by both PCR assays in the biopsy and the stool specimen, thus resulting in a reduction of the PCR specificity to 98% [11]. Culture is only semiquantitative and is time consuming. Histology is also semiquantitative, but its accurateness is relatively weak because of great interobserver variation. Urea breath test has been shown to be uncorrelated to culture-determined bacterial density [10].

5. Epidemiology of clarithromycin resistance

Resistance to clarithromycin is the main predictor of failure of eradication treatments including this compound. Because of an increased use of these macrolides, not only for *H. pylori* eradication, but also for the treatment of respiratory tract infections, the prevalence rate of resistant strains is increasing, and the detection of resistance is becoming of major importance. To render this detection process more effective, results must be available rapidly.

Several studies have shown that the eradication of *H. pylori* plays an important role in the treatment of some gastrointestinal diseases and the results of all currently used tests for bacterial detection can be affected by the treatment [21]. Therefore, a growing attention has been assigned to *H. pylori* antibiotic susceptibility monitoring, due to the increasing prevalence of antibiotic resistance worldwide. Rates of clarithromycin resistance in *H. pylori* strains have been reported in France 21%, Spain 28.3%, Portugal 44.8%, Poland 23.5%, Mexico 21.6%, China 5%, Korea 16.7%, Italy 26.7% and Germany 47% [5, 15, 22-24]. A similar geographical distribution has been observed in Iran, with clarithromycin resistance values ranging from 21% [25] to 35.98% .This relevant discrepancy could be explained not only by the different geographic distribution of resistances, but also by the use of different methodologies to assess clarithromycin resistant status. For example, a study recently performed in the same geographic area (Shahrekord, Iran) has reported clarithromycin resistance rate 22.62% [26] distinctly lower compared with our present experience (35.98%). Nevertheless, it is possible that the different methods used (antibiogram vs. real-time PCR) could have played a role in these discordant data as bacterial culture is hampered by limitations, such as a low sensitivity, even in expert-hands [22].

Although *H. pylori* has two copy of *23S rRNA* gene in own genome, but many authors suggested that more than one strain can present in one patient [11, 27-29]. Also many authors displayed multiple genotypes in one sample because: 1) A troubling aspect of resistance to some antibiotics by *H. pylori* is a phenomenon that has been given the name heteroresistance. This phenomenon has been previously observed for resistance to metronidazole [30]; 2) *H. pylori* is transformable bacterium and the transformation frequency for clarithromycin resistance of *H. pylori* was found to be approximately 2×10^{-6} transformants per viable cell [31]; 3) More importantly, Taylor and et al. suggests that acquisition of antibiotic resistance could result from the horizontal transfer of clarithromycin resistance determinants from resistant cells to susceptible cells of the same strain, probably increasing the population of resistant strains. In addition, such genetic transfer could occur between different strains, since mixed infections with different *H. pylori* strains does occur in some individuals [31].

Country	Year	Technique	Sample No.	Resistance rete	Ref
Australia	2004	Real-time PCR	92	24%	8
France	1994-1999	E-test	150	21%	32
France	1998	Hybridization in Liquid Phase	41	56%	33
France	1999	PCR-DNA Enzyme Immunoassay	61	37.7%	21
France	2000	E-test	61	18%	34
France	2003	Real-time PCR	200	67%	11
France	2003	Real-time PCR	196	18.5%	7
France	2004-2008	Real-time PCR	126	20%	35
Germany	2001	FISH	109	31.2%	36
Germany	1999-2002	E-test	1233	20%	37
Netherland	2001	RAPD-PCR	976	5.2%	8
Italy	2003	PCR-RFLP	283	1.6%	12
Italy	2003	PCR-RFLP & E-test	230	14%	38
Ireland	2001	LiPA	50	26%	39
Spain	2008	E-test	118	35.6%	40
Brazil	2001	Agar Diliution	202	9.85%	41
Brazil	2003	Agar Dilution	155	16%	3
Mexico	1995-1997	E-test	195	24%	42
Peru	1995	Egg Yolk Agar	18	50%	43
Argentina	2000	PCR-RFLP	96	23.9%	44
USA	1996	PCR-OLA	72	55%	45
China	2001	Primer mismatch PCR	96	5%	16
China	200-2009	Agar Dilution	293	8.6%-20.7%	46
Japan	1998	Seminested PCR	85	9%	47
Japan	1999	PCR-RFLP	79	6.3%	22
Japan	2000	PCR-PHFA	412	22%	48
Japan	2001	Real-time PCR	186	21.2%	49
Japan	2001	PCR-RFLP	51	29%	50
Malaysia	2005-2007	E-test	187	2.1%	51
Indonesia	2006	Disk diffusion	126	27.8%	52
Korea	2004	PCR-RFLP	114	20.2%	53
Iran	2007	PCR-RFLP	263	22.6%	54
Iran	2009	PCR-RFLP	200	23.78%	55
Iran	2009	Real-time PCR	200	35.98%	55
Iran	2008-2009	E-test	121	5%	56
Tunisa	2005-2007	Real-time PCR	273	14.6%	57
Cuba	2005	E-test	46	10%	58

Table 2. Prevalence of clarithromycin resistance in the world. Comparison between date, technique and region

Currently, many research aims to evaluation of clarithromycin resistance in *H. pylori* were performed which showed variety of resistance rate around the world, due to 3 main reasons including differences in i: methods, ii: region and iii: date (Table 2).

Many investigators were assessed clarithromycin resistance rate in Europe in 1994 to 2009. In these studies, clarithromycin resistance was more prevalent in France. Also, Fontana et al by PCR-RFLP method showed that clarithromycin resistance was more divers between north (1.6%) and south (14%) of Italy in 2003.

In continent of America, clarithromycin resistance was varies between 9.8% in Brazil to 55% in USA. Less variety were observed in eastern Asia, by 20% to 27% resistance rate. In Iran (Middle East) with variety of customs, Kargar et al showed resistant rate of 23% and 36% in same geographic region in 2009 due to different methods including PCR-RFLP and real-time PCR assays respectively but, PCR-RFLP showed 22% and 23%resistance rate in 2007 and 2009 respectively. Also more variation was observed in 2 near region with different customs and economic level, with 36% in low economic level and 5% in high economic level.

6. Epidemiology of clarithromycin resistance mutations

Many studies aim to assessment of clarithromycin resistance rate were preformed around the world. This studies showed A2144G > A2142G > A2143G > A2142C > A2143C order for clarithromycin resistance point mutations (Table 3).

Researcher	Country	technique	Mutations rate	Ref
Pina	**France**	Hybridization in Liquid Phase	A2144G(56%) A2143G(35%) A2143C(9%)	32
Marais	France	PCR-DNA Enzyme Immunoassay	A2144G(48%) A2143G(24%) A2143C(3%)	21
Russman	Germany	FISH	A2144G(59%) A2143G(35%) A2143C(6%)	36
Maeda	Japan	Seminested PCR	A2144G(87.5%) A2143G(12.5%)	47
Matsuok	Japan	PCR-RFLP	A2144G(80%) A2143G(20%)	22
Matsumura	Japan	Real-time PCR	A2144G(55%) A2143G(5%)	49
Kargar	Iran	PCR-RFLP	A2143G(68.3%) A2142G(15.8%)	54
Kargar	Iran	Real-time PCR	A2144G(5.7%) A2143G(37.1%) A2142G(28.6%) A2143C(21.4%)	55

Table 3. Prevalence of clarithromycin resistance point mutations

7. Problem statement

Following the recognition of the important pathogenic role of *H. pylori* infection in the development of gastroduodenal diseases, there has been a continuous search for improved eradication therapy (Occhilini et al., 1997). *H. pylori* culture, as well as antimicrobial susceptibility studies is difficult to perform as well as labor intensive. Moreover, although the culture method allows antimicrobial susceptibility testing for several antibiotics, only the susceptibilities of macrolides and, in particular, of clarithromycin are really useful since the last is a major predictor of treatment failure. Therefore, detection of clarithromycin-resistant *H. pylori* will facilitate the choice of an appropriate eradication regimen

7.1 Aplication area

The characterization of resistance mechanisms in *H. pylori* and their easy detection will facilitate the choice of appropriate treatment regimens and ultimately the control of infection. PCR-RFLP can be used directly with biopsy specimens, thereby avoiding the requirement for time-consuming culture-based methods. This is particularly important for patients in whom a first eradication attempt has failed.

7.2 Material and methods

Study design

In order to assess the clarithromycin resistance rate, 23S rRNA point mutations responsible for clarithromycin resistance and effect of technique, region and date, 2 separate analyses were performed.

7.3 Analysis 1

Patients

263 consecutive patients with dyspeptic symptoms attending the endoscopy center of the gastroenterology department of the Hajar Hospital, Shahrekord, Iran, were enrolled in this study from July to December 2008. Patient-reported symptoms and endoscopic findings of pathologist were recorded at the time of the consultation by the pathologist help, and these data were obtained retrospectively for analysis. The number of participants who were ineligible or declined participation in the study were not recorded.

For the purpose of analysis, three global variables were created: 1) patient-reported included age, gender and symptoms, 2) clinical signs, and 3) clarithromycin resistance data. Patient-reported symptoms included pain, anorexia, heaviness after meal, early satiety, nausea, vomiting and flatulence. Clinical signs were included gastric ulcer, gastric cancer, non-ulcer disease, gastic erosion, nodularity, gastritis and duodenit. All patients read and signed an 'informed consent' form at the beginning of endoscopy declared their satisfaction for application of their anonymous data for research purpose.

Three biopsy specimens were taken from antrum and corpus of each patient, using a disinfected endoscope. Biopsy samples were placed in 0.1 ml of sterile saline solution and sent to the Biotechnology research center of Shahrekord Azad University. A rapid test for the detection of urease activity was performed by Gastro Urease kit (Bahar-afshan, Iran) according to manufacturer's instructions. DNA was isolated from each tissue with a DNA extraction kit (DNP™, CinnaGen, Iran) according to the manufacturer's instruction and immediately used for molecular analysis.

Bacteria and culture conditions

Biopsy samples were cultured on *Brucella* agar (Merck) supplemented with 7% fresh horse blood, vancomycin (6mg/L, Merck), trimethoprim (5mg/L, Merck) and amphotericin (2mg/L, Merck). For primary culture, plates were incubated at 37°C in a microaerophilic atmosphere (5% O_2, 15% CO_2, 80%N_2) for 3 to 5 days. Strains were identified according to colony morphology, Gram staining and positive reactions with urease, catalase, and oxidase. The *ureC* gene (*glmM*) which encodes urease was used as a DNA target to confirm *H. pylori* strain.

Antimicrobial susceptibility testing

The susceptibilities of the *H. pylori* isolates to clarithromycin were examined by an agar dilution method according to *CLSI* (Clinical and Laboratory Standard Institute) protocol (32). Resistance breakpoint for clarithromycin was defined as the >4 μg/liter.

Conventional PCR assays

A PCR assay targeted at the *ureC* (*glmM*) gene of *H. pylori* was performed with specific primer (Table 4) in an eppendorf mastercycler gradient (eppendorf, Germany). Briefly, the 23 μl PCR mixture, containing 1 μl of extracted DNA, 200 mM (each) deoxynucleoside triphosphates (dNTPs) (dNTP Mix, CinnaGen, Iran), 0.2 mM (each) primer (CinnaGen, Iran), 1.5 mM $MgCl_2$, and 1 U of *Taq* polymerase (CinnaGen, Iran) in PCR buffer (CinnaGen, Iran), was held for 5 min at a denaturation temperature of 95°C, followed by 30 cycles of 1 min each at a denaturation temperature of 95°C, an annealing temperature of 58°C, and an elongation temperature of 72°C and by 5 min at 72°C. The amplified fragment was visualized after electrophoresis on a 1.5% agarose gel stained with ethidium bromide.

PCR-RFLP analysis

A 1,400-bp fragment of the *23S rRNA* gene was amplified with primers Cla-18 and Cla-21 [44] (Table 3). PCR amplification of DNA was performed in a final volume of 24 μl PCR mixture, containing 2 μl of extracted DNA, 200 mM dNTPs, 0.2 mM (each) primer, 1.5 mM $MgCl_2$, and 1 U of *Taq* polymerase in PCR buffer. Amplification was carried out in an eppendorf mastercycler gradient over 30 cycles, each for 1 min at 95°C, 1 min at 62°C, and 1 min at 72°C. These cycles were performed after a denaturation of 5 min at 95°C and a final elongation step at 72°C for 5 min. The amplicon was digested with *BsaI* for 1 h at 37°C and *MboII* (Fermentas GMBH, Germany) for 1 h at 37°C to detect the restriction site occurring when the mutation was A to G transition at 2143 or 2142, respectively (Figure 5). The restriction products were analyzed by electrophoresis on a 2% agarose gel.

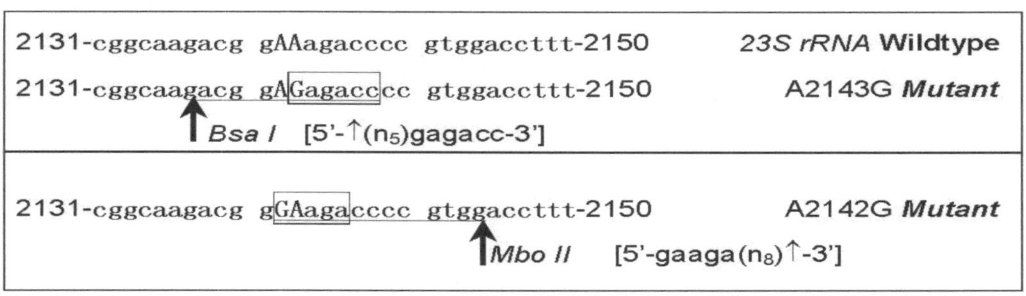

Fig. 5. Schematic diagram for detection of nucleotide alterations of *23S rRNA* by PCR-RFLP assays

7.4 Analysis 2

Sample collection

200 biopsy samples were obtained over a 6-month period (June 2009 to November 2009) from 200 dyspeptic patients referred for endoscopy at Hajar hospital in Iran. All patients read and signed an 'informed consent' form at the beginning of endoscopy declared they are satisfied with application of their anonymous data for research purpose. Every patient history sheet was examined in detail and clinical findings including demographic data were recorded. The mean age of the patients was 52.5 years (range, 17 to 88 years), and 48.1% of the patients were men. Rapid urease test was performed with a Gastro urease kit (bahar-afshan, Iran). DNA was isolated from each tissue with a DNA extraction kit (DNP™, CinnaGen, Iran) according to the manufacturer's instruction and immediately used for molecular analysis. Conventional PCR for detection of *ureC* gene and PCR-RFLP analysis for detection of point mutations were performed as in analysis 1.

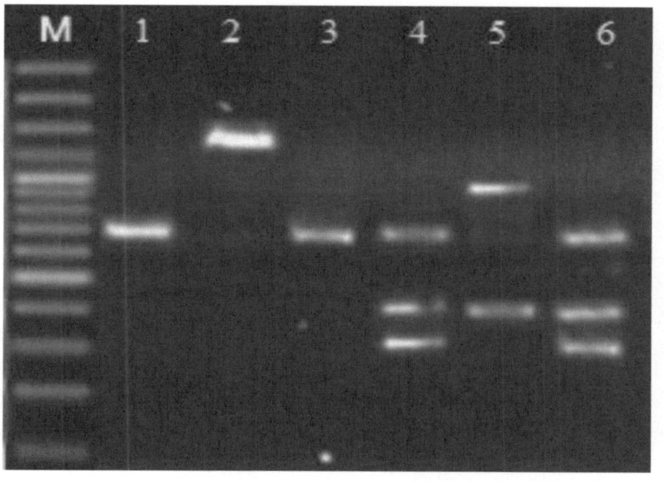

Fig. 6. PCR-RFLP patterns obtained after digestion with *Bsa*I or *Mbo*II. *BsaI* cuts the PCR product of the wild-type sequence into two fragments of 1,000 and 400bp and that of the A2143G sequence into three fragments of 700, 400, and 300bp. *MboII* cuts the PCR product into two fragments of 700bp only when A2142G is present in the sequence: 1)A2142G positive control, 2)A2142G negative control, 3)A2142G positive strain, 4)A2143G positive control, 5)A2143G negative control, 6)A2143G positive strain

Real-time (TaqMan) PCR assay

The real-time PCR was performed by using primer pair HP23S-1 and HP23S-2 and modified probes Pwt, P44G, P43G and P43C that previously reported by Pina et al [33] and newly designed probe P42G according to *23S rRNA* gene sequence (GenBank accession no. U27270) for identification of wild type, A2144G, A2143G, A2143C and A2142G genotypes respectively (Table 3).

The real-time (TaqMan) PCR mixture was prepared until reaching a final solution of 25 µl containing 2 µl of extracted DNA, 200 mM dNTPs, 0.2 mM (each) primer HP23S-1 and HP23S-2, 0.1 mM probe Pwt, 0.2mM probe P44G, 0.1 mM probe P43G, 0.1 mM probe P43C and 0.75 mM probe P42G (Bioneer,Tokyo, Korea) (Table I), 1.5 mM $MgCl_2$, and 1 U of *Taq* polymerase in PCR buffer 1X. Real-time PCR analysis was performed with an Rotor-Gene 6000 (Corbett Research, Australia). The conditions of PCR amplification were 95°C for 5 min and 45 cycles of 95°C for 30 s and 58°C for 40 s. All samples were repeated twice and positive and negative controls were enclosed in each assay. Data were analyzed with rotor-gene 6000 software *ver1.7* (Corbett research). In order to test the specificity of the primers purified DNA of non-*H. pylori* strains was also used as a template for PCR.

Quantification real-time PCR

In order to made standard serial dilution, standard density of bacteria was prepared. After DNA extraction, one 10-fold serial dilution of *H. pylori* DNA was made, with bacterial concentrations ranging from 5×10^2 to 5×10^7 bacteria per 1 µl. Bacterial quantification was performed by TaqMan probe technology of real-time PCR as described above.

Statistical analysis

Statistical analyses were conducted with *chi-square* using the SPSS for Windows (version 17; SPSS, Inc., Chicago, Illinois, USA). *P*-values less than 0.05 were taken to indicate statistical significance.

Target	Sequence (5′→3′)	Primer/Probe
ureC	AAGCTTTTAGGGGTGTTAGGGGTTT	HP-1
	AAGCTTATTTCTAACGC	HP-2
23S rRNA	AGTCGGGACCTAAGGCGAG	Cla-18
	TTCCCGCTTAGATGCTTTCAG	Cla-21
23S rRNA	CCACAGCGATGTGGTCTCAG	HP23S-1
	CTCCATAAGAGCCAAAGCCC	HP23S-2
Wild type	Cy5-GGGGTCTTTCCGTCT-BHQ2	Pwt
A2144G	TAMRA-GGTCCTTCCGTCTTG-Dabcyl	P44G
A2143G	TET-GGTCTCTCCGTCTTG-Dabcyl	P43G
A2143C	HEX-GGTCTGTCCGTCTTG-Dabcyl	P43C
A2142G	FAM-GGTCTTCCCGTCTTG-Dabcyl	P42G

Table 4. Oligonucleotides sequence used in this study

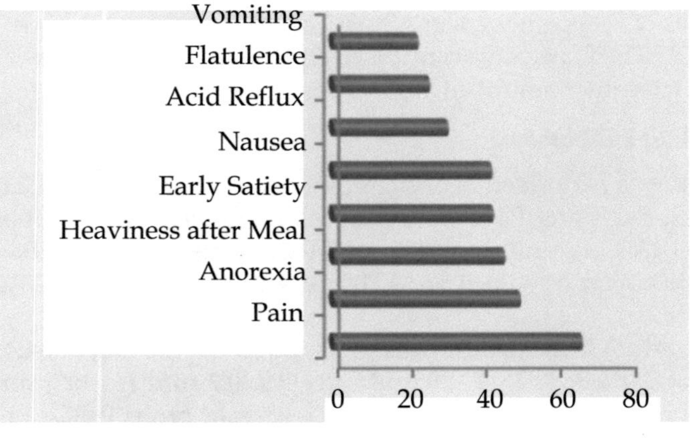

Fig. 7. Prevalence of patients reported symptoms in analysis 1

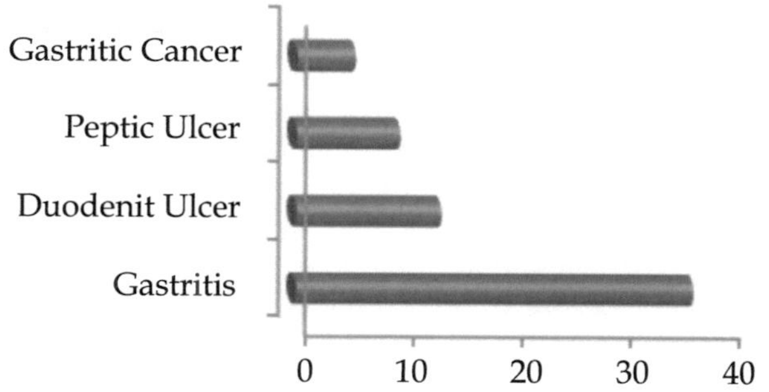

Fig. 8. Prevalence of clinical signs in analysis 1

8. Results

8.1 Analysis 1

Clinical features

Abdominal pain was present in 76% of patients (200/263), dyspepsia in 8%(20/263), vomiting in 6%(16/263), heartburn in 6%(17/263), and weakness 4%(10/263). The main endoscopic findings were 36% gastritis, 13% duodenal ulcer, 10% gastric ulcer, 9% esophagitis, and 5% gastric cancer (Figure 7, 8).

Culture, rapide urease test and PCR

H. pylori could be cultured from 84 of 263 (32%) patients, while a positive RUT or PCR band was observed in 54%(143 of 263) and 85%(223 of 263) of patients, respectively. Of the 84 patients with positive *H. pylori* culture 35/84 (41.7%) were males and 49/84 (58.3%) females. *H. pylori* was successfully cultured from 55 of 135 (41%) patients with non-ulcer dyspepsia and 29 of 62 (47%) with peptic ulcer (PU).
When the PCR was regarded as the "gold standard" of *H. pylori* identification, the sensitivity, specificity, PPV and NPV of RUT were 61%, 87%, 96% and 29% respectively. But for culture method were 36.77%, 95%, 97% and 21.22% respectively [59].

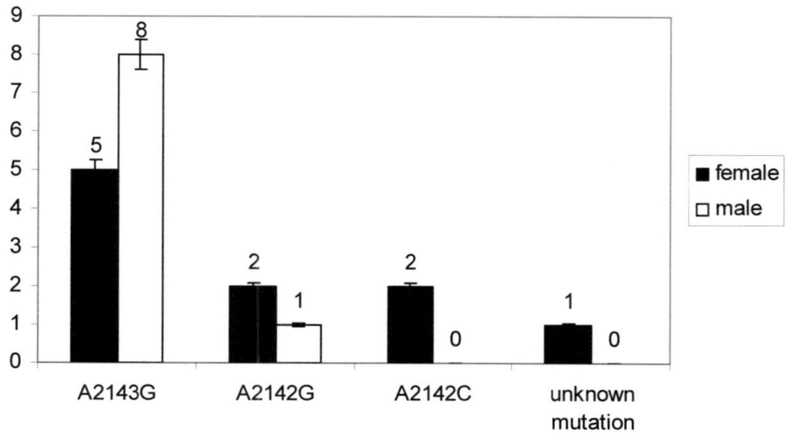

Fig. 9. Frequency of *23S rRNA* mutations in analysis 1 (n=19)

Prevalence of clarithromycin resistance

According to the agar dilution method, 19 of 84 (22.62%) cultured strains were resistant to clarithromycin. A 1.4kb fragment of the *23S rRNA* gene could be amplified in all 19 strains. Furthermore, *MboII* cuts PCR products were obtained from 3 and *BsaI* cuts another 13 amplified fragments of the resistant strains. In one strain, neither *MboII* nor *BsaI* was able to digest the amplicon. However, specially primed mismatched PCR yielded an amplicon, indicating that this strain had the A2142C mutation (Figure 9). No correlation was observed between the clarithromycin resistance, patient gender and clinical findings.

8.2 Analysis 2

Clinical features

164 patients with median age of 51.5 ranged from 15 to 88 years. Pain was present in 103 patient, nausea in 42, anorexia in 40, acid reflux in 33, heaviness after meal in 30, early satiety in 27, vomiting in 31 and flatulence in 42. The main endoscopic findings were 16 gastric ulcer, 3 gastric cancer, 55 non-ulcer disease, 50 gastric erosion, 34 nodularity, 37 gastritis and 3 duodenitis (Table 5).

Age group	Male	Female	Total
10-20	6 (3.66)	4 (2.44)	10 (6.10)
20-30	12 (7.32)	13 (7.93)	25 (15.24)
30-40	13 (7.93)	15 (9.15)	28 (17.07)
40-50	13 (7.93)	14 (8.54)	27 (16.46)
50-60	10 (6.10)	11 (6.71)	21 (12.80)
60-70	12 (7.32)	13 (7.93)	25 (15.25)
70-80	9 (5.49)	6 (3.66)	15 (9.15)
80-90	4 (2.44)	9 (5.49)	13 (7.93)
Total	79 (48.17)	85 (51.83)	164 (100)

Table 5. Distribution of *H. pylori* positive patients according to gender and age group (*n=164*)

Detection of *H. pylori* directly in gastric biopsy samples

RUT results showed that the 164 (82%) of the patients were *H. pylori*-positive. DNA samples derived from gastric biopsy samples of confirmed *H. pylori*-positive patients were positive by the diagnostic PCR assays for the *ureC* targets. The *ureC* PCR assay confirmed the presence of *H. pylori* in all of these 164 biopsy samples (100%) and generated the expected PCR product of 249 bp.

PCR-RFLP

Thirty-nine of 59 resistant strains detected by real-time PCR methods were detected by PCR-RFLP and were distributed as follows: 15 A2143G and 15 A2142G single mutation, 6 wild type/A2143G, one wild type/A2142G and 2 A2143G/A2142G genotypes (Table 6). *BsaI* cuts the PCR product of the wild-type sequence into two fragments of 1,000 and 400bp and that of the A2143G sequence into three fragments of 700, 400, and 300bp. *MboII* cuts the PCR product into two fragments of 700bp only when A2142G is present in the sequence (Figure 6). sensitivity and specificity of PCR-RFLP were 74.68% and 100% respectively when we PCR-RFLP was compared with real-time PCR.

Outcome	sample (%)	Genotype	
		Real-time-PCR	PCR-RFLP
Single genotype 143 (87.19)	105 (64.01)	Wild	Wild
	3 (1.83)	A2144G	Wild
	13(7.93)	A2143G	A2143G
	7(4.27)	A2143C	Wild
	15(9.15)	A2142G	A2142G
Heteroresis tance 21 (12.81)	6(3.66)	A2143G/Wild	A2143G/Wild
	1(0.61)	A2143C/Wild	Wild
	1(0.61)	A2142G/Wild	A2142G/Wild
	1(0.61)	A2143G/A2143C/Wild	Wild
	1(0.61)	A2144G/A2143G/A2143C/ Wild	A2143G
	1(0.61)	A2143G/A2143C	A2143G
	1(0.61)	A2143G/A2143C	Wild
	1(0.61)	A2143G/A2142G	A2143G/A2142G
	1(0.61)	A2143C/A2142G	Wild
	1(0.61)	A2143G/A2143C/A2142G	A2143G/A2142G
	1(0.61)	A2143G/A2143C/A2142G	Wild
	5(3.05)	Not Determined	Wild

Table 6. Frequency of *H. pylori* genotypes determined by real-time PCR and PCR-RFLP methods in analysis 2 (n=164)

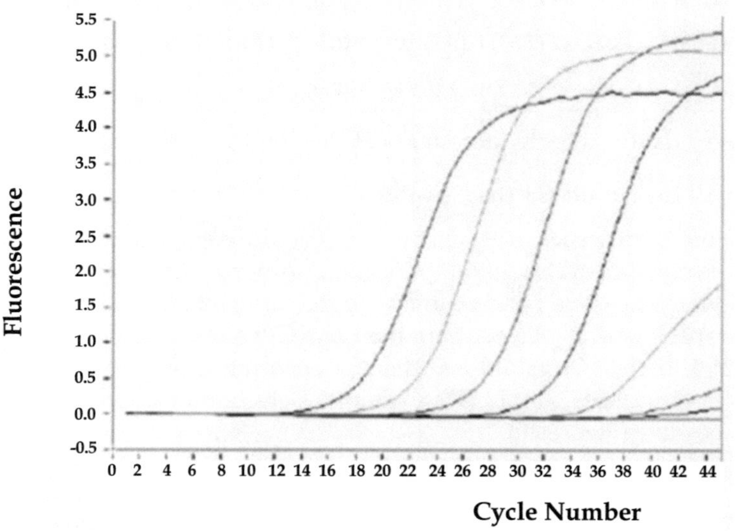

Fig. 10. Graph obtained with real-time PCR for the susceptible and resistant strains isolated from different patients. C_T for pure samples were less than 35 and C_T of mix samples were between 35 and 40. (All graphs obtained by different probes are similar)

Disease	10^4	10^5	10^6	10^7	10^8	10^9	10^{10}	10^{11}	10^{12}	Total
Peptic Ulcer	1 (0.6)	0 (0)	7 (4.27)	4 (2.44)	2 (1.22)	1 (0.6)	0 (0)	0 (0)	0 (0)	15 (9.15)
Gastric Cancer	0 (0)	0 (0)	0 (0)	0 (0)	0 (0)	0 (0)	1 (0.6)	0 (0)	2 (1.22)	3 (1.83)
Gastric Erosion	1 (0.6)	2 (1.22)	20 (12.19)	18 (10.98)	5 (3.05)	1 (0.6)	0 (0)	2 (1.22)	0 (0)	49 (29.88)
Nodularity	2 (1.22)	4 (2.44)	13 (7.93)	11 (6.71)	3 (1.83)	0 (0)	0 (0)	0 (0)	0 (0)	33 (20.12)
Gastritis	3 (1.83)	3 (1.83)	15 (9.15)	13 (7.93)	1 (0.6)	0 (0)	1 (0.6)	0 (0)	0 (0)	36 (21.95)
Duodenitis	0 (0)	1 (0.6)	1 (0.6)	1 (0.6)	0 (0)	0 (0)	0 (0)	0 (0)	0 (0)	3 (1.83)
Atrrophy	0 (0)	0 (0)	0 (0)	2 (1.22)	1 (0.6)	0 (0)	0 (0)	0 (0)	0 (0)	3 (1.83)
Duodenit Ulcer	0 (0)	0 (0)	13 (7.93)	8 (4.88)	1 (0.6)	0 (0)	0 (0)	0 (0)	0 (0)	22 (13.41)

Table 7. Endoscopic finding and frequency of bacterial count of *H. pylori* positive patients (*n=164*)

Symptoms	10^4	10^5	10^6	10^7	10^8	10^9	10^{10}	10^{11}	10^{12}	Total
Pain	3 (1.83)	9 (5.49)	42 (25.61)	32 (19.51)	6 (3.66)	2 (1.22)	2 (1.22)	2 (1.22)	1 (0.6)	99 (60.36)
Nausea	3 (1.83)	1 (0.6)	20 (12.19)	13 (7.93)	3 (1.83)	0 (0)	0 (0)	1 (0.6)	1 (0.6)	42 (25.61)
Anorexia	3 (1.83)	3 (1.83)	18 (10.98)	14 (8.54)	0 (0)	1 (0.6)	0 (0)	0 (0)	0 (0)	39 (23.78)
Acid reflux	4 (2.44)	1 (0.6)	12 (7.32)	9 (5.49)	4 (2.44)	0 (0)	0 (0)	0 (0)	1 (0.6)	31 (18.90)
Heaviness after meal	1 (0.6)	3 (1.83)	9 (5.49)	12 (7.32)	3 (1.83)	0 (0)	1 (0.6)	0 (0)	0 (0)	29 (17.68)
Early satiety	2 (1.22)	1 (0.6)	13 (7.93)	8 (4.88)	1 (0.6)	0 (0)	1 (0.6)	0 (0)	0 (0)	26 (15.85)
Vomiting	3 (1.83)	2 (1.22)	12 (7.32)	10 (6.10)	1 (0.6)	0 (0)	0 (0)	0 (0)	1 (0.6)	29 (17.68)
Flatulence	3 (1.83)	4 (2.44)	19 (11.58)	11 (6.71)	1 (0.6)	0 (0)	1 (0.6)	0 (0)	1 (0.6)	40 (24.39)

Table 8. Interview data and bacterial count of *H. pylori* positive patients (*n=164*)

Determination of the cut-off for the C_T values

The detection of fluorescence was realized in the different channels of the rotor-gene thermocycler during 45 cycles of amplification. Among the 164 biopsy specimens, a detection of fluorescence was positive in one of the different channels in 143 (87.2%) cases. Sixteen biopsy specimens displayed more than one C_T values for mix genotypes. C_T values ranged from 21.4 to 43.6. C_T values less than 35 determined as pure sample DNA and C_T between 35 and 40 indicate as mix DNA sample. Detection of fluorescence over 40 cycles might be false positive (Figure 10).

Development of TaqMan real-time PCR

Concerning amplification of *H. pylori* DNA obtained from a pure culture, linearity was achieved over a 5-log range of input DNA amounts, from 5×10^2 to 5×10^7 bacteria, with 500 bacteria corresponding to 1000 *23S rRNA* gene copies given that there are two gene copies in the genome of *H. pylori*. PCR was also positive for 40 bacteria or 80 copies of the *23S rRNA* gene fragment. The amplification efficiencies obtained with DNA prepared from gastric biopsy specimens were identical to those obtained with DNA samples prepared from bacterial colonies. Thus, the sensitivity of our assay, for DNA samples prepared either from cultures or from gastric biopsy specimens, could quantitatively reach 400 bacteria or 800 copies of the amplicon and qualitatively reach 40 bacteria or 80 copies. The reproducibility of our assay was evaluated with 10-fold serial dilutions of purified *H. pylori* DNA, with no significant difference between runs.

Real-time PCR

Bacterial clarithromycin resistance was assessed on 164 consecutive, *H. pylori*-positive patients. Overall, a clarithromycin susceptible was detected in 105 (64.02%) patients and clarithromycin resistance was detected in 59 (35.98%) which were identified as 4 (6.78%) A2144G, 26 (44.07%) A2143G, 15 (25.42%) A2143C and 20 (33.9%) A2142G point mutations. Purely resistant strains were detected in 38 (64.41%), while a mixture of resistant and susceptible (heteroresistant) bacterial strains were found in the remaining 16 (27.12%) cases. Genotype of 5 (8.47%) strains were not detected (Table 6) [60].

Quantification of bacterial density

Quantification of different genotypes was directly performed on 159 DNA samples with defined genotype by using TaqMan real-time-PCR assay. The bacterial density by this technique could be evaluated for 159 *H. pylori*-positive patients and ranged from 1.53×10^4 to 5.89×10^{12}. In order to evaluate relationship between bacterial concentration and point mutations, samples divided in 9 groups between 1×10^4 to 6×10^{12}, including 10^4, 10^5, 10^6, 10^7, 10^8, 10^9,10^{10}, 10^{11} and 10^{12} groups had 6, 11, 87, 59, 9, 2, 2, 2 and 2 samples respectively (Table 7 and 8).

Bacterial count	Wild type	A2144G	A2143G	A2143C	A2142G
10^4	1	0	2	2	1
10^5	7	0	2	1	1
10^6	39	4	18	12	14
10^7	51	0	4	0	4
10^8	9	0	0	0	0
10^9	2	0	0	0	0
10^{10}	2	0	0	0	0
10^{11}	2	0	0	0	0
10^{12}	2	0	0	0	0
Total	105	4	26	15	20

Table 9. Distribution of 5 different genotypes based on their concentrations

Statistical analysis

Chi-square analysis revealed more relationship between gastritis and age group 30-40 (p=0.007), NUD and 40-50 (p=0.001), early satiety and 10-20 (p=0.05), flatulence and 10-20

(p=0.038), vomiting and 20-30 (p=0.001), pain and 50-60 (p=0.003), heaviness after meal and 50-60 (p=0.018), early satiety and 60-70 (p=0.05).
Also statistical analysis revealed more relationship between wild type and 10^6 (p=0.00) and 10^7 (p=0.00), A2144G and 10^6 (p=0.033), A2143G and 10^6 (p=0.005), A2143C and 10^6 (p=0.005) and A2142G and 10^6 (p=0.015) (Table 9) [61].
Also, results showed relation ships between Ages 10-20 and early satiety (p=0.05) and flatulence (p=0.038), 20-30 and vomiting (p=0.001), 50-60 and pain (p=0.003) and heaviness after meal (p=0.018) and 50-60 and early satiety (p=0.05).

9. Conclusion

In conclusion, we have developed a TaqMan real-time PCR assay that permits accurate, fast, and cost-effective detection of *H. pylori* directly from gastric biopsy specimens as well as detection of clarithromycin resistance. This PCR technique is a good candidate for automated real-time PCR methods allowing simple and rapid detection of *H. pylori* and its resistance to clarithromycin by clinical laboratories which do not practice *H. pylori* culture. Identification of sensitive and resistant strains by using PCR-RFLP method was based on the determination of resistant strains. Therefore, other resistant strains, which mutations cannot be identified by PCR-RFLP method, are considered as sensitive. But, Identification of sensitive and resistant strains by using real-time PCR method was based on the determination of sensitive strains. In the first step, determination of sensitive, resistance and mix of sensitive and resistance strains were done and in the next step, determination of mutations types in resistance and mix strains were done, that leading to accurate diagnosis of the resistant and sensitive strains.
Based on the patterns of competitive growth as well as the individual growth of different clarithromycin resistance mutant strains, Wang and colleagues conclude that the order of preference of competitive accumulation is A2142G A2143G A2142C A2143C (A2142T). If the same is true in vivo, once an A-to-G transient mutation occurs (spontaneously or drug induced), the other types of mutation that exist in the same environment, if any, are likely to be overgrown after a period of time. A-to-C or A-to-T mutants could be isolated only when an A-to-G mutant has not appeared at that particular gastric niche. Their results provide a rational explanation for the mutation pattern observed in clinical isolates [13]. These results are confirmed by Van der Ende and coworkers and discussed that the growth rates of *H. pylori* isolates with the A21423G, A21423C, or A21433G mutation did not differ from that of the wild type, but *H. pylori* isolates with other *23S rDNA* mutations grew more slowly [11].
Based on two opinions, we used real-time PCR for simultaneous identification of *H. pylori*, Clarithromycin resistance point mutations and direct quantification of gastric mucosal density in order to answer to this question; why some clarithromycin resistance point mutations are more prevalent than other mutations. At first; Wang described an additional possible mechanism yet to be identified, by which the A-to-G mutations are preferentially produced in *H. pylori*, may also contribute to the observed predominance of A-to-G mutations [13]. Second; Van der Ende [11] described that; If only a single colony from the primary *H. pylori* populations is used to test for clarithromycin susceptibility, the results can be misinterpreted. Assessment of *23S rRNA* mutations in *H. pylori* directly from biopsy specimens by molecular biological techniques has the advantage that infection with a mixed *H. pylori* population is easily detected. In addition, knowledge of the type of *23S rRNA*

mutation may be important since clarithromycin MICs are associated with the type of *23S rRNA* mutation in *H. pylori* [11].

Several studies which done by Pina [34], Marais [28] and Russmann [36] in Europe revealed that A2144G, A2143G and A2143C were more prevalent in Europe respectively. However, the current study showed that A2143G, A2142G, A2143C and A2144G were more prevalent mutation in Iran respectively. Our data showed that wild type strains more related to 10^6 to 10^7 bacteria in gastric biopsy specimens of patients. Also, strains with clarithromycin resistance mutation assessed in this study are significantly related to 10^6 in gastric biopsy which are equal to density of wild type strain. This data revealed that these mutated strains has a same growth rate to wild type, preferentially produced in populations and selected by natural selection force and they can exist and distributed in *H. pylori* population

10. Acknowledgment

The authors offer their thanks and appreciation to the Islamic Azad University, Jahrom and shahrekord branch for their executive protection of this project.

11. References

[1] Chisholm SA, Owen RJ, Teare EL, and Saverymuttu S. 2001. PCR-Based Diagnosis of *Helicobacter pylori* Infection and Real-Time Determination of Clarithromycin Resistance Directly from Human Gastric Biopsy Samples. *J Clin Microbiol.* 39(4): 1217–1220.

[2] Lottspeich C, Schwarzer A, Panthel K, Koletzko S, and Russmann H. 2007. Evaluation of the Novel *Helicobacter pylori* ClariRes Real-Time PCR Assay for Detection and Clarithromycin Susceptibility Testing of *H. pylori* in Stool Specimens from Symptomatic Children. *J Clin Microbiol.* 45(6): 1718–1722.

[3] Kusters JG, van Vliet AHM, and Kuipers EJ. 2006. Pathogenesis of *Helicobacter pylori* Infection. *Clin Microbiol Reviews.* 19(3): 449–490.

[4] Correa P, Haenszel W, Cuello C, Tannenbaum S, and Archer M. 1975. A model for gastric cancer epidemiology. *Lancet.* ii:58–59.

[5] Cirak MY, Akyön Y, and Mégraud F. 2007. Diagnosis of *Helicobacter pylori. Helicobacter.* 12 (Suppl. 1): 4–9.

[6] Godoy APO, Ribeiro ML, Benvengo YHB, Vitiello L, Miranda MCB, Mendonça S and Pedrazzoli Jr J. 2003. Analysis of antimicrobial susceptibility and virulence factors in *Helicobacter pylori* clinical isolates. *BMC Gastroenterology.* 3(20): Available: http://www.biomedcentral.com/1471-230X/3/20.

[7] Goldman RC, Zakula D, Flamm R, Beyer J, and Capobianvo J. 1994. Tight Binding of Clarithromycin, Its 14-(R)-Hydroxy Metabolite, and Erythromycin to *Helicobacter pylori* Ribosomes. *Antimicrob Agents Chemother.* 38(7):1496-1500.

[8] Liu Z, Shen J, Zhang L, Shen L, Li Q, Zhang B, Zhou J, Gu L, Feng G, Ma J, You WC and Deng D. 2008. Prevalence of A2143G mutation of *H. pylori-23S rRNA* in Chinese subjects with and without clarithromycin use history. *BMC Microbiology,* 8(81): Available: http://www.biomedcentral.com/1471-2180/8/81.

[9] Yilmaz Ö and Demiray E. Clinical role and importance of fl uorescence in situ hybridization method in diagnosis of *H. pylori* infection and determination of

clarithromycin resistance in *H pylori* eradication therapy. *World J Gastroenterol* 2007;13(5):671-675.

[10] Lascols C, Lamarque D, Costa JM, Copie-Bergman C, Glaunec JML, Deforges L, Soussy CJ, Petit JC, Delchier JC, and Tankovic J. 2003. Fast and Accurate Quantitative Detection of *Helicobacter pylori* and Identification of Clarithromycin Resistance Mutations in *H. pylori* Isolates from Gastric Biopsy Specimens by Real-Time PCR. *J Clin Microbiol.* 41(10): 4573–4577.

[11] Van Der Eede A, Van Doorn LJ, Rooijakkers S, Feller M, Tytgat GNJ, and Dankert J. 2001. Clarithromycin-Susceptible and -Resistant *Helicobacter pylori* Isolates with Identical Randomly Amplified Polymorphic DNA-PCR Genotypes Cultured from Single Gastric Biopsy Specimens Prior to Antibiotic Therapy. *J Clin Microbiol.* 39(7): 2648–2651.

[12] Fontana C, Favaro M, Minelli S, Criscuolo AA, Pietroiusti A, Galante A, and Favalli C. 2002. New Site of Modification of *23S rRNA* Associated with Clarithromycin Resistance of *Helicobacter pylori* Clinical Isolates. *Antimicrob Agents Chemother.* 46(12): 3765–3769.

[13] Wang GE and Taylor DE. 1998. Site-Specific Mutations in the 23S rRNA Gene of *Helicobacter pylori* Confer Two Types of Resistance to Macrolide-Lincosamide-Streptogramin B Antibiotics. *Antimicrob Agents Chemother.* 42(8): 1952–1958.

[14] Pfister P, Corti N, Hobbie S, Bruell C, Zarivach R, Yonath A, and Bottger EC. 2005. 23S rRNA base pair 2057–2611 determines ketolide susceptibility and fitness cost of the macrolide resistance mutation 2058A→G. *PNAS.* 102(14): 5180–5185.

[15] Woo HY, Park DI, Park H, Kim MK, Kim DH, Kim IS, and Kim YJ. 2009. Dual-Priming Oligonucleotide-Based Multiplex PCR for the Detection of *Helicobacter pylori* and Determination of Clarithromycin Resistance with Gastric Biopsy Specimens. *Helicobacter.* 14:22–28.

[16] Oleastro M, Menard A, Santos A, Lamouliatte H, Monteiro L, Barthelemy P, and Me´graud F. 2003. Real-Time PCR Assay for Rapid and Accurate Detection of Point Mutations Conferring Resistance to Clarithromycin in *Helicobacter pylori. J Clin Microbiol.* 41(1): 397–402.

[17] Chisholm SA, Owen RJ, Teare EL, and Saverymuttu S. 2001. PCR-Based Diagnosis of *Helicobacter pylori* Infection and Real-Time Determination of Clarithromycin Resistance Directly from Human Gastric Biopsy Samples. *J Clin Microbiol.* 39(4): 1217–1220.

[18] Trebesius K, Panthel K, Strobel S, Vogt K, Faller G, Kirchner T, Kist M, Heesemann J, and Haas R. 2000. Rapid and specific detection of *Helicobacter pylori* macrolide resistance in gastric tissue by fluorescent in situ hybridization. *Gut.* 46:608–614.

[19] Burucoa C, Garnier M, Silvain C, and Fauchere JL. Quadruplex Real-Time PCR Assay Using Allele-Specific Scorpion Primers for Detection of Mutations Conferring Clarithromycin Resistance to *Helicobacter pylori. J Clin Microbiol* 2008; 46(7):2320–2326.

[20] Espy MJ, Uhl JR, Sloan LM, Buckwalter SP, Jones MF, Vetter EA, Yao JDC, Wengenack NL, Rosenblatt JE, Cockerill FR, and Smith TF. 2006. Real-Time PCR in Clinical Microbiology: Applications for Routine Laboratory Testing. *Clin Microbiol Reviews.* 19(1): 165–256.

[21] Kargar M, Baghernejad M, and Doosti A. 2010. Role of *NADPH-insensitive nitroreductase* gene to metronidazole resistance of *Helicobacter pylori* strains. *DARU*. 18(2):137-140.

[22] De Francesco V, Margiotta M, Zullo A, Hassan C, Valle ND, Burattini O, Cea U, Stoppino G, Amoruso A, Stella F, Morini S, Panella C, and Ierardi E. 2006. Primary clarithromycin resistance in Italy assessed on *Helicobacter pylori* DNA sequences by TaqMan real-time polymerase chain reaction. *Aliment Pharm Ther*. 23:429–435.

[23] Pan ZJ, Su WW, Tytgat GNJ, Dankert J, and Van Der Ende A. 2002. Assessment of Clarithromycin-Resistant *Helicobacter pylori* among Patients in Shanghai and Guangzhou, China, by Primer-Mismatch PCR. *J Clin Microbiol*. 40(1): 259–261.

[24] Taneike I, Suzuki K, Nakagawa S, and Yamamoto T. 2004. Intrafamilial Spread of the Same Clarithromycin-Resistant *Helicobacter pylori* Infection Confirmed by Molecular Analysis. *J Clin Microbiol*. 42(8): 3901–3903.

[25] Falsafi T, Mobasheri F, Nariman F, and Najafi M. 2004. Susceptibilities to Different Antibiotics of *Helicobacter pylori* Strains Isolated from Patients at the Pediatric Medical Center of Tehran, Iran. *J Clin Microbiol*. 42(1): 387–389.

[26] Kargar M, Baghernejad M, Doosti A, and Ghodsi M. "Evaluation and prevalence of clarithromycin resistance point mutations in *Helicobacter pylori* in Shahrekord," in Proceedings of the 17th Iranian congress on infectious disease and tropical medicine, Tehran, Iran, 2008 December 20-22:

[27] Kato S, Fujimura S, Udagawa H, Shimizu T, Maisawa S, Ozawa K, and Iinuma K. 2002. Antibiotic Resistance of *Helicobacter pylori* Strains in Japanese Children. *J Clin Microbiol*. 40(2): 649–653.

[28] Marais A, Monteiro L, Occhialini A, Pina M, Lamouliatte H, Mégraud F. 1999. Direct detection of *Helicobacter pylori* resistance to macrolides by a polymerase chain reaction/DNA enzyme immunoassay in gastric biopsy specimens. *Gut*. 44:463–467.

[29] Matsuoka M, Yoshida Y, Hayakawa K, Fukuchi S, Sugano K. 1999. Simultaneous colonisation of *Helicobacter pylori* with and without mutations in the *23S rRNA* gene in patients with no history of clarithromycin exposure. *Gut*. 45:503–507.

[30] Taylor DE, Ge Z, and Purych D, Lo T, and Hiratsuka K. 1997. Cloning and Sequence Analysis of Two Copies of a *23S rRNA* Gene from *Helicobacter pylori* and Association of Clarithromycin Resistance with *23S rRNA* Mutations. *Antimicrob Agents Ch*. 41(12): 2621–2628.

[31] Washington WJ, Stephen A, William J, Koneman E, Procop G, Scheckenberger P, (2006). Color atlas and textbook of diagnostic microbiology. 6th ed. Philadelphia: Lippincott Williams & Wilkins. 765-773.

[32] Pina M, Occhialini A, Monteiro L, Doermann HP, and Megraud F. 1998. Detection of Point Mutations Associated with Resistance of *Helicobacter pylori* to Clarithromycin by Hybridization in Liquid Phase. *J Clin Microbiol*. 36(11): 3285–3290.

[33] Kalach N, Bergeret M, Benhamou PH, Dupont C, and Raymond J. 2001. High Levels of Resistance to Metronidazole and Clarithromycin in *Helicobacter pylori* Strains in Children. *J Clin Microbiol*. 39(1): 394–397.

[34] Kalach N, Benhamou PH, Campeotto F, Bergeret M, Dupont C, and Raymond J. 2001. Clarithromycin Resistance and Eradication of *Helicobacter pylori* in Children. *Antimicrob Agents Chemother*. 45(7): 2134–2135.

[35] Cambau E, Allerheiligen V, Coulon C, Corbel C, Lascols C, Deforges L, Soussy CJ, Delchier JC, and Megraud F. 2009. Evaluation of a New Test, GenoType HelicoDR, for Molecular Detection of Antibiotic Resistance in *Helicobacter pylori*. *J Clin Microbiol*. 47(11): 3600–3607.

[36] Russmann H, Adler K, Haas R, Gebert B, Koletzko S, and Heesemann J. 2001. Rapid and Accurate Determination of Genotypic Clarithromycin Resistance in Cultured *Helicobacter pylori* by Fluorescent in Situ Hybridization. *J Clin Microbiol*. 39(11): 4142–4144.

[37] Koletzko S, Richy F, Bontems P, Crone J, Kalach N, Monteiro ML, Gottrand F, Celinska-Cedro D, Roma-Giannikou E, Orderda G, Kolacek S, Urruzuno P, Martı´nez-Go´mez MJ, Casswall T, Ashorn M, Bodanszky H, Me´graud F. 2006. Prospective multicentre study on antibiotic resistance of Helicobacter pylori strains obtained from children living in Europe. *Gut*. 55:1711–1716.

[38] Fontana C, Favaro M, Pietroiusti A, Pistoia ES, Galante A, and Favalli C. 2003. Detection of Clarithromycin-Resistant *Helicobacter pylori* in Stool Samples. *J Clin Microbiol*. 41(8): 3636–3640.

[39] Ryan KA, Van Doorn LJ, Moran AP, Glennon M, Smith T, and Maher M. 2001. Evaluation of Clarithromycin Resistance and *cagA* and *vacA* Genotyping of *Helicobacter pylori* Strains from the West of Ireland Using Line Probe Assays. *J Clin Microbiol*. 39(5): 1978–1980.

[40] Agudo S, Perez-Perez G, Alarcon T, and Lopez-Brea M. 2010. High Prevalence of Clarithromycin-Resistant *Helicobacter pylori* Strains and Risk Factors Associated with Resistance in Madrid, Spain. *J Clin Microbiol*. 48(10): 3703–3707.

[41] Magalhães PP, Queiroz DMM, Barbosa DVC, Rocha GA, Mendes EN, Santos A, Corrêa PRV, Rocha AMC, Teixeira LM, and de Oliveira CA. 2002. *Helicobacter pylori* Primary Resistance to Metronidazole and Clarithromycin in Brazil. *Antimicrob Agents Chemother*. 46(6): 2021–2023.

[42] Torres J, Camorling-Ponce M , Perez-Perez G , Garza AMD, Dehesa M, Gonzalez-Valencia G, and Munoz O. 2001. Increasing Multidrug Resistance in *Helicobacter pylori* Strains Isolated from Children and Adults in Mexico. *J Clin Microbiol*. 39(7): 2677–2680.

[43] Vasquez A, Valdez Y, Gilman RH, Mcdonald JJ, Westblom TU, Berg D, Mayta H, Gutierrez V, and The Gastrointestinal Phisiology Working Group Of Universidad Peruana Cayetano Heredia and The John Hopkins University. 1996. Metronidazole and Clarithromycin Resistance in *Helicobacter pylori* Determined by Measuring MICs of Antimicrobial Agents in Color Indicator Egg Yolk Agar in a Miniwell Format. *J Clin Microbiol*. 34(5): 1232–1234.

[44] Alarcon T, Vega AE, Domingo D, Martínez MJ, and Lopez-Brea M. 2003. Clarithromycin Resistance among *Helicobacter pylori* Strains Isolated from Children: Prevalence and Study of Mechanism of Resistance by PCR-Restriction Fragment Length Polymorphism Analysis. *J Clin Microbiol*. 41(1): 486–488.

[45] Stone GG, Shortridge D, Versalovich J, Beyer J, Flamm RK, Graham DY, Ghoneim AT, and Tanaka SK. 1997. A PCR-Oligonucleotide Ligation Assay To Determine the Prevalence of *23S rRNA* Gene Mutations in Clarithromycin-Resistant *Helicobacter pylori*. *Antimicrob Agents Chemother*. 41(3): 712–714.

[46] Sun QJ, Liang X, Zheng Q, Gu WQ, Liu WZ, Xiao SD, Lu H. 2010. Resistance of *Helicobacter pylori* to antibiotics from 2000 to 2009 in Shanghai. *World J Gastroenterol*. 16(40): 5118-5121.

[47] Maeda S, Yoshida H, Ogura K, Kanai F, Shiratori Y and Omata M. 1998. *Helicobacter pylori* specific nested PCR assay for the detection of *23S rRNA* mutation associated with clarithromycin resistance. *Gut*. 43:317–321.

[48] Maeda S, Yoshida H, Matsunaga H, Ogura K, Kawamata O, Shiratori Y, and Omata M. 2000. Detection of Clarithromycin-Resistant *Helicobacter pylori* Strains by a Preferential Homoduplex Formation Assay. *J Clin Microbiol*. 38(1): 210–214.

[49] Matsumura M, YOKO Hikiba Y, KEIJI Ogura K, GOICHI Togo G, Tsukud I, Ushikawa K, Shiratori Y, and Omata M. 2001, Rapid Detection of Mutations in the *23S rRNA* Gene of *Helicobacter pylori* That Confers Resistance to Clarithromycin Treatment to the Bacterium. *J Clin Microbiol*. 39(2): 691–695.

[50] Kato S, Fujimura S, Udagawa H, Shimizu T, Maisawa S, Ozawa K, and Iinuma K. 2002. Antibiotic Resistance of *Helicobacter pylori* Strains in Japanese Children. *J Clin Microbiol*. 40(2): 649–653.

[51] Ahmad N, Zakaria WR, Abdullah SA, Mohamed R. 2009. Characterization of clarithromycin resistance in Malaysian isolates of *Helicobacter pylori*. *World J Gastroenterol*. 15(25): 3161-3165.

[52] Kumala W, and Rani A. 2006. Pattern Of *Helicobacter pylori* Isolate Resistance To Fluoroquinolones, Amoxicilin, Clarithromycin and Metronidazoles. *Southeast Asian J Trop Med Public Health*. 37(5):970-974.

[53] Lee JH, Shin JH, Roe IH, Sohn SG, Lee JH, Kang GH, Lee HK, Jeong BC, and Lee SH. 2005. Impact of Clarithromycin Resistance on Eradication of *Helicobacter pylori* in Infected Adults. *Antimicrob Agents Chemother*. 49(4): 1600–1603.

[54] Kargar M, Baghernejad M, Doosti A, Ghorbani-Dalini S. 2011. Clarithromycin resistance and *23S rRNA* Mutations in *Helicobacter pylori* isolates from Iran. *Afr J Microbiol Res*. 2011. In Press

[55] Ghorbani-Dalini S. 2010. Direct detection and identification of Clarithromycin resistance point mutations in *Helicobacter pylori* strains isolated from biopsy specimens by Real-Time PCR assay. Department of Biology, Jahrom Branch, Islamic Azad University.

[56] Farshad S, Alborzi A, Japoni A, Ranjbar R, Hosseini-Asl K, Badiee P, Amin-Shahidi M, Hosseini M. 2010.Antimicrobial susceptibility of Helicobacter pylori strains isolated from patients in Shiraz, Southern Iran. *World J Gastroenterol*. 16(45): 5746-5751.

[57] Ben Mansour K, Burucoa C, Zribi M, Masmoudi A, Karoui S, Kallel L, Chouaib S, Matri S, Fekih M, Zarrouk S, Labbene M, Boubaker J, Cheikh I, Ben Hriz M, Siala N, Ayadi A, Filali A, Ben Mami N, Najjar T, Maherzi A, Sfar MT, Fendri C. 2010. Primary resistance to clarithromycin, metronidazole and amoxicillin of *Helicobacter pylori* isolated from Tunisian patients with peptic ulcers and gastritis: a prospective multicentre study. *Annals of Clin Microbiol and Antimicrob*. 2010, 9:22. Available: http://www.ann-clinmicrob.com/content/9/1/22.

[58] Llanes R, Soria C, Nagashima S, Kobayashi N, Gala A, Guzmán D, Feliciano O, Valdés L, Gutiérrez O, Fernández H, Llop A, and Wada A. 2010. Phenotypic and Genetic Characterization of Antimicrobial Profiles of *Helicobacter pylori* Strains in Cuba. *J Health Popul Nutr*. 28(2):124-129.

[59] Kargar M, Baghernejad M and Doosti A. 2010. Comparison of three methods of polymerase chain reaction, culture and rapid urease test in diagnosis of helicobacter pylori in gastric biopsy specimen. *Journal of Semnan University of Medical Sciences*. 11(3): 191-203. [Persian]

[60] Kargar M, Ghorbani-Dalini S, Doosti A, and Souod N. 2011. Real-Time PCR Assay Using Allele-Specific TaqMan probe for Detection of Clarithromycin Resistance and Its Point Mutations in *Helicobacter Pylori*. *Journal of Isfahan Medical School*. 29(126): 1-9. [Persian]

[61] Kargar M, Ghorbani-Dalini S, Doosti A, Souod N, and Abbasi P. Quantitation of bacteria in gastric biopsy specimen from patients with gastrointestinal disorders: relationship between counts and 23S rRNA point mutations. *Clin. Microbial. and infection*. 17 (Suppl. 4): S129.

10

Heterotopic Gastric Mucosal Patch of the Proximal Esophagus

Vui Heng Chong
Division of Gastroenterology and Hepatology, Department of Medicine, Raja Isteri Pengiran Anak Saleha (RIPAS) Hospital, Bandar Seri Begawan BA 1710, Brunei Darussalam

1. Introduction

Heterotopic gastric mucosa (HGM) is abnormally placed gastric mucosa outside of the stomach and can be found almost anywhere within the gastrointestinal tract (von Rahden et al., 2004). HGM is most commonly found in the esophagus. The most widely known HGM in the gastrointestinal tract is in the Meckel's diverticulum. However, HGM is also found in the other part of the gastrointestinal tract including the tongue (Melato & Ferlito, 1975; Ortiz, 1982; Surana, 1993), duodenum (Kibria et al., 2009; Mann, 2000), gallbladder (Hayama et al., 2010; Popkharitoy et al., 2008), jejunum (Boybeyi et al., 2008; Nowak & Deppisch, 1998), ileum (Chan et al., 1999; Erez et al., 1991), rectum (Garmendia et al., 2007; Vieth et al., 2005) and anus (Steele et al., 2004). Interestingly, HGM of the umbilicus, a part of remnant alimentary tract has also been report (Heo et al., 2010).

HGM patch (HGMP) of the proximal esophagus, also referred to as cervical inlet patch (CIP) is typically found in the proximal esophagus. It can also be found in the other part of the esophagus (Borhan-Manesh & Franum, 1991; Katsanos et al., 2010). On endoscopy, HGMP/CIP is clearly distinct from the esophageal squamous mucosa. HGMP/CIP is widely considered to be congenital in nature. However, it has also been proposed to be an acquired condition (Avidan et al., 2001; Meining & Baubouj, 2010). In clinical practice, HGMP/CIP is an under-recognized condition. The incidence reported in the literature varies with lower estimates in the earlier endoscopic studies (von Rahden et al., 2004). Later studies reported higher incidence (Ohara, 2010). The highest incidence was reported in an autopsy study (von Rahden et al., 2004). Use of newer endoscopic modalities has been reported to increase the pick up rates of HGMP/CIP.

HGMP/CIP is largely asymptomatic and is incidental findings during endoscopy evaluations for other gastrointestinal complaints. Commonly reported symptoms are those symptoms complex referred to as extra-esophageal manifestations of gastro-esophagael reflux disorders. Other common upper aero-digestive disorders have also been linked to HGMP/CIP. Despite the benign nature of HGMP/CIP, serious and important complications have been reported (von Rahden et al., 2004). Furthermore, associations with higher frequencies of laryngopharyngeal malignancies have also been reported (Basseri et al., 2009). A clinico-pathologic classification has been proposed which categorized HGMP/CIP into five distinct groups based on clinical, endoscopic and histological findings (von Rahden et

al., 2004). The management strategies of HGMP/CIP are not well defined and are dependent on the severity of symptoms. However, other newer treatment modalities have also been reported.
This chapter discusses the pathogenesis, the endoscopic features, clinical symptoms and the management of HGMP/CIP, an entity that is still under-recognised and is frequently missed during upper gastrointestinal endoscopy examinations.

2. Pathogenesis

HGMP is widely considered to be congenital in nature, as result of incomplete esophageal squamous epithelization during the embryogenic development stage (von Rahden et al., 2004). Reports of HGMP in the esophagus of young children and even babies support this theory (Boybeyi et al., 2008; Georges et al., 2011; Macha et al., 2005; Surana et al., 1993). However, it has also been proposed to be acquired in nature, similar to Barrett's esophagus (Avidan et al., 2001; Lauwers et al., 2005). There are based on similarities in the mucin and staining characteristics with CK7 and CK20 (Bogomoletz et al., 1988; Lauwers et al., 2005) between Barrett's esophagus and HGMP/CIP. Reports of higher incidence of Barrett's esophagus in patients with HGMP/CIP also suggested a link. Some has even proposed that the origins of HGMP/CIP may be different, congenital in children and acquired in adult (Lauwers et al., 2005). A recently proposed hypothesis suggested that HGMP/CIP developed from rupture retention cyst of the proximal esophagus (Meining & Baubouj, 2010).

2.1 Origin of heterotopic gastric mucosal patch of the proximal esophagus

2.1.1 Congenital origin theory

Embryogenesis of the esophagus

The development of the esophagus starts at the beginning of embryogenesis (Lieberman-Meffert et al., 2002). The upper aerodigestive tract (oro, naso and largyngopharynx), respiratory tract, esophagus and stomach and duodenum arise from the same embryogenic segment. The stages of development are correlated with the length of the embryo. At 3 mm crown-rump length, the esophagus is mainly lined with columnar mucosa and during development at 110 CR length (equivalent to 24 weeks gestation), the squamous lining begin to replace the columnar lining starting at the mid esophagus, migrating in both directions. The cervical region of the esophagus is the last area to get stratification and this account for the common findings of HGMP in the proximal esophagus. The embryogenic development of the esophagus is shown in Figure 1.

2.1.2 Acquired origins theories

Metaplastic transformation of squamous mucosa to columnar mucosa from chronic acid injury

It has also been proposed that the HGMP/CIP is an acquired condition as result of chronic inflammation from exposure to acid as part of gastroesophageal reflux disorders (Avidan et al., 2001; Lauwers et al., 2005). It is postulated that chronic acid exposure results in inflammation that leads to reactivation or proliferation of remnant columnar mucosa. These remnants columnar mucosa are present as microscopic foci in the esophageal lining or are covered by squamous mucosa. With chronic irritations, these foci develop into larger patch resulting in the formation of island of columnar mucosa, HGMP (Figure 2).

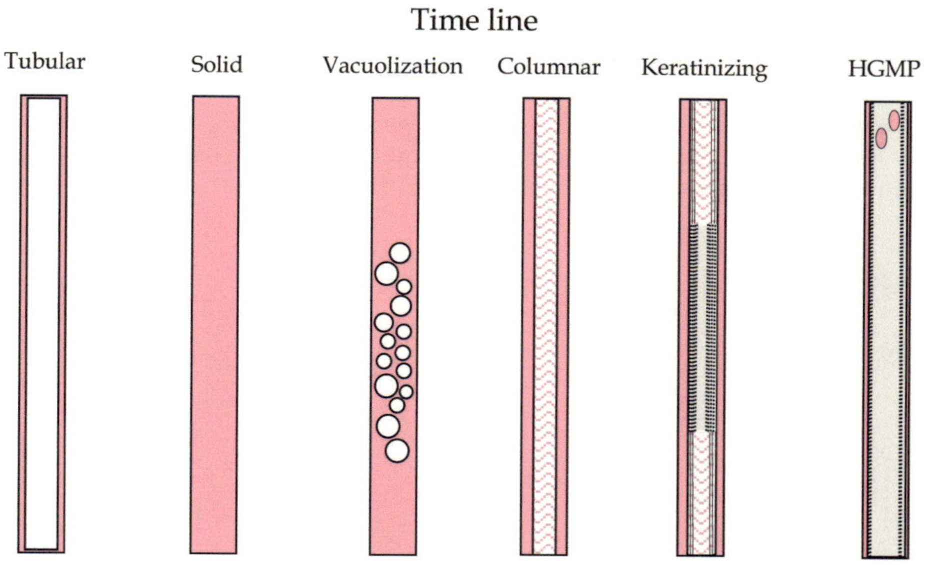

Fig. 1. Embryogenesis of the esophagus: solidification of the hollow tubular esophagus occur with rapid cellular proliferation followed by vacuoles formations (recanalization), columnarization (cilia phase shaded rippled pink) and the final stage of squamous cell mucosa formation (keratinizing followed by dekeratinizing phase-shaded gray). HGMP form when the final phase is incomplete

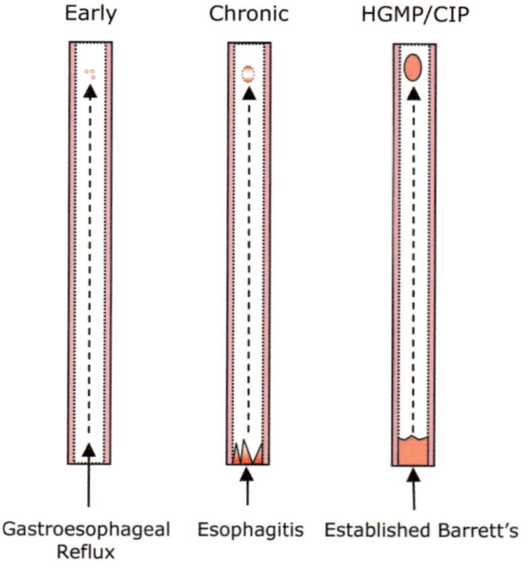

Fig. 2. Proposed acquired pathway through chronic reflux injury: Chronic acid (+/- pepsin and bile injury) leads to reflux esophagitis and reflux may reach the proximal esophagus resulting in similar changes. Chronic esophagitis leads to adaptive changes resulting in metaplasia metaplasia of the distal esophagus. Chronic injury in the proximal esophagus lead to reactivation of buried columnar cells resulting in formation of HGMP

Formation from ruptured retention cyst of the proximal esophagus

This proposed theory suggested that HGMP/CIP formed from ruptured proximal esophageal glandular retention cysts (Meining & Baubouj, 2010). The initial process starts with occlusion of esophageal glands in the proximal esophagus resulting in formation of retention cysts which is internally covered by columnar epithelium. With further enlargement of the cysts, they eventually rupture resulting in the formation of HGMP (Figure 3).

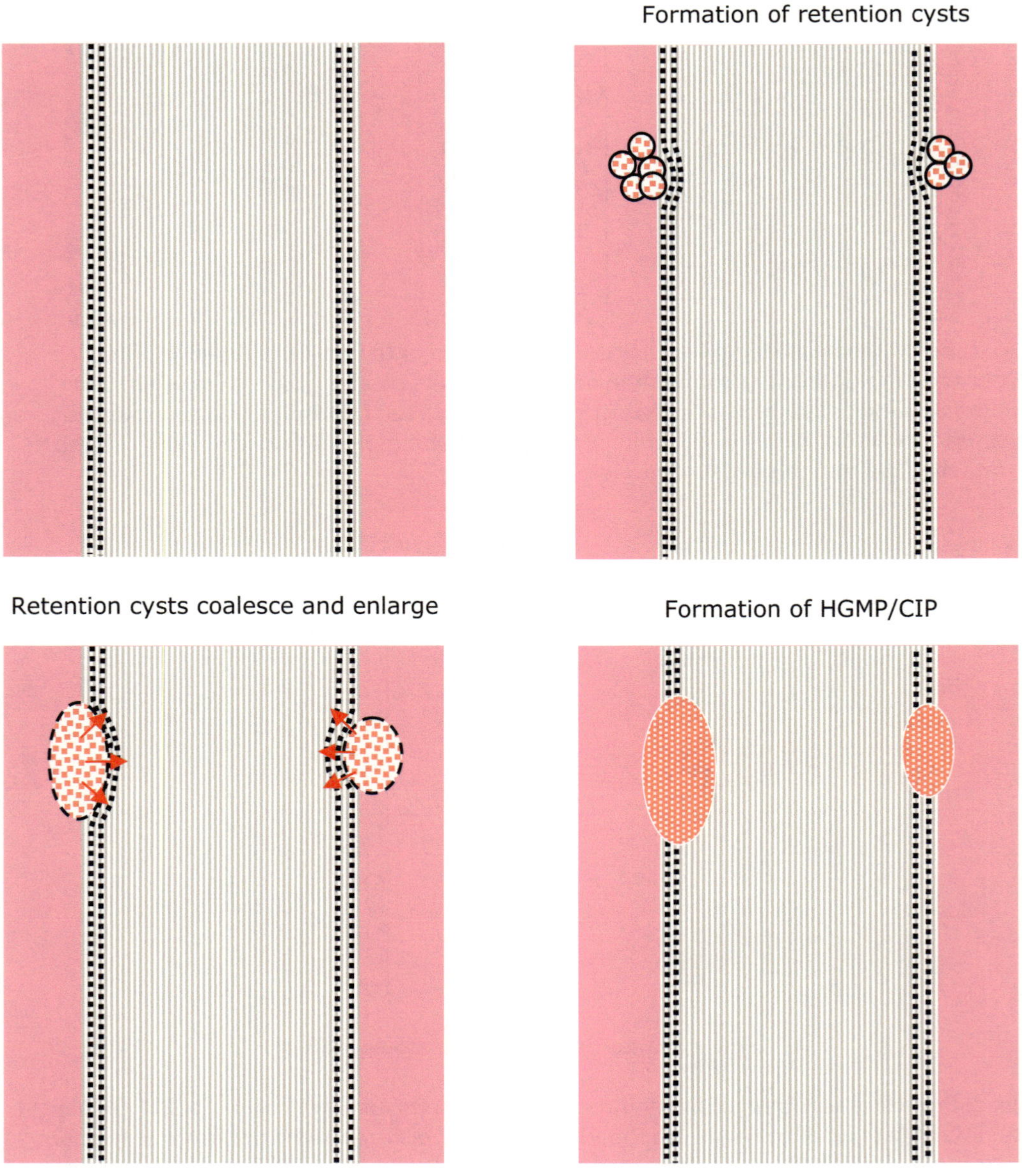

Fig. 3. Proposed acquired pathway through rupture of esophageal glandular retention cysts in the proximal esophagus

2.1.3 Others

Others have proposed that development of HGMP/CIP in adult and children may be different based on differences in the mucin protein (MUC) staining. It has been suggested that two pathogenetic pathways maybe involved: focal upper esophageal mucosal misdevelopment in pediatric population and patchy metaplastic replacement of squamous mucosa in adults with gastroesophageal reflux disease. (Lauwers et al., 2005)

3. Histology

HGMP/CIP consists of columnar mucosa found in the stomach (Figure 4). HGMP/CIP can contain glandular mucosa of different types similar to those found in the stomach. One study showed that the body or fundus mucosa type parietal cells is the most common accounting for 50 to 65% with the antral type and mixed transition type accounting for 20 to 25% respectively (Borhan-Manesh & Franum, 1991). Presence of acid producing parietal mucosa have been associated with acid production (Galan et al., 1998; Hamilton et al., 1986; Korkut et al., 2010; Yüksel et al., 2008). Mucin is also secreted (Bajbouj et al., 2009; Bogomoletz et al., 1988). The cytokeratin staining pattern of HGMP/CIP is similar to those seen with Barrett's esophagus with surface epithelium staining for CK7 and CK20 (Figure 5). The staining pattern of the esophagus and stomach is shown in Figure 6 (Latchford et al., 2001).

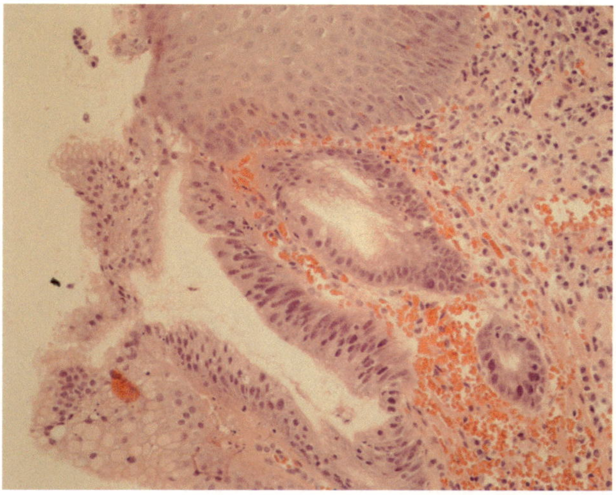

Fig. 4. High power view showing boundary between squamous esophageal mucosa and the glandular mucosa of the HGMP/CIP

Apart from CK, only one study had assessed the MUC protein profiles (Lauwers et al., 2005). This study showed that MUC5AC was strongly expressed on the surface and pits but not in the glands of HGMP/CIP and antral mucosa. In contrast, MUC5AC positivity was noted on the surface, pits and the glands of Barrett's esophagus. MUC6 similarly decorated the glands of HGMP/CIP and Barrett's esophagus. MUC2 was expressed rarely in HGMP/CIP with goblet cells but conspicuously on the surface and pits of Barrett's esophagus. MUC5B was seen in both HGMP/CIP and Barrett's esophagus and rarely in the antral mucosa. The authors concluded that the similarities between HGMP/CIP and Barrett's esophagus but not with normal antral mucosa fit with the hypothesis that both lesions may originate from sub-mucosal esophageal mucous glands. Despite this, there are differences seen between HGMP/CIP and Barrett's esophagus. Staining pattern was also different between HGMP/CIP and the embryogenic esophagus. The authors of this study suggested that HGMP/CIP etiology may be different, congenital in children or babies and acquired in adult.

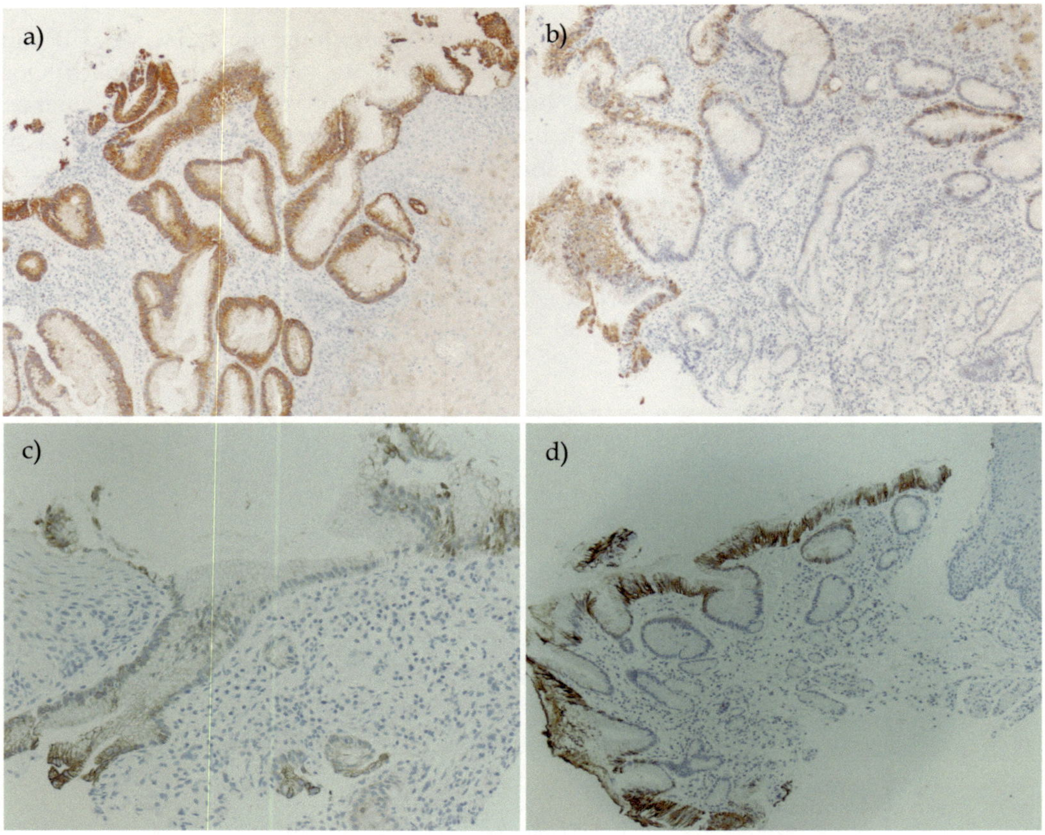

Fig. 5. (a) Cytokeratin (CK) 7 staining of HGMP/CIP showing uptake in the surface glandular tissue similar to that seen in Barrett's esophagus (b). CK20 staining uptakes are similar in HGMP/CIP (c) and Barrett's esophagus (d)

The HGMP/CIP can also be colonized by *Helicobacter pylori* and the patches are subjected to changes that are seen in the stomach (Akbayir et al., 2004; Alagozlu et al., 2010; Borhan-Manesh & Franum, 1991 & 1993; Gutierrez et al., 2003; Jacobs et al., 1997; Maconi et al., 2000; Poyrazoglu et al., 2009; Tang et al., 2004; Yüksel et al., 2008). Chronic inflammatory changes can be seen and progression to atrophy, intestinal metaplasia, dysplasia and malignant transformation have been reported (Borhan-Manesh & Franum, 1991). The surrounding squamous cell mucosa can also show inflammatory changes similar to those seen in reflux esophagitis (Borhan-Manesh & Franum, 1991).

4. Classification

A clinico-pathologic classification has been proposed by von Rahden *et al.* (von Rahden et al., 2004) which categorized patients with HGMP into five groups (I to V) based on the clinical, endoscopic and histological findings (Table 1). This classification also takes into account of small patches that may be only visible microscopically. Based on this classification, majority of the HGMP/CIP are categorized into types I and II, asymptomatic and mildly symptomatic respectively. One study found that the most common lesions are types I (73%) and II (27%) lesions.

Category	Description	Symptoms/findings	Frequency
I	Asymptomatic	None	Common
II	Symptomatic	Laryngopharyngeal reflux	Common
III	Symptomatic with benign complications	Strictures/webs/fistula/bleeding * Polyps	Uncommon
IV	Intra-epithelial dysplasia	None/non-specific	Uncommon
V	Malignant transformation	Asymptomatic/dysphagia	Reported
Suffix			
a	inlet patch (macroscopically visible patch of HGMP/CIP)		
b	microscopic foci (only microscopically visible HGMP/CIP)		

Adapted from von. Rahden *et al.* Heterotopic gastric mucosa of the esophagus: literature-review and proposal of a clinicopathologic classification. Am J Gastroenterol. 2004; 99:543-51.
* Not included in the original classification

Table 1. Clinico-pathological classification for HGMP/CIP

5. Clinical manifestations

The majority of patients found to have HGMP/CIP are asymptomatic and the HGMP/CIP are usually detected incidentally while being evaluated with endoscopy for other gastrointestinal complaints. The clinical importance of HGMP/CIP remains controversial with some authors believe that they are benign and of no clinical relevance. Others have shown HGMP/CIP to be clinically important especially for a subset of patients with HGMP/CIP. For those who have symptoms attributable to the HGMP/CIP, most are mild and are detected only on direct inquiries. For a small proportion of patients, the symptoms can be prominent and patients may have many consultations before a diagnosis is made. The prevalence of any symptoms, typically those considered extra-esophageal symptoms complex of gastroesophageal reflux such as chronic cough, throat irritation or sore throat, regurgitation, globus pharyngeus, dysphagia or hoarseness ranges from very low to as high as 75% (Chong & Jalihal, 2010; Maconi et al., 2000).

HGMP/CIP like other ectopic gastric mucosal have been proven to be able to secrete acid in sufficient quantity to induce inflammatory changes and acid related symptoms (Baudet et al., 2006; Galan et al., 1998; Hamilton et al., 1986; Korkut et al., 2010; Nakalima et al., 1993; Yüksel et al., 2008). Acid is the main cause of symptoms in patients with HGMP/CIP. Given the proximity of the HGMP/CIP to the laryngopharyngeal area, it is not surprising that

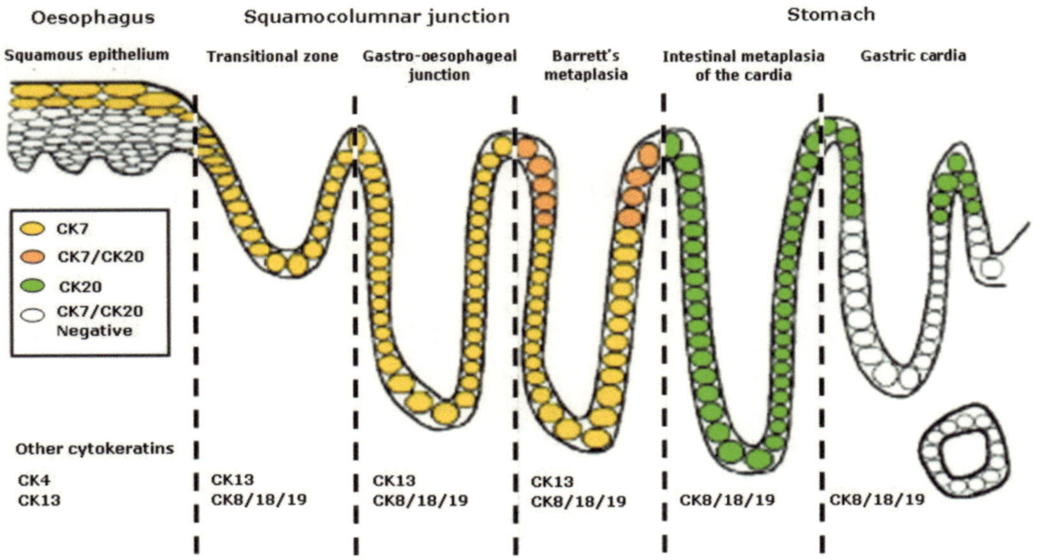

Fig. 6. Schematic illustration of cytokeratin (CK) 7 and 20 expression in the normal esophagus, Barrett's metaplasia, squamocolumnar junction, and proximal stomach. LATCHFORD A et al. Gut 2001; 49:746-747 (*Reprinted with permission from GUT BMJJournal*) (Latchford et al., 2001).

even weakly acidic secretion can cause symptoms. Others have proposed that mucin secretion can also cause symptoms (Bajbouj et al., 2009). Proximal esophagus dysmotility has also been shown to be associated with HGMP/CIP (Korkut et al., 2010).

Studies that had looked at specific groups of patients, such as those with laryngopharyngeal complaints, have found mixed results. The overall prevalence of HGMP/CIP was in the similar range compared to studies that had been carried out on patients coming for routine endoscopy. One study that had looked specifically at patients with laryngopharyngeal reflux found significantly more HGMP/CIP in patients than controls, those without LPR symptoms (11.4% vs. 1.6%, $p<0.05$). These patients also had significantly more laryngeal acid reflux documented on pH study (Akbayir N. et al., 2004). Similarly, other studies have found more laryngopharyngeal reflux symptoms in patients with HGMP/CIP (Akbayir et al, 2004; Baudet et al., 2006; Borhan-Manesh & Franum, 1993; Tang et al., 2004). Another study looking at patients who had undergone fundoplications for gastroesophageal reflux with laryngeal reflux only found one patient (3.4%) to have HGMP/CIP (Salminen & Ovaska, 2009). This patient had a small HGMP/CIP and the authors concluded that HGMP/CIP does not have a significant role in laryngopharyngeal reflux in patients with gastroesophageal reflux disease.

Unfortunately, all these studies have not inquired on the same symptoms complex and hence make comparison difficult.

Interestingly, only one study had assessed the size of HGMP/CIP on clinical symptoms and did not find significant differences (Chong & Jalihal, 2010). This study categorized HGMP/CIP to small/moderate (<15mm) and large (>15mm). Only cough was significantly more (50% vs. 8.3%, p=0.022) common in patients with larger patch. Interestingly, patients with smaller HGMP/CIP were found to have more globus and regurgitation. Several explanations were given for the lack of correlations between size of HGMP/CIP and symptoms and these include; a) missed patches, b) the mucosal types of HGMP/CIP and c) the underlying degree of inflammatory changes that can affect acid output. Patients with predominant antral mucosal type HGMP/CIP may not have or minimal acid related symptoms. Patients with severe inflammatory changes approaching atrophy may have reduce acid output, hence minimal symptoms. Interestingly, more patients with HGMP/CIP also experienced heartburn compared to those with HGMP/CIP. This patients either had non erosive gastroesophageal reflux or symptoms induced by acid secreted by the patch flowing down. One study showed that greater acid production was found in those with larger HGMP/CIP patch (Baudet et al., 2006).

6. Diagnosis

6.1 Endoscopic features

On endoscopy, HGMP/CIP appears as salmon or velvety colored patch that is clearly distinct to the slatey white esophageal squamous cell mucosa (Figure 7). A majority of HGMP/CIP is round or ovoid. Some can be elongated with the maximal dimension in the longitudinal direction. Rarely, HGMP/CIP can be so big that they cover almost or the entire circumference of the esophagus. Smaller patches tend to be round or oval, are usually elevated or flat with smooth texture and white edges. Larger patches tend to be depressed on maximal insufflations during endoscopic examination and are ovoid or elongated with jagged edges and nodular surface textures. Occasionally, inflammatory changes similar to those observed in reflux esophagitis can be seen at the edges. Most are single patch and

Authors [Ref]	Symptoms	Prevalence
Jacob et al [1997]	Symptoms inquired Pharyngeal discomfort, Globus, burning sensation in throat, odynophagia & dysphagia to liquid/solid	Overall, 9.1% (p=ns)
Maconi et al [2000]	Symptoms Dysphagia, throat discomfort and heartburn	Overall, 5.5% (p=ns) Overall, 22.2% (milder symptoms included)
Akbayir et al [2004]	Upper esophageal and laryngopharyngeal symptoms Individual symptoms not defined	Overall, 45% vs. 21.5% (p=0.07)
Baudet et al [2006]	Dysphagia	21 vs. 4.0, p<0.001
Poyrazoglu et al [2007]	Symptoms (not defined) Dysphagia	Overall not defined 39.4% vs. 0% (p<0.05)
Chong & Jalihal [2010]	Symptoms Chronic cough Sore throat/hoarseness Globus Regurgitation Heartburn	Overall, 73.1% (p<0.05) 29.2 vs. 10.6% (p<0.01) 54.2 vs. 11.7% (p<0.01) 23.1 vs. 7.1% (p<0.01) 42.3 vs. 13.1% (p<0.01) 50.0 vs. 22.5% (p<0.01)

Table 2. Prevalence of symptoms reported to be associated with HGMP/CIP

in patients with multiple patches, they tend to be found in close proximity, above or below forming columns or on the opposite side (kissing patches). It is uncertain whether the size of HGMP/CIP may change with time. One study reported that the size of a HGMP/CIP decreased during subsequent endoscopy whilst on acid suppression treatment (Chong & Jalihal, 2006). Healing of surrounding inflammation may account for this observation. Associated findings include elevated whitish nodules that do not have the characteristic salmon colored mucosa. In elderly patients, venous bled or hematoma can also be found. To date, the profiles of HGMP/CIP have not been properly studied. Interestingly, HGM can also be found in other parts of the esophagus, mid esophagus and above the gastro-esophageal junction (Borhan-Manesh & Franum, 1991; Katsanos et al., 2010) (Figure 7e).
It is likely that the overall acid production from the HGMP/CIP is less than that seen in gastroesophageal reflux disease affecting the gastroesophageal junction. Acid related injuries can be seen in the patch and the surrounding esophageal squamous mucosa. Inflammatory macroscopic changes visible during endoscopy or microscopic changes only visible on histological examinations resembling those seen in reflux esophagitis have been described.

7. Modalities for detection of HGMP

7.1 High definition endoscopy

Use of high definition endoscopy will improve the clarity and definition and can differentiate HGMP/CIP from the squamous mucosa.

7.2 Narrow band imaging

Narrow band imaging (NBI) which utilizes different light wavelengths has been reported to improve the detection rate of HGMP/CIP (Hori et al., 2010; Ohara, 2010). NBI allows better visualization of the more superficial features of mucosa. In NBI, the HGMP/CIP appears a grayish pink patch surrounded by greenish hued squamous cell mucosa. Occasionally area where the thickness of squamous cell layer is less, it can also give the similar appearance but in this case, mucosal vessels, greenish in appearance, can still be seen coursing through the area. In HGMP/CIP, vessels are not seen.

7.3 Chromoendoscopy

HGMP/CIP can also be visualized with chromoendoscopy. Both Lugol's solution and methylene blue can be used to identify HGMP/CIP. Lugol's solution is iodine based and has affinity that has affinity for glycogen in non-keratinized squamous cell epithelium of the esophagus. HGMP/CIP will not stain and appear lighter shade compared to the surrounding esophagus. Methylene blue will stain HGMP/CIP blue in colour. However, this procedure requires the spraying of dye and to do this in the proximal esophagus may induce cough reflex causing discomfort to the patient (Dib & Ortiz, 2009).

7.4 Wired guided examination

Use of wire guided examination has also been reported to improve the yield. The endoscope is withdrawn into the mid-esophagus and a guide wire is threaded through into the esophagus. The endoscope is then slowly withdrawn while examining the proximal esophagus and crico-pharyngeal area (Bhasin et al., 2006).

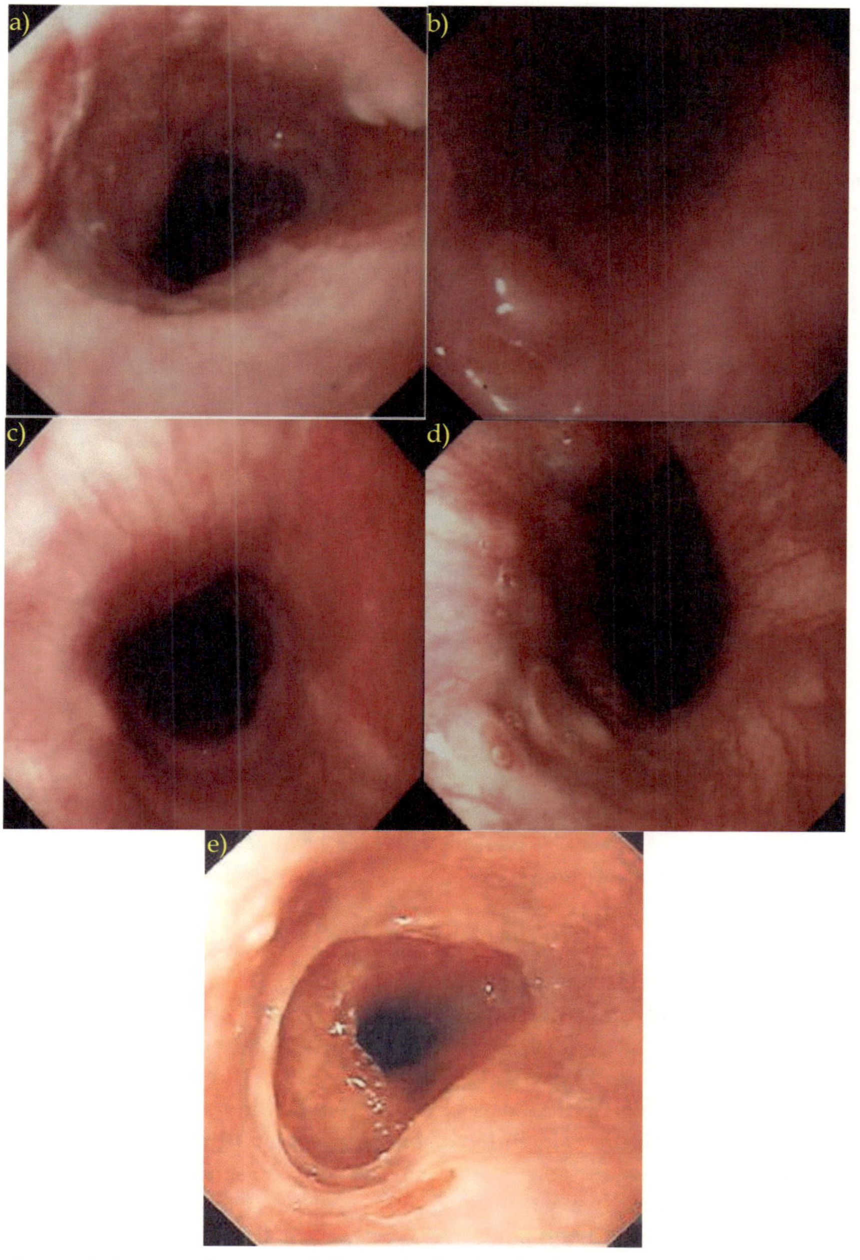

Fig. 7. Endoscopic images showing different HGMPs; a) a large depressed patch with coarse surface texture with another patch located on the opposite wall, b) two small patch with smooth surface texture, one elevated and the other flat, c) a large slightly depressed patch with coarse surface texture on the right lateral wall, d) two round elevated patch with white edges and smooth surface and associated venous bled, and e) a small flat round patch with smooth surface texture located above the gastroesophageal junction. All the patches shown stained positive for CK7 and CK20 with characteristics pattern

7.5 Radio-nuclear imaging

Radio nuclear scan has been widely used for the detection of ectopic gastric mucosa especially in cases suspected to have Meckel's diverticulum (Kiratli et al., 2009). Technetium-99m pertechnetate scintigraphy can accurately localize the location of HGMP. The role and use of nuclear imaging in detecting HGMP/CIP remains unknown. One study reported its use in five patients with patches of gastric fundal type columnar epithelium in the proximal esophagus at the level of the upper esophageal sphincter diagnosed by upper endoscopy (Chen et al., 1989). In all instances, the patches contained both chief cells and mucus-secreting cells. Two cases of HGMP/CIP were demonstrated by TcO4-. Unfortunately, TcO4- accumulation in the thyroid glands of three patients caused overlapping activity between the thyroid gland and HGMP/CIP. It was concluded that TcO4- scintigraphy is only suitable for patients who have had a total thyroidectomy or are on suppressive thyroid therapy.

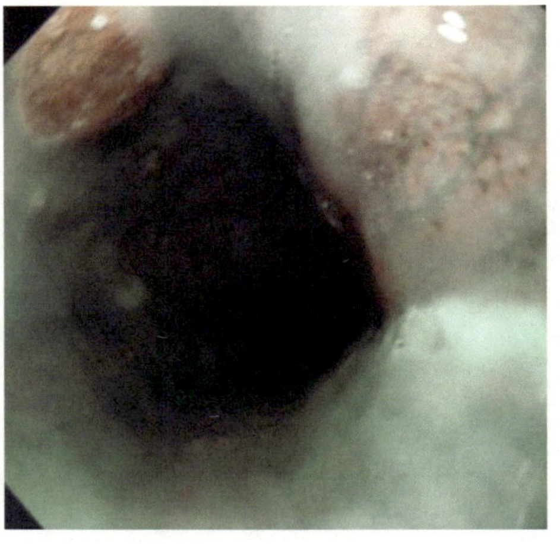

Fig. 8. Narrow band imaging showing an ectopic gastric mucosal patch as salmon coloured patch with greenish background

7.6 Contrast fluoroscopy/Barium swallows

One study showed that careful fluoroscopy study can detect subtle abnormalities that may be due to HGMP/CIP (Takeji et al., 1995). This study detected 27 cases of HGMP/CIP confirmed on endoscopy and biopsy in 1,142 patients undergoing annual health check. The most common radiographic finding was a pair of small indentations on the wall of the esophagus (n=18). Other findings included a rim-like shadow (three patches), a pair of large indentations with a shallowly depression (two patches), one indentation (five patches), a small flat elevation (one patch), a serrated irregular outline (five radiologic lesions consisted of 11 patches), other various irregular outlines (two patches), and a polypoid area (one patch). One study using barium contrast swallow showed features similar to those described for esophageal webs and suggested that in fact, esophageal webs maybe due to HGMP/CIP (Ainley, 2011). This study clearly showed that HGMP/CIP produced the same imaging features of esophageal web on barium swallow. Chronic acid injuries lead to inflammations and subsequent healing results in a web or stricture formation. This has been referred to as type AA ring in contrast to the A (muscular ring) and B (Schatzki ring) rings in the distal esophagus.

7.7 Others

Use of proximal pH monitoring can also provide clue to the presence of HGMP/CIP. Presence of acid pH detected in the proximal esophagus without acidic pH detected in the distal esophagus suggests the presence of HGMP/CIP. However, both gastroesophageal reflux and proximal acid reflux secondary to HGMP/CIP may co exist. Endoscopic imaging will still be required to confirm the presence of HGMP/CIP. Use of confocal microendoscopy for the diagnosis has also been reported.

8. Complications

Complications of HGMP/CIP are those cases classified under the clinico-pathological classification as types III to V (von Rahden et al., 2004). To date, there have been around thirty cases of cervical esophagus adenocarcinoma (type V) reported (Abe et al., 2004 ; Alaani et al., 2007 ; Alrawi et al., 2005 ; Balon et al., 2003; Berkelhammer et al., 1997; Carrie, 1950; Chatelain et al., 2002; Christensen & Sternberg, 1987; Clemente, 1974; Danoff et al., 1978; Davis et al., 1969; Goëau-Brissonnière et al., 1985; Haruki et al., 2008 ; Hirayama et al., 2003; Ishii et al., 1991; Kammori et al., 1996; Kamiya et al., 1983; Klaase et al., 2001; Lauwers et al., 1998 ; Morson & Belcher, 1952; Noguchi et al., 2001 ; Pai et al., 1997; Pech et al., 2001; Raphael et al., 1966; Sakamoto et al., 1970; Schmidt et al., 1985; Sperling & Grendell, 1995; Takagi et al., 1995; von Rahden et al., 2004 & 2005; Yoshida et al., 1986; Yoshida et al., 2010) in the literature. Other non-malignant complications (types III and IV) have been reported in both children and adults and are shown in Table 1 (Sauvé et al., 2001; Mion et al., 1996; Steadman et al., 1988; Yarborough et al., 1993; Bosher & Taylor, 1951; Powell & Luck, 1988; Karnak et al., 1999; Buse et al., 1993; Waring & Wo, 1997; Weaver, 1979; Bataller et al., 1995; Kohler et al., 1988; Garcia et al., 2002; Daher et al., 2010; Sánchez-Pernaute et al., 1999; Righini et al., 2007 ; Chatelain et al., 1998; Oguma et al., 2005 ; Rana et al., 2006 ; Schulewitz et al., 2007). Proximal esophageal web or stricture associated with Plummer-Vinson or Paterson-Kelly-Brown syndrome associated with sideroblastic anemia is now believed to complication of HGMP/CIP (Ainsley, 2011). Table 3 shows the listed of reported complications associated with HGMP/CIP.

8.1 Other possible associated with HGMP/CIP

Other conditions reported to be associated with laryngopharyngeal reflux include chronic obstructive airway disease exacerbations, obstructive sleep apnea and laryngopharyngeal neoplasms (Eryuksel et al., 2009; Wise et al., 2006; Copper et al., 2000). Indirectly, there may be association with HGMP/CIP (Basseri et al., 2009; Satoh et al., 2007).

9. Treatment/management

The management of patients with HGMP/CIP depends on the presence of symptoms or complications following the clinico-pathological classification proposed by von-Rahden. For the majority of patients, HGMP/CIP are detected incidentally (type I) and as such do not require any treatment, follow up or surveillance. For patients with acid related symptoms, treatment with acid suppression with or without pro-kinetic and antacid will suffice. For majority, a short course of treatment will be adequate. However, for a proportion, prolonged acid suppression similar to patients with significant gastro-esophageal reflux disorders may be required.

Clinico-pathological classification	Conditions		References
Type III	Stricture	Reported	Bosher & Taylor, 1951; Karnak et al., 1999; Powell & Luck, 1988; Steadman et al., 1988; Yarborough et al., 1993.
	Web	Reported	Ainsley, 2011; Buse et al., 1993; Waring & Wo, 1997; Weaver, 1979.
	Bleeding	Reported	Bataller et al., 1995.
	Fistula	Reported	Katsanos et al., 2010 ; Kohler et al., 1988; Garcia et al., 2002 ; Daher et al., 2010.
	Perforation **	Reported	Righini et al., 200 ; Sánchez-Pernaute et al., 1999
	Polyp **	Reported	Chatelain et al., 1998; Oguma et al., 2005 ; Rana et al., 2006 ; Schulewitz et al., 2007
Type IV	Dysplasia		
	Low grade	Unknown	None
	High Grade	Reported	Klaase et al., 2001; Mion et al., 1996; Sauvé G et al., 2001
Type V	Adenocarcinoma		
	Early (pT1 tumor)	Reported	Abe et al., 2004; Alrawi et al., 2005; Balon et al., 2003; Berkelhammer et al., 1997; Davis et al., 1968; Haruki et al., 2008; Hirayama et al., 2003; Kammori et al., 1996; Noguchi et al., 2001; Pech et al., 2001; Schmidt et al., 1985; Takagi et al., 1995; Yoshida et al., 2009.
	Advanced	Reported	Alaani et al., 2007; Carrie, 1950; Chatelain et al., 2002; Christensen & Sternberg, 1987; Clemente, 1974; Danoff et al., 1978; Goëau-Brissonnière et al., 1985; Ishii et al., 1991; Kamiya et al., 1983 ; Klaase et al., 2001; Lauwers et al., 1998; Morson & Belcher, 1952; Pai et al., 1997; Rapheal et al., 1966; Sakamoto et al., 1970; Sperling & Grendell, 1995; von Rahden et al., 2005; Yoshida et al., 1986.

* Number of cases identified through literature searches up till December 2010

** Not included in the original classification proposed by von Rahden (1)

Table 3. Reported complications associated with HGMP/CIP based on literature search to 2010

Other reported modalities for treating symptomatic non neoplastic HGMP/CIP include argon plasma coagulation and endoscopic mucosal resection. However, these modalities have only been reported in small series.
For those cases with complicated HGMP/CIP (type III), apart from acid suppressions, other modalities such as dilatation for stricture and even surgery may be required.
Type IV cases will require close follow up treatment may include argon plasma coagulation (Sauvé et al., 2001; Klaase et al., 2001), endoscopic mucosal resection (EMR) and endoscopic sub-mucosal dissection (ESD). For those with type V HGMP/CIP, treatment will depend on the stages of disease. Early adenocarcinoma can be treated with EMR or ESD. These can be resected after the creation of a polyp by rubber band ligation or with cap assisted EMR. For other cases, surgical resections are indicated.
It remains unknown whether patients detected to have HGMP/CIP requires to be followed up for future complications or progressions to types III to V. Patients found on biopsy to have dysplastic HGMP/CIP mucosa will require surveillance. It is unknown what time interval is recommended. Given that HGMP/CIP is gastric mucosa, following the recommendations for stomach will probably be adequate.

10. Controversies

Currently, there are several controversies regarding HGMP/CIP. First, there is still dispute with regard to the origin of HGMP/CIP. However, it is widely believed to be congenital origin as result of remnant of columnar epithelium due to failure of complete squamization of the esophagus. There are several factors that favor the congenital origin hypothesis. The embryogenesis of esophagus can explain the profiles of HGMP/CIP; proximal location correlating with the last part of the esophagus, the proximal esophagus to transform to keratinized mucosa. Babies and children do not have sufficient duration of acid exposure to induce changes suggested by the acquired theory. Finally, although the staining pattern based on CK7 and CK20 are similar, staining with MUC protein shows differences between HGMP/CIP and Barrett's (Lauwers et al., 2005).
An earlier study had also shown that the HGMP/CIP had cellular component different from Barrett's esophagus, suggesting embryogenic in origin (Fuerle et al., 1990).
The proposed theory on acquired origin was based on similarities between histological findings of HGMP/CIP and Barrett's esophagus. Mucin protein (MUC) and CK7 and CK20 similarities suggested similar origin. Other study based on MUC also suggested HGMP/CIP being acquired in origin. In the future, other staining methods may be identified and may show clear differences between HGMP/CIP and Barrett's esophagus. Weak evidence come from higher incidence of Barrett's esophagus in patients found to have HGMP/CIP. However, the overall reported incidence rates are still too low to lend strong support for this theory.
The latest theory proposed was based on findings of glandular cystic retentions secondary in the proximal esophagus. The evidence to support this theory are lacking given the very few reports of glandular retention cysts encountered in the clinical practice and reported in the literature. Furthermore, the absence of lesions found in the other part of esophagus makes the second and the third proposed theories less likely. Interestingly, it has also been proposed that the origin may be different, congenital in baby or children and acquired in adult (Lauwers et al., 2005).

Second, the actual incidence of HGMP/CIP is not exactly known. Earlier endoscopic studies have reported rates ranging from 0.35 to 10.0% and a latest study that had used NBI reported a rate of 13.8% (Ohara, 2010). An autopsy studies have reported rate as high as 70%. However, autopsy studies on paediatric population in the mid-twentieth century had only reported rates of less than 10%. With the advent of newer imaging modalities that provide superior endoscopic images, this will provide more accurate incidence. The true incidence rates are likely to be close to the rates reported by NBI studies given the clear distinction of HGMP/CIP observed with NBI. In future studies, it is very important that the endoscopists are aware and to look for this lesions. Several studies have already reported that the pick up rates were higher when endoscopist were aware of the entity (Maconi et al., 2000; Azar et al., 2007).

The third controversy relates the clinical significance of HGMP/CIP in clinical practice. While many have found low prevalence of symptoms in associated with HGMP/CIP, it is no doubt that HGMP/CIP have clinical significance given the reported complications that include malignant transformations.

Other controversies include suggested association with extra-esophageal cancers in the aero-digestive tract. Incidence of laryngeal carcinoma has been shown to be higher in patients with laryngopharyngeal reflux disorder (Copper MP et al., 2000).

11. Future areas

HGMP/CIP remains a mysterious entity that have not been well studied compared to other esophageal disorders. Encouragingly, in the last decade, the number of publications on HGMP/CIP has been increasing. However most of these studies have only looked at the clinical and histological profiles without further addressing newer areas that can help to address the controversies that still surround HGMP/CIP. Future areas of interest include addressing the controversies that still surround HGMP/CIP. Other areas of interest are highlighted in Table 4.

12. Overview

Endoscopy is important part of our armamentarium for the evaluation of suspected gastrointestinal pathologies. Significant pathologies commonly encountered in the upper gastrointestinal tract include gastro-esophageal reflux related disorders (esophagitis, ulcers and strictures), varices, esophageal tumor, gastric ulcers, gastric tumor and duodenal ulcers. Most clinicians and endoscopists are aware of these pathologies. The proximal esophagus is frequently neglected during endoscopy with little time spent to examine this area. Pathologies found in or around the proximal esophagus include HGMP/CIP, Zenker's diverticulum, esophageal web, downhill varices and venous blebs or hematoma.

HGMP/CIP is an interesting clinical entity that still hold many mysteries and is still relatively under-recognized and unknown to many clinicians, even those who manage patients with laryngopharyngeal reflux disorders. It was first reported by Schmidt in 1805 (Schidmt, 1805). There are still very few publications compared to other esophageal disorders and only in the last decade the number of publications on this entity has increased, albeit slightly.

The proximal location of the HGMP/CIP contributes to the low detection as this area is difficult to examine. Endoscopists need to be aware and look for this condition. Studies have shown higher pick up rate when the lesions are being looked for. HGMP/CIP can also be found in the other part of the esophagus. On endoscopy, HGMP/CIP appears as a salmon-colored or velvety patch on white light endoscopy that is distinct from the esophageal squamous mucosa. HGMP/CIP may appear different color on other imaging techniques. Use of confocal endoscopy has been reported for the diagnosis of HGMP/CIP (López-Cerón Pinilla M et al., 2011). Majority of HGMP/CIP are solitary but can be multiple and the sizes can range from very small to very large. In patients with multiple patches, they are usually small and are located in close proximity of each other. They are typically found on the right or left lateral esophageal wall but can also be circumferential. They are usually oval, ovoid or round but can be elongated in shape.

Current controversies

- Origin of HGMP/CIP- Congenital/Acquired
- Clinical significance
- Exact incidence

Others

- Best method of detection
  - Magnification endoscopy
  - Narrow band imaging
  - Chromoendoscopy
  - Others
- Role of measuring acid output and clinical correlation with symptoms
- Method of measuring the surface area- Exact size of HGMP/CIP
- Role in clinical symptoms
  - Acid
  - Non acidic secretion
- Surrogate markers of histological activities of HGMP/CIP
- Treatment modalities for the various types of HGMP/CIP
- Role of Helicobacter pylori in histological progression and malignant transformation

Table 4. Future areas to address on HGMP/CIP

HGMP/CIP is reported to cause laryngopharyngeal reflux or extra-esophageal symptoms of gastro-esophageal reflux disorder. The reported frequency of laryngopharyngeal reflux symptoms ranged from very low to as high as 75% in patients with HGMP/CIP (Chong & Jalihal, 2010). Fortunately, most laryngopharyngeal reflux symptoms are mild. However, complications such as ulcerations, strictures, perforation and malignant transformation have been reported (von Rahden et al., 2004). Associations with higher frequency of laryngopharyngeal malignancies in patients with laryngopharyngeal reflux have also been reported.

The current clinico-pathological classification proposed by von-Rahden *et al.* provides a useful classification of the various manifestations of HGMP/CIP (von Rahden et al., 2004). It also guides clinical management which largely depends on the presence and severity of symptoms. Management is mainly with pharmacotherapy and instrumentations (endoscopic) and surgery may be required for complicated cases. Ablative therapies with argon plasma coagulation have been reported to provide symptoms relieve or cure in those with globus pharyngeus (Bajbouj M et al., 2009). Use of argon plasma has also been reported to be effective for dysplasia and early carcinoma. EMR or ESD have been reported to be successful for curative treatment of pT1 lesions whereas surgery is required for more advanced lesions. Controversies remain regarding the origin, clinical significance and the true incidence of HGMP/CIP. From current available evidence, it seems more likely that HGMP/CIP is congenital in origin. Despite the overall benign nature of the condition with most being categorized as type I (asymptomatic), serious complications including malignant transformation have been reported. It remains unknown how malignant transformation occur; whether it follows the established sequence of atrophy, metaplasia, dysplasia to neoplasia for Barrett's adenocarcinoma or *Helicobacter pylori* associated adenocarcinoma sequence.

Interesting future areas include studies to address the controversies mentioned, the role of newer imaging techniques to increase the diagnosis and distinguish the underlying histological profiles of HGMP/CIP, the role and significance *Helicobacter pylori* in symptoms or histological progression (whether it share similarities with gastric and *Helicobacter pylori*), ways of measuring size of patch and acid output, role of acid or mucin secretion in symptoms and possible surrogate markers for assessing histological activities of the HGMP/CIP. Biopsies of the HGMP/CIP can be difficult and it is uncertain whether the histological activities of HGMP/CIP parallel that of the gastric mucosa within the antrum, body or fundus.

13. References

Abe T, Hosokawa M, Kusumi T, Kusano M, Hokari K, Kagaya H, Watanabe A, Fujita M, Sasaki S. Adenocarcinoma arising from ectopic gastric mucosa in the cervical esophagus. *Am J Clin Oncol*. 2004; 27:644-5.

Ainley EJ. High oesophageal web formation in association with heterotopic gastric mucosa (the gastric inlet patch): a small case series. *Frontline Gastroenterology*. 2011; 2:117-23.

Alaani A, Jassar P, Warfield AT, Gouldesbrough DR, Smith I. Heterotopic gastric mucosa in the cervical oesophagus (inlet patch) and globus pharyngeus--an under-recognised association. *J Laryngol Otol*. 2007; 121:885-8.

Alrawi SJ, Winston J, Tan D, Gibbs J, Loree TR, Hicks W, Rigual N, Lorè JM Jr. Primary adenocarcinoma of cervical esophagus. *J Exp Clin Cancer Res*. 2005; 24:325-30.

Akbayir N, Alkim C, Erdem L, Sökmen HM, Sungun A, Başak T, Turgut S, Mungan Z. Heterotopic gastric mucosa in the cervical esophagus (inlet patch): endoscopic prevalence, histological and clinical characteristics. *J Gastroenterol Hepatol*. 2004; 19:891-6.

Alagozlu H, Simsek Z, Unal S, Cindoruk M, Dumlu S, Dursun A. Is there an association between Helicobacter pylori in the inlet patch and globus sensation? *World J Gastroenterol*. 2010; 16:42-7.

Avidan B, Sonnenberg A, Chejfec G, Schnell TG, Sontag SJ. Is there a link between cervical inlet patch and Barrett's esophagus? Gastrointest Endosc. 2001; 53:717-21.

Azar C, Jamali F, Tamim H, Abdul-Baki H, Soweid A. Prevalence of endoscopically identified heterotopic gastric mucosa in the proximal esophagus: endoscopist dependent? *J Clin Gastroenterol*. 2007; 41:468-71.

Balon JM, Mariette C, Fabre S, Tiret E, Triboulet JP. Primary adenocarcinoma of the cervical esophagus arising from heterotopic gastric mucosa. *Gastroenterol Clin Biol.* 2003; 27:836-8. Review. French.

Bajbouj M, Becker V, Eckel F, Miehlke S, Pech O, Prinz C, Schmid RM, Meining A. Argon plasma coagulation of cervical heterotopic gastric mucosa as an alternative treatment for globus sensations. *Gastroenterology.* 2009; 137:440-4.

Bataller R, Bordas JM, Ordi J, Llach J, Elizalde JI, Mondelo F. Upper gastrointestinal bleeding: a complication of "inlet patch mucosa" in the upper esophagus. *Endoscopy.* 1995; 27:282.

Baudet JS, Alarcón-Fernández O, Sánchez Del Río A, Aguirre-Jaime A, León-Gómez N. Heterotopic gastric mucosa: a significant clinical entity. *Scand J Gastroenterol.* 2006; 41:1398-404.

Basseri B, Conklin JL, Mertens RB, Lo SK, Bellack GS, Shaye OA. Heterotopic gastric mucosa (inlet patch) in a patient with laryngopharyngeal reflux (LPR) and laryngeal carcinoma: a case report and review of literature. *Dis Esophagus.* 2009; 22:E1-5. Review.

Berkelhammer C, Bhagavan M, Templeton A, Raines R, Walloch J. Gastric inlet patch containing submucosally infiltrating adenocarcinoma. *J Clin Gastroenterol.* 1997; 25:678-81.

Bhasin DK, Rana SS, Chandail VS. Nanda M, Nadkarni N, Masoodi I, SInha SK, Nagi B. Endoscopic examination of the upper esophagus by withdrawal of endoscope over guide wire. *Trop Gastroenterol.* 2006; 27:172-4.

Bogomoletz WV, Geboes K, Feydy P, Nasca S, Ectors N, Rigaud C. Mucin histochemistry of heterotopic gastric mucosa of the upper esophagus in adults: possible pathogenic implications. *Hum Pathol.* 1988; 19:1301-6.

Borhan-Manesh F, Farnum JB. Incidence of heterotopic gastric mucosa in the upper oesophagus. *Gut.* 1991; 32:968-72.

Borhan-Manesh F, Farnum JB. Study of Helicobacter pylori colonization of patches of heterotopic gastric mucosa (HGM) at the upper esophagus. *Dig Dis Sci.* 1993; 38:142-6.

Bosher LH, Taylor FH. Heterotopic gastric mucosa in the esophagus with ulceration and stricture formation. *J Thorac Surg.* 1951; 21:306-12.

Boybeyi O, Karnak I, Güçer S, Orhan D, Senocak ME. Common characteristics of jejunal heterotopic gastric tissue in children: a case report with review of the literature. *J Pediatr Surg.* 2008 Jul;43(7):e19-22. Review.

Buse PE, Zuckerman GR, Balfe DM. Cervical esophageal web associated with a patch of heterotopic gastric mucosa. *Abdom Imaging.* 1993; 18:227-8.

Carrie A. Adenocarcinoma of the upper end of the oesophagus arising from ectopic gastric epithelium. *Br J Surg.* 1950; 37:474.

Chatelain D, Fléjou JF. [Hyperplastic polyp in heterotopic gastric mucosa. A rare lesion of the cervical esophagus]. *Ann Pathol.* 1998; 18:415-7. French.

Chatelain D, de Lajarte-Thirouard AS, Tiret E, Flejou JF. Adenocarcinoma of the upper esophagus arising in heterotopic gastric mucosa: common pathogenesis with Barrett's adenocarcinoma? *Virchows Arch.* 2002; 441:406-11.

Chan GS, Yuen ST, Chu KM, Ho JW, Leung SY, Ho JC. Helicobacter pylori in Meckel's diverticulum with heterotopic gastric mucosa in a population with relatively high H. pylori prevalence rate. *J Gastroenterol Hepatol.* 1999; 14:313-6.

Chen CH, DeRidder PH, Fink-Bennett D, Alexander TJ. Detection of heterotopic gastric mucosa in the upper esophagus with 99mTc-pertechnetate scintigraphy. *J Clin Gastroenterol*. 1989; 11:23-6.

Chong VH, Jalihal A. Cervical inlet patch: case series and literature review. *South Med J*. 2006; 99:865-9.

Chong VH, Jalihal A. Heterotopic gastric mucosal patch of the esophagus is associated with higher prevalence of laryngopharyngeal reflux symptoms. *Eur Arch Otorhinolaryngol*. 2010; 267:1793-9.

Christensen WN, Sternberg SS. Adenocarcinoma of the upper esophagus arising in ectopic gastric mucosa. Two case reports and review of the literature. *Am J Surg Pathol*. 1987; 11:397-402.

Clemente C. A case of adenocarcinoma of the upper third of the esophagus arising on ectopic gastric tissue (author's transl). *Tumori*. 1974; 60:17-24.

Copper MP, Smit CF, Stanojcic LD, Devriese PP, Schouwenburg PF, Mathus-Vliegen LM. High incidence of laryngopharyngeal reflux in patients with head and neck cancer. *Laryngoscope*. 2000; 110:1007-11.

Daher P, Francis E, Raffoul L, Riachy E. Ectopic gastric mucosa in the cervical esophagus presenting as a recurrent neck abscess: a case report. *J Pediatr Surg*. 2010 Jun;45(6):e15-7.

Danoff B, Cooper J, Klein M. Primary adenocarcinoma of the upper oesophagus. *Clin Radiol*. 1978; 29:519-22.

Davis WM, Goodwin MN Jr, Black HC Jr, Hawk JC. Polypoid adenocarcinoma of the cervical esophagus. *Arch Pathol*. 1969; 88:367-70.

Dib J Jr, Ortiz A. Heterotopic gastric mucosa in the proximal esophagus. Chromoendoscopy dependent? *J Clin Gastroenterol*. 2009; 43:96; author reply 97-8.

Erez I, Kovalivker M, Lew S, Lazar L, Motovic A. Ectopic gastric mucosa in a polyp causing ileo-ileal intussusception: a case report of a three-month-old baby. *Eur J Pediatr Surg*. 1991; 1:118-20.

Eryuksel E, Dogan M, Olgun S, Kocak I, Celikel T. Incidence and treatment results of laryngopharyngeal reflux in chronic obstructive pulmonary disease. *Eur Arch Otorhinolaryngol*. 2009; 266:1267-71.

Feurle GE, Helmstaedter V, Buehring A, Bettendorf U, Eckardt VF. Distinct immunohistochemical findings in columnar epithelium of esophageal inlet patch and of Barrett's esophagus. *Dig Dis Sci*. 1990; 35:86-92.

Galan AR, Katzka DA, Castell DO. Acid secretion from an esophageal inlet patch demonstrated by ambulatory pH monitoring. *Gastroenterology*. 1998; 115:1574-6.

García AO, Mazzadi SA, Raffo L, Bonfanti M, Salis GB, Arra A, Chiocca JC. Heterotopic gastric mucosa in the upper esophagus: report of a case with a fistula. *Dis Esophagus*. 2002; 15:262-5.

Garmendia M, Aparicio JR, Martínez J, Casellas JA. Heterotopic gastric mucosa in the rectum. *Gastrointest Endosc*. 2007; 65:921; discussion 922.

Georges A, Coopman S, Rebeuh J, Molitor G, Rebouissoux L, Dabadie A, Kalach N, Lachaux A, Michaud L. Inlet Patch: Clinical Presentation and Outcome in Children. *J Pediatr Gastroenterol Nutr*. 2011 Jan 12.

Goëau-Brissonnière O, Hannoun L, Huguet C. Adenocarcinoma of the cervical esophagus. Association with a gastric heterotopia. *J Chir (Paris)*. 1985; 122:101-3.

Gutierrez O, Akamatsu T, Cardona H, Graham DY, El-Zimaity HM. Helicobacter pylori and hetertopic gastric mucosa in the upper esophagus (the inlet patch). *Am J Gastroenterol*. 2003; 98:1266-70.

Hamilton JW, Thune RG, Morrissey JF. Symptomatic ectopic gastric epithelium of the cervical esophagus. Demonstration of acid production with Congo red. *Dig Dis Sci*. 1986; 31:337-42.

Haruki S, Kawano T, Nagai K, et al. A case of esophageal adenocarcinoma arising from heterotopic gastric mucosa [Japanese with English abstract]. *Jpn J Gastroenterol Surg*. 2008;41:493–498

Hayama S, Suzuki Y, Takahashi M, Hazama K, Fujita M, Kondo S, Katoh H. Heterotopic gastric mucosa in the gallbladder: report of two cases. *Surg Today*. 2010; 40:783-7.

Heo YS, Jeong SY, Son SW, Kim IH, Seo SH. Heterotopic gastric mucosa in the umbilicus. *Ann Dermatol*. 2010; 22:223-5. Epub 2010 May 18.

Hirayama N, Arima M, Miyazaki S, Shimada H, Okazumi S, Matsubara H, Suzuki T, Ochiai T, Kouzu T. Endoscopic mucosal resection of adenocarcinoma arising in ectopic gastric mucosa in the cervical esophagus: case report. *Gastrointest Endosc*. 2003; 57:263-6.

Hori K, Kim Y, Sakurai J, Watari J, Tomita T, Oshima T, Kondo C, Matsumoto T, Miwa H. Non-erosive reflux disease rather than cervical inlet patch involves globus. *J Gastroenterol*. 2010; 45:1138-45. Epub 2010 Jun 26.

Ishii K, Ota H, Nakayama J, Katsuyama T, Matsuzawa K, Honda T, Akamatsu T. Adenocarcinoma of the cervical oesophagus arising from ectopic gastric mucosa. The histochemical determination of its origin. *Virchows Arch A Pathol Anat Histopathol*. 1991; 419:159-64.

Jacobs E, Dehou MF. Heterotopic gastric mucosa in the upper esophagus: a prospective study of 33 cases and review of literature. *Endoscopy*. 1997; 29:710-5.

Kamiya J, Ishigure H, Akita M, et al. A case of adenocarcinoma of the cervical esophagus arising from ectopic gastric mucosa. *Nippon Geka Gakkai Zasshi*. 1983; 16:1808-11.

Kammori A, Ogawa T, Hashimoto M, et al. A case of early esophageal adenocarcinoma developed from inlet patch of gastric mucosa in the cervical esophagus [Japanese with English abstract]. *Jpn J Gastroenterol Surg* 1996; 29:717-21.

Karnak I, Senocak ME, Akçören Z, Büyükpamukçu N, Hiçsönmez A. Ectopic gastric mucosa causing dysphagia due to strictures in a boy. *Eur J Pediatr Surg*. 1999; 9:413-5.

Katsanos KH, Christodoulou DK, Kamina S, Maria K, Lambri E, Theodorou S, Tsampoulas K, Vasiliki M, Tsianos EV. Diagnosis and endoscopic treatment of esophago-bronchial fistula due to gastric heterotopy. *World J Gastrointest Endosc*. 2010; 2:138-42.

Kibria R, Butt S, Ali SA, Akram S. Heterotropic gastric tissue in duodenal bulb mimicking duodenal cancer: an unusual duodenal lesion. *J Gastrointest Cancer*. 2009; 40:142-3.

Kiratli PO, Aksoy T, Bozkurt MF, Orhan D. Detection of ectopic gastric mucosa using 99mTc pertechnetate: review of the literature. *Ann Nucl Med*. 2009; 23:97-105.

Klaase JM, Lemaire LC, Rauws EA, Offerhaus GJ, van Lanschot JJ. Heterotopic gastric mucosa of the cervical esophagus: a case of high-grade dysplasia treated with argon plasma coagulation and a case of adenocarcinoma. *Gastrointest Endosc*. 2001; 53:101-4.

Kohler B, Köhler G, Riemann JF. Spontaneous esophagotracheal fistula resulting from ulcer in heterotopic gastric mucosa. *Gastroenterology*. 1988; 95:828-30.

Korkut E, Bektaş M, Alkan M, Ustün Y, Meco C, Ozden A, Soykan I. Esophageal motility and 24-h pH profiles of patients with heterotopic gastric mucosa in the cervical esophagus. *Eur J Intern Med.* 2010; 21:21-4.

Latchford A, Eksteen B, Jankowski J. The continuing tale of cytokeratins in Barrett's mucosa: as you like it. *Gut.* 2001; 49:746-7.

Lauwers GY, Scott GV, Vauthey JN. Adenocarcinoma of the upper esophagus arising in cervical ectopic gastric mucosa: rare evidence of malignant potential of so-called "inlet patch". *Dig Dis Sci.* 1998; 43:901-7.

Lauwers GY, Mino M, Ban S, Forcione D, Eatherton DE, Shimizu M, Sevestre H. Cytokeratins 7 and 20 and mucin core protein expression in esophageal cervical inlet patch. *Am J Surg Pathol.* 2005; 29:437-42.

Lieberman-Meffert D, Duranceau A, Stein HJ. Anatomy and embryology. In: Orringer MB, Heitmiller R, eds. The Esophagus, Vol I. Zuidema GD, Yeo ChJ. Sheckford's surgery of the alimentary tract. 5th Ed., Philadelphia: WB Saunders, 2002: pg 3-39.

López-Cerón Pinilla M, Jimeno Ramiro M, Rodríguez de Miguel C, Pellisé Urquiza M. Heterotopic gastric mucosa diagnosed by confocal endomicroscopy. *Rev Esp Enferm Dig.* 2011; 103:40-1.

Macha S, Reddy S, Rabah R, Thomas R, Tolia V. Inlet patch: heterotopic gastric mucosa--another contributor to supraesophageal symptoms? *J Pediatr.* 2005; 147:379-82.

Maconi G, Pace F, Vago L, Carsana L, Bargiggia S, Bianchi Porro G. Prevalence and clinical features of heterotopic gastric mucosa in the upper oesophagus (inlet patch). *Eur J Gastroenterol Hepatol.* 2000; 12:745-9.

Mann NS, Mann SK, Rachut E. Heterotopic gastric tissue in the duodenal bulb. *J Clin Gastroenterol.* 2000; 30:303-6. Review.

Melato M, Ferlito A. Heterotopic gastric mucosa of the tongue and the oesophagus. *ORL J Otorhinolaryngol Relat Spec.* 1975; 37:244-54.

Meining A, Bajbouj M. Erupted cysts in the cervical esophagus result in gastric inlet patches. *Gastrointest Endosc.* 2010; 72:603-5.

Mion F, Lambert R, Partensky C, Cherkaoui M, Berger F. High-grade dysplasia in an adenoma of the upper esophagus developing on heterotopic gastric mucosa. *Endoscopy.* 1996; 28:633-5.

Morson BC, Belcher JR. Adenocarcinoma of the oesophagus and ectopic gastric mucosa. *Br J Cancer.* 1952; 6:127-30.

Nakajima H, Munakata A, Sasaki Y, Yoshida Y. pH profile of esophagus in patients with inlet patch of heterotopic gastric mucosa after tetragastrin stimulation. An endoscopic approach. *Dig Dis Sci.* 1993; 38:1915-9.

Noguchi T, Takeno S, Takahashi Y, Sato T, Uchida Y, Yokoyama S. Primary adenocarcinoma of the cervical esophagus arising from heterotopic gastric mucosa. *J Gastroenterol.* 2001; 36:704-9.

Nowak M, Deppisch L. Giant heterotopic gastric polyp in the jejunum. *Arch Pathol Lab Med.* 1998; 122:90-3. Review.

Oguma J, Ozawa S, Omori T, Kitagawa Y, Saikawa Y, Mikami S, Kitajima M. EMR of a hyperplastic polyp arising in ectopic gastric mucosa in the cervical esophagus: case report. *Gastrointest Endosc.* 2005; 61:335-8.

Ohara M. Incidence of heteroptopic gastric mucosa in the upper esophagus in first time narrow banding image endoscopy of consecutive 900 patients. *Gastrointest Endosc.* 2010; 71:AB316-17.

Ortiz MJ, Fay JT, Weir GT. Heterotopic gastric mucosa of the tongue. *J Oral Maxillofac Surg.* 1982; 40:667-70.

Pai S, Deshpande R, Naresh KN. Adenocarcinoma of cervical esophagus arising in aberrant gastric mucosa. *Indian J Gastroenterol.* 1997; 16:157-8.

Pech O, May A, Gossner L, Vieth M, Trump F, Stolte M, Ell C. Early stage adenocarcinoma of the esophagus arising in circular heterotopic gastric mucosa treated by endoscopic mucosal resection. *Gastrointest Endosc.* 2001; 54:656-8.

Popkharitov AI, Gulubova MV, Dandov AD, Sivrev DP. Heterotopic gastrointestinal cyst mimicking chronic cholecystitis: a case report. *J Med Case Reports.* 2008; 2:173.

Powell RW, Luck SR. Cervical esophageal obstruction by ectopic gastric mucosa. *J Pediatr Surg.* 1988; 23:632-4.

Poyrazoglu OK, Bahcecioglu IH, Dagli AF, Ataseven H, Celebi S, Yalniz M. Heterotopic gastric mucosa (inlet patch): endoscopic prevalence, histopathological, demographical and clinical characteristics. *Int J Clin Pract.* 2009; 63:287-91.

Rana SS, Panda N, Sinha SK, Nada R, Nagi B, Bhasin DK. Heterotopic gastric mucosa in the upper esophagus manifesting as a polypoidal mass causing dysphagia. *Gastrointest Endosc.* 2006; 63:185-7.

Raphael HA, Ellis FH Jr, Dockerty MB. Primary adenocarcinoma of the esophagus: 18-year review and review of literature. *Ann Surg.* 1966; 164:785-96.

Righini CA, Faure C, Karkas A, Schmerber S, Reyt E. Spontaneous perforation in the upper oesophagus resulting from ulcer in heterotopic gastric mucosa. *Rev Laryngol Otol Rhinol (Bord).* 2007; 128:197-200.

Sakamoto G, Nakamura K, Saito K, Sato M, Sugahara T. Primary adenocarcinoma of the esophagus arising from heterotopic gastric glands. *Gan No Rinsho.* 1970; 16:1105-10.

Salminen P, Ovaska J. Heterotopic gastric mucosal patch in patients with reflux laryngitis: an entity of clinical interest? *Surg Laparosc Endosc Percutan Tech.* 2009; 19:361-3.

Sánchez-Pernaute A, Hernando F, Díez-Valladares L, González O, Pérez Aguirre E, Furió V, Remezal M, Torres A, Balibrea JL. Heterotopic gastric mucosa in the upper esophagus ("inlet patch"): a rare cause of esophageal perforation. *Am J Gastroenterol.* 1999; 94:3047-50.

Satoh S, Nakashima T, Watanabe K, Toda S, Kuratomi Y, Sugihara H, Inokuchi A. Hypopharyngeal squamous cell carcinoma bordering ectopic gastric mucosa "inlet patch" of the cervical esophagus. *Auris Nasus Larynx.* 2007 Mar;34(1):135-9.

Sauvé G, Croué A, Denez B, Boyer J. High-grade dysplasia in heterotopic gastric mucosa in the upper esophagus after radiotherapy: successful eradication 2 years after endoscopic treatment by argon plasma coagulation. *Endoscopy.* 2001; 33:732.

Schmidt FA. De mammalium oesophagus atque ventriculo. Inaugural dissertation; Halle, Bethenea, 1805.

Schmidt H, Riddell RH, Walther B, Skinner DB, Riemann JF, Groitl H. [Adenocarcinoma of heterotopic gastric mucosa in the proximal esophagus]. *Leber Magen Darm.* 1985; 15:144-7. German.

Schmulewitz N, Tobias J, Singh P. Hyperplastic polyp arising from heterotopic gastric epithelium in the esophagus. *Gastrointest Endosc.* 2007; 66:1221-2; discussion 1222.

Sperling RM, Grendell JH. Adenocarcinoma arising in an inlet patch of the esophagus. *Am J Gastroenterol.* 1995; 90:150-2.

Steadman C, Kerlin P, Teague C, Stephenson P. High esophageal stricture: a complication of "inlet patch" mucosa. *Gastroenterology.* 1988; 94:521-4.

Steele SR, Mullenix PS, Martin MJ, Ormseth E, Weppler E, Graham J, Place RJ. Heterotopic gastric mucosa of the anus: a case report and review of the literature. *Am Surg.* 2004; 70:715-9. Review.

Surana R, Losty P, Fitzgerald RJ. Heterotopic gastric cyst of the tongue in a newborn. *Eur J Pediatr Surg.* 1993; 3:110-1.

Takagi A, Ema Y, Horii S, Morishita M, Miyaishi O, Kino I. Early adenocarcinoma arising from ectopic gastric mucosa in the cervical esophagus. *Gastrointest Endosc.* 1995; 41:167-70.

Takeji H, Ueno J, Nishitani H. Ectopic gastric mucosa in the upper esophagus: prevalence and radiologic findings. *AJR Am J Roentgenol.* 1995; 164:901-4.

Tang P, McKinley MJ, Sporrer M, Kahn E. Inlet patch: prevalence, histologic type, and association with esophagitis, Barrett esophagus, and antritis. *Arch Pathol Lab Med.* 2004; 128:444-7.

Vieth M, Kushima R, de Jonge JP, Borchard F, Oellig F, Stolte M. Adenoma with gastric differentiation (so-called pyloric gland adenoma) in a heterotopic gastric corpus mucosa in the rectum. *Virchows Arch.* 2005; 446:542-5.

von Rahden BH, Stein HJ, Becker K, Liebermann-Meffert D, Siewert JR. Heterotopic gastric mucosa of the esophagus: literature-review and proposal of a clinicopathologic classification. *Am J Gastroenterol.* 2004; 99:543-51.

von Rahden BH, Stein HJ, Becker K, Siewert RJ. Esophageal adenocarcinomas in heterotopic gastric mucosa: review and report of a case with complete response to neoadjuvant radiochemotherapy. *Dig Surg.* 2005; 22:107-12. Epub 2005 Apr 20. Review.

Waring JP, Wo JM. Cervical esophageal web caused by an inlet patch of gastric mucosa. *South Med J.* 1997; 90:554-5.

Weaver GA. Upper esophageal web due to a ring formed by a squamocolumnar junction with ectopic gastric mucosa (another explanation of the Paterson-Kelly, Plummer-Vinson syndrome). *Dig Dis Sci.* 1979; 24:959-63.

Wise SK, Wise JC, DelGaudio JM. Gastroesophageal reflux and laryngopharyngeal reflux in patients with sleep-disordered breathing. *Otolaryngol Head Neck Surg.* 2006; 135:253-7.

Yarborough CS, McLane RC. Stricture related to an inlet patch of the esophagus. *Am J Gastroenterol.* 1993; 88:275-6.

Yoshida M, Ide H, Yamada A, Endo M. Early detection of adenocarcinoma of the esophagus. *Endoscopy.* 1986;18 Suppl 3:44-8.

Yoshida T, Shimizu Y, Kato M. Image of the month. Use of magnifying endoscopy to identify early esophageal adenocarcinoma in ectopic gastric mucosa of the cervical esophagus. *Clin Gastroenterol Hepatol.* 2010; 8:e91-3.

Yüksel I, Usküdar O, Köklü S, Başar O, Gültuna S, Unverdi S, Oztürk ZA, Sengül D, Arikök AT, Yüksel O, Coban S. Inlet patch: associations with endoscopic findings in the upper gastrointestinal system. *Scand J Gastroenterol.* 2008; 43:910-4.

11

Endoscopic Detection and Eradication of Dysplastic Barrett's Oesophagus

L. Max Almond and Hugh Barr
Biophotonics Unit (Cranfield Health), Gloucestershire Hospitals NHS Foundation Trust, United Kingdom

1. Introduction

Over the past four decades the incidence of oesophageal cancer has increased more rapidly than that of any other solid tumour in the Western World. This rise reflects the emergence of oesophageal adenocarcinoma as the most common pathological type. Despite this growing incidence, progress towards early detection and treatment has been slow and mortality figures have remained dismal - Cancer Research UK quotes overall one and five year survival rates of just 28% and 8% respectively.(CrUK, 2010) As a result, oesophageal cancer repreasents a real and growing public health problem and urgent action is required to improve detection and facilitate early intervention, ideally at a pre-malignant stage.

Most oesophageal adenocarcinoma develops following a well recognised series of cellular changes secondary to a multifactorial aetiology. In the classically described pathway there is initially a metaplastic change in the epithelial lining of the oesophagus (Barrett's oesophagus) which then progresses to 'low-grade' and then 'high-grade' dysplasia. As many as 30% of patients newly diagnosed with high-grade dysplasia may already have a coexistent invasive cancer, and between 5-60% of patients will develop cancer during surveillance over 1-7 years.

To date there is no early diagnostic test which can enable instantaneous accurate diagnosis of dysplasia. Clinicians are advised to take random biopsies from areas of Barrett's oesophagus in order to identify dysplasia, but even histological assessment of dysplasia is subjective and can be unreliable. As a result, significant dysplastic change (or even intramucosal cancer) may be missed. In addition, as dysplasia (the premalignant lesion) is difficult to identify, screening for early oesophageal cancer / high-grade dysplasia cannot currently be recommended, and as a consequence, oesophageal tumours present late and so have a poor prognosis.

The early recognition of high-grade dysplasia is paramount to enabling a successful treatment strategy. Surgery is one option for patients with confimred HGD, however the emergence of multiple endotherapies over the past 20 years have demonstrated the ability to cure focal high-grade dysplasia, thus preventing progression to invasive malignancy. In this chapter we will discuss the accuracy of endoscopic and histological diagnosis of dysplasia and will consider novel endoscopic adjuncts which may improve endoscopic sensitivity. We will then discuss the endoscopic therapeutic options that are available for management of dysplastic Barrett's oesophagus and will propose a endotherapy algorithm for use in specialist Barrett's surveillance centres.

2. Endoscopic detection of Barrett's oesophagus

Barrett's oesophagus is most often identified incidentally in patients who are undergoing an upper endoscopy for investigation of reflux symptoms. Barrett's oesophagus has a classical endoscopic appearance of 'salmon pink' columnar mucosa arising proximally from the oesophago-gastric junction (OGJ), often with characteristic 'tongue' extensions. There may also be readily identifiable islands of columnar mucosa. Following endoscopic recognition, the extent of proximal extension above the OGJ should be measured and documented, taking care to accurately identify any sliding hiatus hernia which may confuse this measurement. The diagnosis must then be confirmed / corroborated histologically by multiple pinch biopsies of the affected segment. When biopsies are obtained it is crucial that they originate from the oesophagus and that their site is recorded as accurately as possible.

The 'Prague C and M criteria', defined by an International Working Group on Barrett's oesophagus, offers a validated method of classifying Barrett's based on its endoscopic appearance. (Sharma et al., 2006b) The extent of circumferential involvement in centimetres from the OGJ should be recorded, as should the maximum length of the Barrett's segment (including tongues of Barrett's but excluding isolated 'islands').

Difficulties arise in diagnosis particularly in 'ultra-short' segment Barrett's oesophagus. The original description of Barrett's oesophagus was of columnar metaplasia extending for at least 3cm from the OGJ. Although the risk of malignant progression is greater in long Barrett's segments (>8cm), it is now recognised that shorter lengths, even below 3cm have malignant potential. (Hirota et al., 1999; Schnell et al., 1992; Sharma et al., 1997; May et al., 2002) However, what appears endoscopically to be a short segment of Barrett's oesophagus in the distal oesophagus or an irregular z-line may in fact represent intestinal metaplasia of the gastric cardia known as cardia intestinal metaplasia (CIM). (BSG Working Party, 2005) This can lead to misclassification of CIM as short segment Barrett's. For this reason, the endoscopist has a crucial role in defining the exact position from which biopsies are taken to prevent misdiagnosis.

3. Definition and clinical significance of Barrett's dysplasia

Dysplasia is defined as "an unequivocal neoplastic alteration of epithelium which has the potential to progress to invasive malignancy but remains confined within the basement membrane of the epithelium within which it arose." (Shaheen and Ransohoff, 2002; Riddell et al., 1983) Dysplasia is classified as either low grade (LGD), or high grade (HGD) (often also termed high-grade intraepithelial neoplasia HGIN)), based on its histological appearances. As already described, HGD has a higher malignant potential than LGD and malignant transformation classically occurs through a stepwise progression of pathology from metaplastic Barrett's oesophagus, to LGD, then HGD, and finally invasive adenocarcinoma.

Understanding the pathogenesis and natural history of Barrett's oesophagus is key to understanding the malignant potential and clinical significance of the various dysplastic stages. Surveillance studies have shown that the risk of developing adenocarcinoma varies between 0.4% and 1% per year (in the US and UK respectively). However, it is clear from cohort studies that not all Barrett's oesophagus progresses to dysplasia. In fact, in most long-term studies fewer than 10% of patients show evidence of progressive disease. (Schnell et al., 2001a) Patients with Barrett's oesophagus are thought to have a lifetime risk of developing oesophageal adenocarcinoma of 3-14% (approximately 0.5-1% per year following diagnosis).

(Shaheen et al., 2000; Drewitz et al., 1997) (Jankowski et al., 2000; Spechler et al., 2010; Shaheen and Richter, 2009; Jankowski et al., 2002) This represents an increased risk of 30-100 fold compared to the general population. However, cancer rates in excess of 10% per year have been described in patients with HGD. (Shaheen and Richter, 2009)
Several studies have also noted regression of disease in patients treated with acid suppression, and even complete resolution has been described. Similarly there is some data suggesting that anti-reflux surgery can improve the histological appearance of Barrett's oesophagus, although it is not currently recommended for this purpose. (BSG Working Party, 2005).

4. Endoscopic recognition of dysplasia

Endoscopic recognition of dysplasia within Barrett's oesophagus is difficult and unreliable, even for skilled endoscopists. A rigorous biopsy protocal such as that recommended by the British Society of Gastroenterologists (Box 1) is therefore necessary to identify any dysplastic change so that apropriate surveillance / endotherapy / surgery can be considered. Sites of biospy must be accurately recorded and when possible macroscopic lesions should be classified using the Paris classification (Box 2).

Box 1. Biopsying Barrett's oesophagus

Dysplasia is often macroscopically invisible. In patients with Barrett's oesophagus, endoscopists are therefore advised to follow a rigorous biopsy protocol. The British Society of Gastroenterologists recommends the following:

- Quadrantic biopsies for every 2cm of columnar lined oesophagus
- Additional biopsies of macroscopically suspicious areas

NB/ Even with strict adherence to this policy <5% of oesophageal mucosa is sampled.

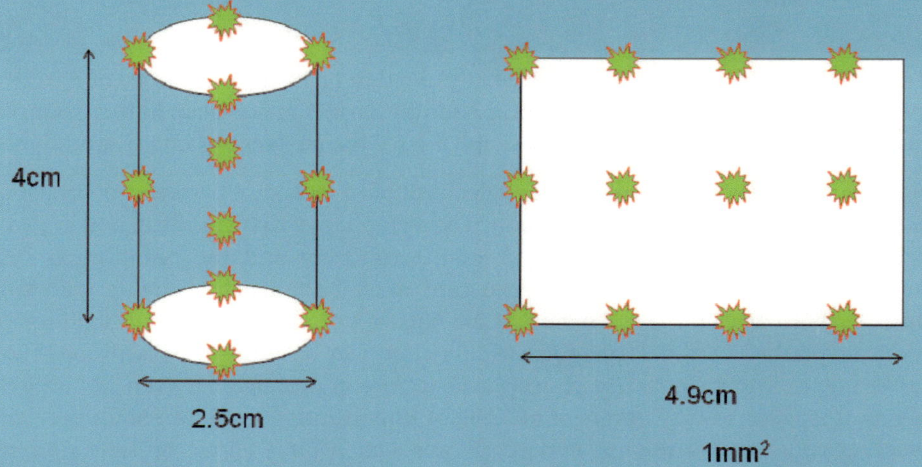

Relative sampling volume = 0.05%

Endoscopic recognition of gross mucosal abnormalities such as ulceration, nodularity, and erythema is relatively straightforward. The problem is that early neoplastic lesions are frequently flat and often have little or no visible mucosal abnormality. Only 50-70% of HGD can be identified by experienced endoscopists using white light endoscopy. This figure is lower for non-specialists and is considerably lower for the detection of LGD. In addition, more than 20% of intramucosal cancers may be missed endoscopically, even in specialist units. This is particularly concerning when it is considered that routine biopsy protocols used for Barrett's surveillance have been shown to miss up to 57% of early neoplastic lesions. (Vieth et al., 2004)
As early neoplasia in Barrett's oesophagus is a relatively rare finding, the lack of familiarity of most endoscopists with its typical appearances is a significant limiting factor in its detection. Knowledge of the appearance of these early lesions is therefore key to their early recognition. Figure 1 illustrates a range of mucosal abnormalities within segments of Barrett's oesophagus which are consistent with early neoplastic change.

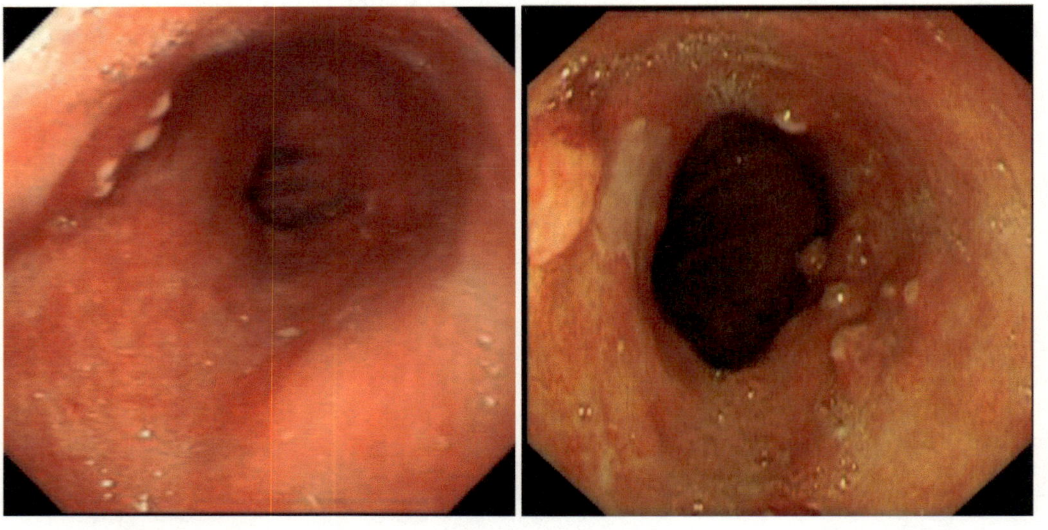

Fig. 1a (left) illustrates a nodular area of what proved to be HGD in a tongue of Barrett's oesophagus. 1b (right) illustrates multifocal nodular Barrett's neoplasia. In this example clinicians must have a very high level of suspicion for the presence of invasive malignancy

Another factor critical to endoscopic detection of dysplastic Barrett's oesohagus is a systematic approach to mucosal inspection. The oesophagus may be cleaned using water or 1% acetylcysteine to remove saliva and gastric refluxate and the oesophagus must be adequately distended by inflation. Special care must be taken in patients with a hiatus hernia as in these cases the distal extent of the Barrett's segments can be difficult to identify meaning dysplasia at the oesophagogastric junction can be missed. In addition, clinicains should be aware that the majority of neoplastic lesions are located between 12 and 6 o'clock in the endoscopists view. (Curvers et al., 2008b) Importantly clinicians should also commit to investing considerable time to endoscopic inspection (as well as the time required for multiple biopsies), and endoscopy lists should be planned accordingly when patients with known Barrett's oesophagus are attending for surveillance.

Biopsies should be taken (as per the BSG guidelines described in Box 1) and should start distally and work proximally to minimise any obstruction to the endoscopic view caused by bleeding. A description of the Barrett's segment should then be recorded using the Prague C&M classification (see section 2) and positions of random biopsies and suspicious areas recorded meticulously. Where possible, visible macroscopic neoplasia should also be classified according to the Paris classification (Box 2).

Box 2. Classification of visible early Barrett's neoplasia

Visible macroscopic early neoplastic lesions in Barrett's oesophagus are classified using the Paris classification. A description of the superficial (0) lesions is detailed below.

0	**Superficial lesions**		
	0-I		Protruding / polypoid lesions
		0-Ip	Pedunculated
		0-Is	Sessile lesions
	0-II		Non-protruding / non-excavated lesions
		0-IIa	Slightly elevated
		0-IIb	Completely flat
		0-IIc	Slightly depressed
	0-III		Excavated / ulcerated lesions

Most dysplastic Barrett's lesions are of superficial type (0-II).

Several techniques have been developed to improve endoscopic recognition of dysplasia and intramucosal carcinoma in Barrett's oesophagus. These aim to minimise sampling randomness and also facilitate targetted endoscopic resection in patients with histologically confirmed HGD / IMC. In addition, they aim to improve assessment of disease extent and minimise the incidence of missed synchronous tumours.

4.1 High resolution endoscopy by expert endoscopists

Modern high resolution endoscopes which generate up to one million pixel images (compared to the 300,000 pixel images of traditional scopes) have been shown to have a higher sensitivity for the detection of early Barrett's neoplasia provided they are used by expert endoscopists.(Kara et al., 2005a; Kara et al., 2005c) These high definition endoscopes should be used in conjunction with a high definition television to further enhance the projected image quality and enable projection onto a larger screen without loss of image resolution.

Studies have shown that up to 80% of patients referred to specialist units with biopsy proven HGD without visible abnormality will be found to have 1 or more visible abnormalities when endoscopy is repeated by an expert endoscopist using a high resolution endoscope. (10,12 from endoscopic work-up) (Kara et al., 2005a; Curvers et al., 2008d)

4.2 Chromoendoscopy

Chromoendoscopy utilises stains which bind selectively to different oesophageal mucosa and so can enable discrimination between non-dysplastic Barrett's oesophagus and HGD /

adenocarcinoma. Staining and lesion defining agents utilised include methylene blue, indigo carmine, and acetic acid. Results from studies utilising this technique have been mixed citing problems such as an inability to uniformly coat the oesophageal mucosa with the stain, and excessive time necessary for stain spraying as particular concerns.(Shaheen and Richter, 2009; Lim et al., 2006; Ragunath et al., 2003) None of these techniques has been shown to consistently out-perform high resolution endoscopy in the detection of early neoplastic lesions.(Curvers et al., 2008c) Chromoendoscopy is often both labour-intensive and operator-dependent and therefore although it may have a role when used in specialist centres by expert users, it is unlikely to develop a wider role in routine clinical practice.

4.3 Narrow band imaging (NBI)

NBI filters white light into blue and green wavelengths (at the push of a button) giving more accurate images of the mucosal and vascular patterns in the oesophageal lining. This increased superficial imaging of the oesophagus (without the need for staining) can be used to identify dysplastic lesions within Barrett's segments.(Kara et al., 2006a) In the hands of experienced users the technique has shown promise however, results have been mixed.(Sharma et al., 2006a; Curvers et al., 2008a) A recent trial from Holland shows no diagnostic benefit from either NBI or chromoendoscopy.(Curvers et al., 2008a) However, data on the accuracy of NBI is still inconclusive and results of ongoing mulitcentre randomised controlled trials are awaited.

4.4 Autofluorescence imaging (AFI)

Following excitation with short wavelengths of light many endogenous tissues emit fluorescence radiation which can be measured using fluorescence spectroscopy. Metaplastic and dysplastic Barrett's oesohagus have been shown to emit slightly different fluorescence spectra enabling the technique to be used as a mechanism to discriminate between the two pathologies. AFI appears to improve the detection of early Barrett's neoplasia when used in combination with high resolution endoscopy, although the false positive rate is relatively high.(Curvers et al., 2008b; Kara et al., 2005b; Kara et al., 2006b) Further studies are clearly indicated to truely assess the potential long-term role for AFI.

4.5 Optical coherence tomography (OTC)

OCT is analogous to ultrasound but can produce higher quality images as it relies on scattering of near infrared light as opposed to reflection of sound waves. OCT can obtain cellular images of sub-epithelial tissue through differences in their light scattering properties and avoids the need for exogenous contrast material.

In a study of 55 patients with Barrett's oesophagus, OCT was shown to delineate between HGD and oesophageal adenocarcinoma with a sensitivity of 83% and a specificity of 75%.(Evans et al., 2006) Similarly, a study of 33 patients demonstrated a diagnostic accuracy of 78% for the identification of dysplastic Barrett's oesophagus but with considerable user discrepency (56% to 98%). (Isenberg et al., 2005) Further clinical evaluation is required to fully assess the performance of OCT and assess the feasibility of introducing this promising diagnostic tool into routine clinical practice.

4.6 Confocal microscopy (CM)

CM magnifies the mucosa by more than 1000 fold producing images with 1-2 μm spatial resolution and allowing real time visualisation of cellular structures. Kiesslich et al studied

63 patients with Barrett`s oesophagus using white light endoscopy and confocal microscopy. Intravenous fluorescein was administered to generate vascular contrast and at sites of neoplasia could be seen to disperse within the lamina propria due to irregular neovascularisation. Accuracy of CM was found to be 97.4% (sensitivity 93%, specificity 98%). (Kiesslich et al., 2006) In another study by Dunbar et al, CM was shown to help target biopsies to areas of neoplasia, doubling diagnostic yield per biopsy taken, and avoiding the need for biopsy in two thirds of patients undergoing surveillance. However, no overall increase in neoplasia was identified when CM targetted biopsying was compared to random quadrantic random biopsies every 2cm.

Confocal microscopy is an expensive technique and requires the use of exogenous contrast. It has already demonstrated potential in early diagnosis of Barrett`s neoplasia although the excellent results reported by some studies have not been universally matched. (Pohl et al., 2008) Further studies are required before this technique can be reccommended for widespread use.

4.7 Labelling of biomarkers

Molcular biomarkers associated with neoplastic cells can be labelled using a specifically targetted probe molecule which has been tagged with a visual agent such as a fluoresecent dye. (Pierce et al., 2008) (Thekkek et al., 2011) The probe molecule selectively binds to the biomarker so that areas of neoplasia can be visualised with a high signal to noise ratio.

Lu et al identified a cell surface peptide specific to adenocarcinoma which they labelled using a fluorescein-tagged antibody delivered topically. The oesophagus was then washed to remove any unbound antibody and a fluorescence endoscope was used to visualise neoplastic disease. (Lu and Wang, 2008)

Other similar studies have used a range of potential biomarkers with similar effect. This is clearly a very promising technique for the detection of early neoplasia but further on-going work is necessary to identify novel molecular targets in order to improve sensitvity and specificity before widespread implementation of the technique can be contemplated.

4.8 Raman spectroscopy

Raman spectroscopy is an optical diagnostic technique which has shown considerable potential for early diagnosis of a variety of malignant disease states including oesophageal neoplasia. Raman spectroscopy measures the molecular-specific, inelastic scattering of laser light within tissue in order to generate a unique molecular 'fingerprint'. Normal, dysplastic and cancerous tissues have differing biochemical cellular components leading to characteristic spectral differences which can be analysed. Laboratory based Raman spectrometers are capable of discriminating between eight pathological groups in the distal oesophagus (including Barrett's metaplasia, HGD and adenocarcinoma) with sensitivities between 73% and 100%. (Kendall et al., 2003) Several groups are currently investigating the potential for endoscopic Raman spectroscopy using a fibre-optic Raman probe. Fibre-optic Raman sectroscopy has already demonstrated encouraging results following in vivo trials in the stomach, bladder and cervix. Although some way off clinical implementation in the oesohagus, in vivo and ex vivo results are promissing and this technique may become widely available in the short to medium term to enable instant endoscopic diagnosis of dyslasia (without the need for biopsy) and to facilitate immediate, targetted endotherapy.

5. Barrett's oesophagus surveillance

As endoscopic recognition of dysplasia remains limited at present, a policy of regular endoscopic surveillance, in conjunction with a rigourous biopsy regimen, is recommeded. The frequency of surveillance endoscopy depends predominantly on the presence and degree of dysplasia identified, and also to a lesser extent on patient age, comorbidity and patient preference.

Several retrospective studies have demonstrated a survival benefit for patients with cancers detected by surveillance endoscopy rather than following symptom investigation. (Streitz et al., 1993; Peters et al., 1994; van Sandick et al., 1998; Fountoulakis et al., 2004; Corley et al., 2002) However, many other studies have failed to show this. (Wong et al., 2010) The Barrett's Oesophagus Surveillance Study (BOSS) is a multi-centre randomised control trial currently recruiting patients throughout the UK. In this study patients are randomised to either 'endoscopy at need' (no routine surveillance), or repeat OGD combined with BSG biopsy regimen every two years for a total of ten years. The study aims to define the objective value of endoscopic surveillance and the most appropriate surveillance protocol.

Despite the current lack of high level evidence, most clinicians elect to follow up patients with Barrett's oesophagus provided the pros and cons of surveillance have been fully discussed with the patient and they subsequently wish to proceed with surveillance endoscopy. Clearly, this approach is not suitable for all-comers, and management should therefore be individualised appropriately. For example, long-term follow-up of elderly patients who are unfit for intervention is not usually recommended.

Where surveillance is deemed appropriate BSG guidelines recommend 2-yearly endoscopy using a comprehensive biopsy protocol. (BSG Working Party, 2005) Quadrantic biopsies are recommended every 2cm of Barrett's oesophagus, with more targeted biopsies of any raised or suspicious looking areas (Box 1). Patients should have their reflux treated with a proton pump inhibitor so that the presence of oesophagitis does not complicate the histological identification of dysplasia. Patients with Barrett's oesophagus who are not enrolled in endoscopic surveillance should also receive proton pump inhibitor (PPI) therapy The effectiveness and dosage of PPI therapy with and without aspirin for the prevention of progression of Barrett's oesophagus is being addressed in the Aspirin Esomeprazole Chemotherapy Trial (ASPECT) in the united Kingdom.

For those patients undergoing routine endoscopic surveillance, the risk of developing adenocarcinoma is approximately 1% a year in the UK, and about half this figure in the US. (Jankowski et al., 2002) Critcially when dysplasia has been identified on endoscopy every effort must be made to ensure that the correct diagnosis has been reached and an appropriate management strategy should then be formulated.

6. Importance of histological / radiological assessment

Accurate histological diagnosis is essential when assigning treatment strategies for Barrett's dysplasia and early Barrett's malignancies. Histopathologists can have difficulty differentitating HGD from LGD, and also HGD from early invasive (T1) carcinoma based on point biopsy appearances alone. In recent years endoscopic resection (ER) has become recognised as not only a potentially curative therapy, but also a vital diagnostic technique (section 7.1.1). The role of 'diagnostic' ER is expanding as pathologists realise the importance of accurate assessment and grading of early tumours.

The current BSG guidelines from 2005 do not recognise the diagnostic role of ER. However, new guidelines are currently being formulated by an international consensus group the 'Barrett's Dysplasia and Cancer Taskforce' (BAD CAT). These will stress the need for extremely accurate assessment of the presence and depth of invasive cancer and will recommend confirmation using ER, as well as (when indicated) further staging using endoscopic ultrasound (EUS) (which is known to be poor at differentiating between T1a and T1b tumours but is sensitive for lymph node metastases), and possibly PET-CT.

Recent studies have demonstrated the importance of accurate staging of early (T1) tumours. T1a lesions (confined to the mucosa) have a very low incidence of lymphatic invasion (<5%) whereas, invasion into the submucosa (T1b) is associated with lymphatic spread in 20-45% of cases. New evidence has suggested that the distinction between $T1sm_1$ and $T1sm_2$ (i.e. between the upper 1/3 and lower 2/3 of the submucosa) may be particularly significant as the risk of lymphatic spread appears to significantly increase in $T1sm_2$ tumours. This distinction is vital as surgical oesophagectomy and lymphadenectomy provide the only chance of cure for patients with lymphatic spread, whereas endoscopic therapy is potentially curative in those without lymphatic invasion.

As histopathological diagnosis and grading of dysplasia is difficult and subjective, any suggestion of dysplasia should be reviewed by expert pathologists at an MDT prior to initiation of a management plan. In cases where exact histopathological diagnosis proves difficult clinicians should have a low threshold for 'diagnostic' endoscopic resection to aid histological classification. This may be of particular benefit in distinguishing between HGD and early invasive (T1) carcinoma, and in accurately T-staging these early cancers.

7. Endoscopic therapies for HGD and IMC

Once an accurate diagnosis has been made and corroborated by consensus opinion in an MDT, a management plan can be formulated. All patients should be commenced on high dose PPI therapy. Subsequent management is currently subject to significant debate but is largely dependent on the degree of dysplasia, patient comorbidity and patient preference.

Recent developments have led to potentially curative endoscopic treatments for HGD and early mucosal cancer. Many of these techniques are relatively novel and are not supported by highest level evidence (RCTs). BSG and American College of Gastroenterology (ACG) guidelines from 2005 and 2008 respectively are now somewhat out-of-date when considering the management of advanced dysplasia / early cancer. However, the management of LGD has not altered in recent years as a simple 'number needed to treat' analysis confirms that the limited risks posed by LDG (in isolation), do not warrant the cost and morbidity imposed by endoscopic therapies.

The management of HGD and intramucosal cancer (T1a) is currently hotly debated and new guidelines are awaited (BAD CAT consensus). It is clear that management policies must be individualised according to the nature and severity of disease and the age and comorbidity of the patient being treated, and all management decisions must be discussed at a specialist cancer MDT.

There are two main forms of endoscopic therapy available to treat HGD and intramucosal tumours - endoscopic resection and endoscopic ablation. These techniques aim to destroy the lining of the oesophagus and promote regenerative re-growth of normal squamous mucosa. In order for this to occur, (as opposed to columnar re-growth) some of the superficial squamous lined ducts must survive the process. Techniques for mucosal ablation include photodynamic therapy, thermal ablation, radiofrequency ablation and argon plasma coagulation.

8. Endoscopic resection

Endoscopic mucosal resection (EMR) describes any technique which removes a complete area of mucosa. However, the term is somewhat misleading and many authors recommend a switch to the term 'endoscopic resection' (ER), as the aim of EMR should involve complete excision of the mucosal and submucosal layers down to the muscularis propria.
The technique involves raising an area of mucosa using suction or by submucosal injection, and then snaring it off (in a similar manner to a colonic polyp). It is a useful technique for removing focal areas of HGD or early cancer, and as well as being therapeutic, can provide important diagnostic information.

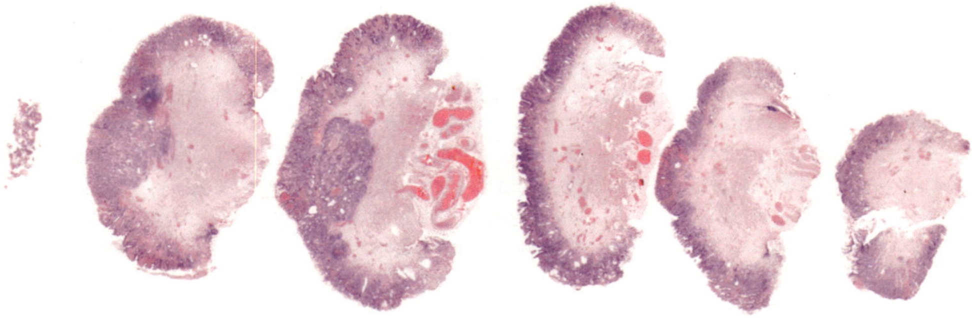

Fig. 2. Endoscopic resection of an early invasive cancer

8.1 Diagnostic endoscopic resection

Although not yet recognised by BSG guidelines, ER has now become an important diagnostic technique in patients with HGD / early cancer. ER preserves tissue architecture so that a full histopathological assessment can be made. (Odze and Lauwers, 2008) An ER specimen can be more easily orientated than a mucosal point biopsy and should contain a significant portion of submucosa allowing accurate assessment of the depth of invasion of IMC. A retrospective study of 150 EMR specimens (focal lesions) found that following analysis of EMR specimens, initial diagnoses (based on point mucosal biopsies) where changed in 49% of cases, leading to a change in management plan in 30%. (Peters et al., 2008) Mino-Kenudson et al recently demonstrated that interobserver reporting agreement between pathologists was improved when reporting EMR specimens rather than point biopsies, particularly when differentiating between intramucosal and submucosal carcinoma - a key distinction when planning a treatment strategy. (Mandal et al., 2009) ER specimens also enable improved assessment of other important prognostic factors such as the grade of cellular differentiation and the presence of lymphovascular invasion. ER has been shown to be the best technique for assessment of visible mucosal abnormalities within Barrett's oesophagus. However, the technique does have complications, and these must be considered when performing an ER for diagnostic purposes.

8.1.1 Therapeutic ER

As a therapeutic technique, oesophageal ER has been assessed in a number of large studies, although no randomised controlled trials currently exist. Its first description in HGD and early mucosal cancers in Barrett's oesophagus was published in 2000, although ER was described for early oesophageal SCC as far back as the early 1990s.

A recent study reported that ER achieved remission in 82.5% of patients with HGD. However, over a 12 month period of follow-up, metachronous lesions or disease recurrence were identified in 14% of patients, necessitating re-treatment. A further study using ER, photodynamic therapy (PDT) or a combination, showed overall complete disease remission in 98% of patients, but metachronous cancer was identified in 31% over a 34 month post treatment surveillance period. (Pech et al., 2007)

Extensive, multifocal disease is more difficult to manage endoscopically using ER. Several studies have described circumferential ER of extensive Barrett's segments but, despite experienced hands, these extensive resections have been associated with significant complication rates (bleeding 33%, strictures 17-26% and perforation 3%) and large studies with prolonged follow-up have not been conducted. (Pech et al., 2007; Seewald et al., 2003)In addition, significant recurrence rates have been reported and in up to 25% of cases, complete resection of the Barrett's segment was impossible despite several staged attempts at treatment. (Pech et al., 2007)

As discussed previously, oesophageal lesions that invade into the lamina propria but are confined to it (do not invade the submucosa) T1m1-3 (T1a) lesions have a 5% chance or less of nodal involvement. Recent data have suggested that shallow mucosal invasion $T1_{sm1}$ also has a significantly lower risk of nodal metastases than other grades of submucosal invasion. (Prasad et al., 2007; Gondrie et al., 2008) Whereas deeper invasion into the submucosa (T1sm2-3) sees this risk rise to 20-45%. (Peyre et al., 2008) In early cancers with a low risk of lymphatic spread, ER offers a curative, minimally invasive treatment option, which may be particularly appropriate in older patients at higher risk of operative morbidity / mortality. Average 3-year survival rates of more than 80% have been reported for IMC treated by ER.

In recent years there has been a move towards combination therapy in an attempt to reduce recurrence rates. Areas of focal dysplasia (or IMC) could be treated with ER, followed by complete ablation of the entire Barrett's segment using APC, PDT, or RFA.

8.2 Mucosal ablation therapy

Ablation techniques aim to destroy the lining of the oesophagus and promote regenerative growth of normal squamous mucosa. Techniques for mucosal ablation include photodynamic therapy, thermal ablation, radiofrequency ablation and argon plasma coagulation, all of which must be used in combination with acid suppression.

There are so far no randomised trials comparing these treatments against each other. In addition, the natural history of regenerated squamous epithelium is not fully known, (although there certainly appears to be a substantial reduction in malignant potential) so further long-term studies are still awaited. (Overholt et al., 2005)

8.2.1 Radiofrequency ablation

RFA is a relatively new technique which can be used to ablate circumferential ($HALO^{360}$) or focal ($HALO^{90}$) Barrett's oesophagus. Circumferential ablation is performed using a balloon to apply radiofrequency energy evenly to the oesophageal lining.

The length of the Barrett's segment is first measured endoscopically. N-acetylcysteine is then used to wash saliva, mucus and gastric juice from the oesophagus and a guidewire is placed into the gastric antrum. The endoscope is removed and a sizing balloon is inserted over the guide wire and inflated once in the distal oesophagus. In long segment Barrett's oesophagus several measurements are taken and subsequently, an appropriately sized ablation catheter is selected (based on the smallest oesophageal diameter measurement). The catheter is then passed over the guide wire and positioned at the proximal extent of the Barrett's segment. The endoscope is re-passed to ensure correct positioning of the catheter and the balloon is then inflated and a standardised dose of energy is delivered (which has a power density sufficient to ablate down to the muscularis mucosae, 700-1000μm deep). After a short period of treatment (<5s) the catheter is passed distally to the next portion of the oesophagus to be treated, trying to minimise overlap between zones by endoscopic visualisation. Once the entire Barrett's segment has been ablated the catheter is removed and the endoscope is reinserted in order to debride the ablated mucosa. The procedure is then repeated so that the whole Barrett's segment receives two treatments.

Complications are rare but include significant bleeding (1-2%), stricture formation (6%) and perforation (very rare). (Shaheen et al., 2009) Repeat OGD is recommended after 2 - 3 months and any residual focal Barrett's oesophagus can then be treated using $HALO^{90}$ RFA.

The only RCT, by Shaheen et al in 2009, demonstrated successful resolution of dysplastic Barrett's oesophagus following treatment with RFA.(Shaheen et al., 2009) Complete eradication of LGD was seen in 90.5% (ablation group) compared to 22.7% (control group) (P<0.001). Complete eradication of HGD occurred in 81.0% (ablation group) versus 19.0% (control group) (P<0.001). RFA also decreased the likelihood of disease progression (3.6% vs. 16.3%, P=0.03) and cancer (1.2% vs. 9.3%, P=0.045).

Recent NICE guidelines (June 2010) recommend that clinicians in the UK consider endoscopic ablation therapy (preferentially RFA) along with EMR, for treatment of HGD and IMC, particularly in patients not suitable for oesophagectomy.

8.2.2 Photodynamic therapy

Porfimer sodium photodynamic therapy (PDT) has been approved by the US Food and Drug Administration (FDA) and (provisionally) by NICE for treatment of HGD in Barrett's oesophagus.

The procedure involves systemic (intravenous) administration of a photosensitising agent (porfimer sodium) which is retained selectively by dysplastic cells. After about 48 hours the patient undergoes an upper endoscopy and a laser is used to excite a cytotoxic reaction in dysplastic Barrett's cells, leading to their destruction. There is now strong evidence that PDT can prevent the progression of disease in patients with Barrett's HGD. (Overholt et al., 2007) A five year randomised multicentre trial by Overholt et al demonstrated that PDT was significantly more effective at eradicating HGD than omeprazole only (odds ratio 2±0.7). It also significantly lengthened the time taken to progress to malignancy and reduced the overall risk of malignant progression by half. (Overholt et al., 2007) Following PDT, patients are required to continue life-long surveillance, and repeat ablation may become necessary.

Side-effects of PDT include nausea and chest pain in the first day or two after treatment. In the longer term, oesophageal strictures may occur in up to a quarter of patients. Oesophageal perforation has also been described (very rarely). In addition, due to the photosensitising affect of porfimer sodium, patients are required to minimise light exposure to their skin for up to 4-6 weeks after the treatment.

Several trials in Europe have used 5-ALA as the photosensitising agent in an effort to reduce skin sensitivity and oesophageal strictures. However, additional blood pressure and cardiac complications have been reported with 5-ALA and further work is therefore required to clarify the most effective drug with the least side-effects.

8.2.3 Argon plasma coagulation

APC (the most commonly used form of thermal ablation) uses a jet of ionized argon gas (plasma) directed through an endoscopic probe to ablate short segments of Barrett's or areas of persistent disease following other ablative treatment. A trial by Pech et al retrospectively assessed disease recurrence in patients treated by EMR with or without subsequent APC ablation of the residual Barrett's segment. Rates of recurrence fell from 33.3% to 17.6% with the inclusion of APC ablation. Other studies support these results and confirm low complication rates.

9. Buried glands

In some cases following ablative therapy for Barrett's oesophagus, a normal squamous epithelium may re-grow over a portion of Barrett's tissue. Endoscopically this appears normal, but these buried Barrett's glands may retain malignant potential. Endoscopists must be aware of this when surveying patients who have previously undergone ablative endotherapy and for this reason life-long endoscopic surveillance is recommended for these patients, even in the absence of residual Barrett's oesophagus.

10. Oesophagectomy

HGD is associated with early invasive malignancy in up to 30% of cases, and carries a significant long-term chance of malignant progression. In addition, recurrence rates following ablative therapies are significant and endoscopic surveillance must be lifelong. For these reasons, surgical excision of the entire Barrett's segment must still be considered the 'gold standard' treatment for young, fit patients with multifocal HGD.

Oesophagectomy is the only potentially curative treatment once lymph nodes are involved. It also aims to remove the entire Barrett's segment minimising the chance of recurrence or missed metachronous lesions. Recent centralisation of cancer services has improved operative mortality to 5% or less in most specialist units. However, for patients without proven invasive cancer, this still remains a considerable risk. In addition, morbidity following oesophagectomy remains considerable although minimally invasive and vagal sparing surgery aims to minimise this and improve long-term functional outcomes. (Ell et al., 2007)

11. Management of low-grade dysplasia

Patients with LGD should undergo repeat endoscopy with adherence to a 'gold standard' biopsy regimen 8-12 weeks after the commencement of PPI therapy. A repeat endoscopy should then be performed at 6 months, and if LGD persists, endoscopy should be repeated 6-monthly unless regression to normal Barrett's or squamous epithelium occurs, at which time surveillance can be reduced to 2 yearly intervals. (BSG Working Party, 2005)

In some cases of multifocal, persistent LGD, endoscopic mucosal ablation therapy could be considered, particularly if there is a strong patient desire for intervention (BSG Working Party, 2005) (although evidence for this statement is limited and widespread treatment of LGD is not cost-effective and is not recommended).

12. Management of high-grade dysplasia / intramucosal cancer

Data from case series suggest that up to 10% of patients with Barrett's oesophagus develop HGD, and that HGD may be associated with a focus of adenocarcinoma in up to 30% of patients. Several studies also have described high rates of progression to malignancy – annual rates of progression of 2.2%, 4% and 11.8% have been described recently. (Schnell et al., 2001b; Buttar et al., 2001; Reid et al., 2000b) In addition, the average time to progression from HGD to cancer is known to be short, typically around 24 months, (ranging from 6-43 months), (although, in most cases, HGD remains stable without progression, or may even regress). (BSG Working Party, 2005)

In confirmed cases of IMC, clinicians must not only consider T-stage, but also other important prognostic indicators including the grade of cellular differentiation and the presence of lymphatic or vascular invasion, when formulating a management strategy.

It is now clear that ER has an important diagnostic role in the determining these important prognostic indicators. Endoscopic ultrasound (EUS) is also important in intramucosal cancer to assess for the presence of early nodal metastases. EUS has been shown to be substantially more accurate than CT for detecting nodal metastases and the role of CT in investigation of intramucosal tumours is probably limited. PET-CT is a more reliable means of assessing the presence of distant metastasis which would circumvent the need for surgery and necessitate palliative therapy.

EUS is known to be poor at distinguishing between T1a and T1b tumours (33-85% accuracy) and importantly, under-diagnosis of T1b lesions is common. (May et al., 2004; Zuccaro et al., 2005). ER assessment is much more reliable but may fail to completely excise the submucosa making exact distinction between $T1_{sm1}$ and $T1_{sm2}$ difficult. Frequently pathologists use the measured depth of invasion in micrometers to differentiate the two. However, there is a paucity of published data correlating measured depth of submucosal invasion with likelihood of lymph node metastasis. Currently the role of endoscopic submucosal dissection (ESD) in the oesophagus is unclear and further trials are awaited.

If endoscopic therapy is to be considered ahead of surgery for early oesophageal tumours and HGD, a number of important considerations should be satisfied (Box 3). Similarly, if surgery is to be considered in cases where there is no overt evidence of lymphatic spread, complication rates must be low. Many papers continue to quote historic rates of mortality following oesophagectomy. It is important when contemplating treatment options to compare up-to-date data which reflects recent improvements in operative outcomes (mortality and morbidity) since surgical centralisation took place.

Box 3. Important considerations when considering the role of endoscopic therapy.

- There must be no (or minimal) under-staging of disease.
- Practitioners must be adequately skilled.
- Recurrence must be identified early and there must be a means of treating it.
- Patients must understand that endoscopic therapy is less likely to provide a "cure" than surgical treatment.
- Patients must understand that they will require long-term surveillance, (unlike following surgery).
- Complication rates (morbidity and mortality) must be low.

12.1 Multifocal HGD

Patients with multifocal disease are at a significant risk (up to 30%) of an undetected metachronous cancer and therefore warrant definitive treatment. Surgical oesophagectomy should still be considered as the first line treatment option for patients with persistent HGD provided they are deemed low operative risk and have a long life expectancy. Surgery must be carried out in specialist centres where mortality rates do not exceed 5%.

Those patients with confirmed persistent multifocal HGD who are deemed unfit for an oesophagectomy should receive ER to visible areas of HGD and subsequent ablation of the entire Barrett's segment. Several ablative treatments (using different modalities) may be required to establish complete remission. Patients will subsequently require lifelong endoscopic surveillance.

12.2 Focal HGD

Patients should be initially managed by ER of the affected area to confirm the diagnosis and exclude early malignancy. Those with a limited area of histologically confirmed HGD should undergo subsequent mucosal ablation of the whole Barrett's segment. Young patients who are fit for major surgery should be considered for oesophagectomy.

Clinicians should have a high level of suspicion for cancer and if suspected appropriate investigations e.g. endoscopic ultrasound and PET-CT should be considered. Nodularity on endoscopy should particularly raise concern although occult intramucosal tumours can occur with no visible mucosal abnormality.

Patients with HGD should initially undergo three monthly endoscopy with quadrantic biopsies every 1cm - shown to half the chance of missing oesophageal adenocarcinoma compared to 2cm biopsies. (Reid et al., 2000a) Jumbo biopsies (using large capacity forceps) can also be taken in this setting.

12.3 Intramucosal carcinoma

All patients with confirmed oesophageal cancer should undergo formal tumour staging to establish the presence or absence of distant or locoregional metastases. Surgery should be regarded as the treatment of choice for patients deemed fit enough to tolerate oesophagectomy. Patients with high operative risk with T1a (and possibly $T1_{sm1}$) tumours confirmed on ER should be considered for endoscopic therapy (ER followed by ablation).

13. Summary

All treatment decisions should be discussed in a multidisciplinary team meeting once every effort has been made to ensure the correct diagnosis has been reached. Patients (and families) should be fully informed and involved in the decision making process. All surgical and endoscopic procedures should be performed by specialists in recognised cancer units.

ER should be used as a potentially curative treatment for IMC and focal HGD, and also has an emerging role in aiding histological diagnosis. Following ER the goal should be to ablate the entire Barrett's segment. Due to the technical difficulties and costs associated with PDT, its role is increasingly being superseded by that of RFA. Following initial ablative therapy, further treatments (using the same or different treatment modalities) should be given in an attempt to destroy any remaining metaplastic / dysplastic epithelium. The aim should be complete squamous regeneration, however even if successful, surveillance should be life-long as glands with malignant potential may persist burried beneathe the regenerated mucosa.

This combination of endoscopic resection and ablation of high-grade dysplasia and intramucosal cancer offers alternative therapeutic options to those unsuitable or unwilling to contemplate radical surgical excision. This combination endotherapy has been shown to provide long-term survival in patients with HGD and IMC and it is possible that this management strategy may soon become the treatment of choice for all patients with HGD.

14. References

Buttar, N. S., Wang, K. K., Sebo, T. J., Riehle, D. M., Krishnadath, K. K., Lutzke, L. S., Anderson, M. A., Petterson, T. M. and Burgart, L. J. (2001), "Extent of high-grade dysplasia in Barrett's esophagus correlates with risk of adenocarcinoma", *Gastroenterology,* vol. 120, no. 7, pp. 1630-1639.

BSG Working Party: A Report of the Working Party of the British Society of Gastroenterology, principal authors: A Watson, RC Heading, NA Shepherd (2005), "Guidelines for the diagnosis and management of Barrett's columnar-lined oesophagus".

Cancer Research UK. (2010*), Oesophageal cancer - UK incidence statistics.* http://info.cancerresearchuk.org/cancerstats/types/oesophagus/incidence/

Corley, D. A., Levin, T. R., Habel, L. A., Weiss, N. S. and Buffler, P. A. (2002), "Surveillance and survival in Barrett's adenocarcinomas: a population-based study", *Gastroenterology,* vol. 122, no. 3, pp. 633-640.

Curvers, W., Baak, L., Kiesslich, R., Van Oijen, A., Rabenstein, T., Ragunath, K., Rey, J. F., Scholten, P., Seitz, U., Ten Kate, F., Fockens, P. and Bergman, J. (2008a), "Chromoendoscopy and narrow-band imaging compared with high-resolution magnification endoscopy in Barrett's esophagus", *Gastroenterology,* vol. 134, no. 3, pp. 670-679.

Curvers, W. L., Bansal, A., Sharma, P. and Bergman, J. J. (2008b), "Endoscopic work-up of early Barrett's neoplasia", *Endoscopy,* vol. 40, no. 12, pp. 1000-1007.

Curvers, W. L., Kiesslich, R. and Bergman, J. J. (2008c), "Novel imaging modalities in the detection of oesophageal neoplasia", *Best practice & research.Clinical gastroenterology,* vol. 22, no. 4, pp. 687-720.

Curvers, W. L., Singh, R., Song, L. M., Wolfsen, H. C., Ragunath, K., Wang, K., Wallace, M. B., Fockens, P. and Bergman, J. J. (2008d), "Endoscopic tri-modal imaging for detection of early neoplasia in Barrett's oesophagus: a multi-centre feasibility study using high-resolution endoscopy, autofluorescence imaging and narrow band imaging incorporated in one endoscopy system", *Gut,* vol. 57, no. 2, pp. 167-172.

Drewitz, D. J., Sampliner, R. E. and Garewal, H. S. (1997), "The incidence of adenocarcinoma in Barrett's esophagus: a prospective study of 170 patients followed 4.8 years", *The American Journal of Gastroenterology,* vol. 92, no. 2, pp. 212-215.

Ell, C., May, A., Pech, O., Gossner, L., Guenter, E., Behrens, A., Nachbar, L., Huijsmans, J., Vieth, M. and Stolte, M. (2007), "Curative endoscopic resection of early esophageal adenocarcinomas (Barrett's cancer)", *Gastrointestinal endoscopy,* vol. 65, no. 1, pp. 3-10.

Evans, J. A., Poneros, J. M., Bouma, B. E., Bressner, J., Halpern, E. F., Shishkov, M., Lauwers, G. Y., Mino-Kenudson, M., Nishioka, N. S. and Tearney, G. J. (2006), "Optical coherence tomography to identify intramucosal carcinoma and high-grade dysplasia in Barrett's esophagus", *Clinical gastroenterology and hepatology : the official clinical practice journal of the American Gastroenterological Association,* vol. 4, no. 1, pp. 38-43.

Fountoulakis, A., Zafirellis, K. D., Dolan, K., Dexter, S. P., Martin, I. G. and Sue-Ling, H. M. (2004), "Effect of surveillance of Barrett's oesophagus on the clinical outcome of oesophageal cancer", *The British journal of surgery,* vol. 91, no. 8, pp. 997-1003.

Gondrie, J. J., Pouw, R. E., Sondermeijer, C. M., Peters, F. P., Curvers, W. L., Rosmolen, W. D., Krishnadath, K. K., Ten Kate, F., Fockens, P. and Bergman, J. J. (2008), "Stepwise circumferential and focal ablation of Barrett's esophagus with high-grade dysplasia: results of the first prospective series of 11 patients", *Endoscopy,* vol. 40, no. 5, pp. 359-369.

Hirota, W. K., Loughney, T. M., Lazas, D. J., Maydonovitch, C. L., Rholl, V. and Wong, R. K. (1999), "Specialized intestinal metaplasia, dysplasia, and cancer of the esophagus and esophagogastric junction: prevalence and clinical data", *Gastroenterology,* vol. 116, no. 2, pp. 277-285.

Isenberg, G., Sivak, M. V.,Jr, Chak, A., Wong, R. C., Willis, J. E., Wolf, B., Rowland, D. Y., Das, A. and Rollins, A. (2005), "Accuracy of endoscopic optical coherence tomography in the detection of dysplasia in Barrett's esophagus: a prospective, double-blinded study", *Gastrointestinal endoscopy,* vol. 62, no. 6, pp. 825-831.

Jankowski, J. A., Harrison, R. F., Perry, I., Balkwill, F. and Tselepis, C. (2000), "Barrett's metaplasia", *Lancet,* vol. 356, no. 9247, pp. 2079-2085.

Jankowski, J. A., Provenzale, D. and Moayyedi, P. (2002), "Esophageal adenocarcinoma arising from Barrett's metaplasia has regional variations in the west", *Gastroenterology,* vol. 122, no. 2, pp. 588-590.

Kara, M. A., Ennahachi, M., Fockens, P., ten Kate, F. J. and Bergman, J. J. (2006a), "Detection and classification of the mucosal and vascular patterns (mucosal morphology) in Barrett's esophagus by using narrow band imaging", *Gastrointestinal endoscopy,* vol. 64, no. 2, pp. 155-166.

Kara, M. A., Peters, F. P., Fockens, P., ten Kate, F. J. and Bergman, J. J. (2006b), "Endoscopic video-autofluorescence imaging followed by narrow band imaging for detecting early neoplasia in Barrett's esophagus", *Gastrointestinal endoscopy,* vol. 64, no. 2, pp. 176-185.

Kara, M. A., Peters, F. P., Rosmolen, W. D., Krishnadath, K. K., ten Kate, F. J., Fockens, P. and Bergman, J. J. (2005a), "High-resolution endoscopy plus chromoendoscopy or narrow-band imaging in Barrett's esophagus: a prospective randomized crossover study", *Endoscopy,* vol. 37, no. 10, pp. 929-936.

Kara, M. A., Peters, F. P., Ten Kate, F. J., Van Deventer, S. J., Fockens, P. and Bergman, J. J. (2005b), "Endoscopic video autofluorescence imaging may improve the detection of early neoplasia in patients with Barrett's esophagus", *Gastrointestinal endoscopy,* vol. 61, no. 6, pp. 679-685.

Kara, M. A., Smits, M. E., Rosmolen, W. D., Bultje, A. C., Ten Kate, F. J., Fockens, P., Tytgat, G. N. and Bergman, J. J. (2005c), "A randomized crossover study comparing light-induced fluorescence endoscopy with standard videoendoscopy for the detection of early neoplasia in Barrett's esophagus", *Gastrointestinal endoscopy,* vol. 61, no. 6, pp. 671-678.

Kendall, C., Stone, N., Shepherd, N., Geboes, K., Warren, B., Bennett, R. and Barr, H. (2003), "Raman spectroscopy, a potential tool for the objective identification and classification of neoplasia in Barrett's oesophagus.", *Journal of Pathology,* vol. 200, no. 5, pp. 602-609.

Kiesslich, R., Gossner, L., Goetz, M., Dahlmann, A., Vieth, M., Stolte, M., Hoffman, A., Jung, M., Nafe, B., Galle, P. R. and Neurath, M. F. (2006), "In vivo histology of Barrett's esophagus and associated neoplasia by confocal laser endomicroscopy", *Clinical gastroenterology and hepatology : the official clinical practice journal of the American Gastroenterological Association,* vol. 4, no. 8, pp. 979-987.

Lim, C. H., Rotimi, O., Dexter, S. P. and Axon, A. T. (2006), "Randomized crossover study that used methylene blue or random 4-quadrant biopsy for the diagnosis of dysplasia in Barrett's esophagus", *Gastrointestinal endoscopy,* vol. 64, no. 2, pp. 195-199.

Lu, S. and Wang, T. D. (2008), "In vivo cancer biomarkers of esophageal neoplasia", *Cancer biomarkers : section A of Disease markers,* vol. 4, no. 6, pp. 341-350.

Mandal, R. V., Forcione, D. G., Brugge, W. R., Nishioka, N. S., Mino-Kenudson, M. and Lauwers, G. Y. (2009), "Effect of tumor characteristics and duplication of the muscularis mucosae on the endoscopic staging of superficial Barrett esophagus-related neoplasia", *The American Journal of Surgical Pathology,* vol. 33, no. 4, pp. 620-625.

May, A., Gossner, L., Pech, O., Muller, H., Vieth, M., Stolte, M. and Ell, C. (2002), "Intraepithelial high-grade neoplasia and early adenocarcinoma in short-segment Barrett's esophagus (SSBE): curative treatment using local endoscopic treatment techniques", *Endoscopy,* vol. 34, no. 8, pp. 604-610.

May, A., Gunter, E., Roth, F., Gossner, L., Stolte, M., Vieth, M. and Ell, C. (2004), "Accuracy of staging in early oesophageal cancer using high resolution endoscopy and high resolution endosonography: a comparative, prospective, and blinded trial", *Gut,* vol. 53, no. 5, pp. 634-640.

Odze, R. D. and Lauwers, G. Y. (2008), "Histopathology of Barrett's esophagus after ablation and endoscopic mucosal resection therapy", *Endoscopy,* vol. 40, no. 12, pp. 1008-1015.

Overholt, B. F., Lightdale, C. J., Wang, K. K., Canto, M. I., Burdick, S., Haggitt, R. C., Bronner, M. P., Taylor, S. L., Grace, M. G., Depot, M. and International Photodynamic Group for High-Grade Dysplasia in Barrett's Esophagus (2005), "Photodynamic therapy with porfimer sodium for ablation of high-grade dysplasia in Barrett's esophagus: international, partially blinded, randomized phase III trial", *Gastrointestinal endoscopy,* vol. 62, no. 4, pp. 488-498.

Overholt, B. F., Wang, K. K., Burdick, J. S., Lightdale, C. J., Kimmey, M., Nava, H. R., Sivak, M. V.,Jr, Nishioka, N., Barr, H., Marcon, N., Pedrosa, M., Bronner, M. P., Grace, M., Depot, M. and International Photodynamic Group for High-Grade Dysplasia in Barrett's Esophagus (2007), "Five-year efficacy and safety of photodynamic therapy with Photofrin in Barrett's high-grade dysplasia", *Gastrointestinal endoscopy,* vol. 66, no. 3, pp. 460-468.

Pech, O., May, A., Rabenstein, T. and Ell, C. (2007), "Endoscopic resection of early oesophageal cancer", *Gut,* vol. 56, no. 11, pp. 1625-1634.

Peters, F. P., Brakenhoff, K. P., Curvers, W. L., Rosmolen, W. D., Fockens, P., ten Kate, F. J., Krishnadath, K. K. and Bergman, J. J. (2008), "Histologic evaluation of resection specimens obtained at 293 endoscopic resections in Barrett's esophagus", *Gastrointestinal endoscopy,* vol. 67, no. 4, pp. 604-609.

Peters, J. H., Clark, G. W., Ireland, A. P., Chandrasoma, P., Smyrk, T. C. and DeMeester, T. R. (1994), "Outcome of adenocarcinoma arising in Barrett's esophagus in endoscopically surveyed and nonsurveyed patients", *The Journal of thoracic and cardiovascular surgery,* vol. 108, no. 5, pp. 813-21; discussion 821-2.

Peyre, C. G., Hagen, J. A., DeMeester, S. R., Van Lanschot, J. J., Holscher, A., Law, S., Ruol, A., Ancona, E., Griffin, S. M., Altorki, N. K., Rice, T. W., Wong, J., Lerut, T. and DeMeester, T. R. (2008), "Predicting systemic disease in patients with esophageal cancer after esophagectomy: a multinational study on the significance of the number of involved lymph nodes", *Annals of Surgery,* vol. 248, no. 6, pp. 979-985.

Pierce, M. C., Javier, D. J. and Richards-Kortum, R. (2008), "Optical contrast agents and imaging systems for detection and diagnosis of cancer", *International journal of cancer.Journal international du cancer,* vol. 123, no. 9, pp. 1979-1990.

Pohl, H., Rosch, T., Vieth, M., Koch, M., Becker, V., Anders, M., Khalifa, A. C. and Meining, A. (2008), "Miniprobe confocal laser microscopy for the detection of invisible neoplasia in patients with Barrett's oesophagus", *Gut,* vol. 57, no. 12, pp. 1648-1653.

Prasad, G. A., Wang, K. K., Buttar, N. S., Wongkeesong, L. M., Krishnadath, K. K., Nichols, F. C.,3rd, Lutzke, L. S. and Borkenhagen, L. S. (2007), "Long-term survival following endoscopic and surgical treatment of high-grade dysplasia in Barrett's esophagus", *Gastroenterology,* vol. 132, no. 4, pp. 1226-1233.

Ragunath, K., Krasner, N., Raman, V. S., Haqqani, M. T. and Cheung, W. Y. (2003), "A randomized, prospective cross-over trial comparing methylene blue-directed biopsy and conventional random biopsy for detecting intestinal metaplasia and dysplasia in Barrett's esophagus", *Endoscopy,* vol. 35, no. 12, pp. 998-1003.

Reid, B. J., Blount, P. L., Feng, Z. and Levine, D. S. (2000a), "Optimizing endoscopic biopsy detection of early cancers in Barrett's high-grade dysplasia", *The American Journal of Gastroenterology,* vol. 95, no. 11, pp. 3089-3096.

Reid, B. J., Levine, D. S., Longton, G., Blount, P. L. and Rabinovitch, P. S. (2000b), "Predictors of progression to cancer in Barrett's esophagus: baseline histology and flow cytometry identify low- and high-risk patient subsets", *The American Journal of Gastroenterology,* vol. 95, no. 7, pp. 1669-1676.

Riddell, R. H., Goldman, H., Ransohoff, D. F., Appelman, H. D., Fenoglio, C. M., Haggitt, R. C., Ahren, C., Correa, P., Hamilton, S. R. and Morson, B. C. (1983), "Dysplasia in inflammatory bowel disease: standardized classification with provisional clinical applications", *Human pathology,* vol. 14, no. 11, pp. 931-968.

Schnell, T. G., Sontag, S. J. and Chejfec, G. (1992), "Adenocarcinomas arising in tongues or short segments of Barrett's esophagus", *Digestive diseases and sciences,* vol. 37, no. 1, pp. 137-143.

Schnell, T. G., Sontag, S. J., Chejfec, G., Aranha, G., Metz, A., O'Connell, S., Seidel, U. J. and Sonnenberg, A. (2001a), "Long-term nonsurgical management of Barrett's esophagus with high-grade dysplasia", *Gastroenterology,* vol. 120, no. 7, pp. 1607-1619.

Schnell, T. G., Sontag, S. J., Chejfec, G., Aranha, G., Metz, A., O'Connell, S., Seidel, U. J. and Sonnenberg, A. (2001b), "Long-term nonsurgical management of Barrett's esophagus with high-grade dysplasia", *Gastroenterology,* vol. 120, no. 7, pp. 1607-1619.

Seewald, S., Akaraviputh, T., Seitz, U., Brand, B., Groth, S., Mendoza, G., He, X., Thonke, F., Stolte, M., Schroeder, S. and Soehendra, N. (2003), "Circumferential EMR and complete removal of Barrett's epithelium: a new approach to management of Barrett's esophagus containing high-grade intraepithelial neoplasia and intramucosal carcinoma", *Gastrointestinal endoscopy,* vol. 57, no. 7, pp. 854-859.

Shaheen, N. and Ransohoff, D. F. (2002), "Gastroesophageal reflux, Barrett esophagus, and esophageal cancer: clinical applications", *JAMA : the journal of the American Medical Association,* vol. 287, no. 15, pp. 1982-1986.

Shaheen, N. J., Crosby, M. A., Bozymski, E. M. and Sandler, R. S. (2000), "Is there publication bias in the reporting of cancer risk in Barrett's esophagus?", *Gastroenterology,* vol. 119, no. 2, pp. 333-338.

Shaheen, N. J. and Richter, J. E. (2009), "Barrett's oesophagus", *Lancet,* vol. 373, no. 9666, pp. 850-861.

Shaheen, N. J., Sharma, P., Overholt, B. F., Wolfsen, H. C., Sampliner, R. E., Wang, K. K., Galanko, J. A., Bronner, M. P., Goldblum, J. R., Bennett, A. E., Jobe, B. A., Eisen, G. M., Fennerty, M. B., Hunter, J. G., Fleischer, D. E., Sharma, V. K., Hawes, R. H., Hoffman, B. J., Rothstein, R. I., Gordon, S. R., Mashimo, H., Chang, K. J., Muthusamy, V. R., Edmundowicz, S. A., Spechler, S. J., Siddiqui, A. A., Souza, R. F., Infantolino, A., Falk, G. W., Kimmey, M. B., Madanick, R. D., Chak, A. and Lightdale, C. J. (2009), "Radiofrequency ablation in Barrett's esophagus with dysplasia", *The New England journal of medicine,* vol. 360, no. 22, pp. 2277-2288.

Sharma, P., Bansal, A., Mathur, S., Wani, S., Cherian, R., McGregor, D., Higbee, A., Hall, S. and Weston, A. (2006a), "The utility of a novel narrow band imaging endoscopy system in patients with Barrett's esophagus", *Gastrointestinal endoscopy,* vol. 64, no. 2, pp. 167-175.

Sharma, P., Dent, J., Armstrong, D., Bergman, J. J., Gossner, L., Hoshihara, Y., Jankowski, J. A., Junghard, O., Lundell, L., Tytgat, G. N. and Vieth, M. (2006b), "The development and validation of an endoscopic grading system for Barrett's esophagus: the Prague C & M criteria", *Gastroenterology,* vol. 131, no. 5, pp. 1392-1399.

Sharma, P., Morales, T. G., Bhattacharyya, A., Garewal, H. S. and Sampliner, R. E. (1997), "Dysplasia in short-segment Barrett's esophagus: a prospective 3-year follow-up", *The American Journal of Gastroenterology,* vol. 92, no. 11, pp. 2012-2016.

Spechler, S. J., Fitzgerald, R. C., Prasad, G. A. and Wang, K. K. (2010), "History, molecular mechanisms, and endoscopic treatment of Barrett's esophagus", *Gastroenterology,* vol. 138, no. 3, pp. 854-869.

Streitz, J. M.,Jr, Andrews, C. W.,Jr and Ellis, F. H.,Jr (1993), "Endoscopic surveillance of Barrett's esophagus. Does it help?", *The Journal of thoracic and cardiovascular surgery,* vol. 105, no. 3, pp. 383-7; discussion 387-8.

Thekkek, N., Anandasabapathy, S. and Richards-Kortum, R. (2011), "Optical molecular imaging for detection of Barrett's-associated neoplasia", *World journal of gastroenterology : WJG,* vol. 17, no. 1, pp. 53-62.

van Sandick, J. W., van Lanschot, J. J., Kuiken, B. W., Tytgat, G. N., Offerhaus, G. J. and Obertop, H. (1998), "Impact of endoscopic biopsy surveillance of Barrett's oesophagus on pathological stage and clinical outcome of Barrett's carcinoma", *Gut,* vol. 43, no. 2, pp. 216-222.

Vieth, M., Ell, C., Gossner, L., May, A. and Stolte, M. (2004), "Histological analysis of endoscopic resection specimens from 326 patients with Barrett's esophagus and early neoplasia", *Endoscopy,* vol. 36, no. 9, pp. 776-781.

Wong, T., Tian, J. and Nagar, A. B. (2010), "Barrett's surveillance identifies patients with early esophageal adenocarcinoma", *The American Journal of Medicine,* vol. 123, no. 5, pp. 462-467.

Zuccaro, G.,Jr, Rice, T. W., Vargo, J. J., Goldblum, J. R., Rybicki, L. A., Dumot, J. A., Adelstein, D. J., Trolli, P. A. and Blackstone, E. H. (2005), "Endoscopic ultrasound errors in esophageal cancer", *The American Journal of Gastroenterology,* vol. 100, no. 3, pp. 601-606.

12

Atrophic Body Gastritis: A Challenge for the Presumptive Endoscopic and Histologic Diagnosis of Autoimmune Gastritis

Alfredo J. A. Barbosa and Camila G. Miranda
Laboratory of Digestive and Neuroendocrine Pathology, Faculty of Medicine, Federal University of Minas Gerais (UFMG), Belo Horizonte Brazil

1. Introduction

The diagnosis of glandular atrophy of the gastric mucosa (gastric atrophy) remains a challenge in the areas of gastrointestinal endoscopy and pathology. The importance of an endoscopic suspicion of this regressive tissue change is the possibility of alerting the pathologist to its presence. Patients with gastric atrophy, especially in more advanced stages, are more prone to develop intestinal metaplasia, dysplasia and gastric carcinoma, known as the Correa cascade (Correa, 1984, 1992). The most common type of gastric atrophy is that associated with *Helicobacter pylori* (*H. pylori*) infection. In such cases, the glandular atrophy usually occurs in parallel to the course of the inflammatory process that takes place in the gastric antrum (antral gastritis, multifocal gastritis) or in both gastric antrum and body (pangastritis, multifocal gastritis). In contrast, in most cases the chronic atrophic gastritis selective of the gastric body and sparing the antral mucosa is a consequence of an autoimmune inflammatory process. For the purpose of this chapter, the chronic gastritis presenting this histopathological pattern will be called atrophic body gastritis (ABG). Exceptionally, some patients with *H. pylori*-associated gastritis develop gastric lesions with histological pattern very similar to that of ABG which can lead to uncertainty about the differential histologic diagnosis with chronic gastritis of autoimmune origin.
Therefore, the two most important inflammatory diseases of the gastric mucosa, multifocal chronic gastritis and autoimmune gastritis, tend to progress to glandular atrophy of the gastric mucosa. In the first case, gastric atrophy may not occur or it develops more slowly, becoming conspicuous usually in later stages of life. In the second case, which is also more frequent with advancing age, gastric atrophy progresses more rapidly and may induce severe gastric changes also in the younger age groups. This differential course of the development of gastric atrophy in these two inflammatory diseases of the stomach involves different clinical and pathophysiological consequences. Those associated with *H. pylori* infection usually do not involve important pathophysiological changes, while the atrophy resulting from autoimmune disease often leads to well-known pathophysiological changes of the gastric mucosa, often culminating in pernicious anemia. Furthermore, the *H. pylori*-dependent glandular atrophy is considered to be a condition predisposing to gastric adenocarcinoma, which has high rates of morbidity and mortality, while the autoimmune-

dependent glandular atrophy is considered to be a condition predisposing to gastric carcinoids, which, unlike the adenocarcinomas, have low rates of morbidity and mortality. Due to the different regional involvement of the stomach by these two types of chronic gastritis, their histological recognition is relatively easy when tissue samples are properly collected and processed. However, this is not always the case.
Thus, the importance of the differential diagnosis of ABG within this group of chronic gastritis resides in the possibility of its autoimmune origin and in its major clinical consequence, i.e., pernicious anemia. Pernicious anemia and autoimmune gastritis progress in an insidious manner and are usually diagnosed when they have reached florid clinical and morphological characteristics after years of evolution. However, a number of patients with dyspeptic complaints and patients with ABG and pernicious anemia undergo endoscopy in tertiary care settings without a prior knowledge of major illness. (Carmel, R., 1996) Therefore, for some patients seeking a first endoscopy service, the collection of biopsies from the gastric mucosa may be the first opportunity to establish the initial diagnosis of ABG, with or without pernicious anemia. This is important because the evolution of subclinical gastric lesions and systemic symptoms may result in undesirable consequences that become established in a gradual manner. These consequences mainly result from achlorhydria, vitamin B12 deficiency, and the development of hyperplastic polyps and neuroendocrine tumors of the gastric mucosa. For this reason, the diagnosis of ABG acquires importance since it establishes an appropriate clinical and endoscopic follow-up of the patient.
The objective of this article is to present some data on this topic obtained from a tertiary care unit of gastrointestinal endoscopy and to discuss some pitfalls linked to the routine histopathologic diagnosis of atrophic body gastritis.

2. Methods and results

For the purpose of evaluating the outcomes of endoscopic examination of patients with a final histopathological diagnosis of ABG we surveyed all cases of upper gastrointestinal endoscopy with biopsy sampling of gastric antrum and gastric body performed from 2007 to 2009 at a referral center for digestive endoscopy in the city of Belo Horizonte, Brazil.
A total of 6,005 consecutive gastroesophageal endoscopies with gastric biopsies of the antral and body mucosa of the stomach were reviewed. Among these cases 2,564 (42.7%) had the diagnosis of chronic gastritis as the main pathological condition of the gastric mucosa. Of these, 141 (5.5%) had a diagnosis of atrophic body gastritis (type A gastritis) suggestive of an autoimmune nature. However, a conclusive diagnosis could not be made in the remaining 230 patients (9.0%) whose histology report was mainly descriptive, stating the presence of "chronic gastritis of the body with areas of atrophy" or "body-predominant chronic atrophic gastritis ". Therefore, in most cases of chronic gastritis with body mucosa atrophy it seems that the pathologists did not find sufficient morphological evidence for a more conclusive diagnosis.
All histological slides of the 141 cases of atrophic body gastritis as well as those of the 230 patients with inconclusive diagnosis of gastritis were re-examined by an expert gastrointestinal pathologist (AJAB). When necessary the corresponding paraffin blocks were recovered for new histological sections. After reviewing all cases, the previous diagnosis of the 141 patients with atrophic body gastritis was confirmed. Among the 230 patients with an inconclusive diagnosis, 55 (24%) could be confirmed as cases of atrophic body gastritis

(Table 1). The 196 patients with a final histologic diagnosis of ABG ranged in age from 11 to 94 years, with a significant predominance of females (76.0%) over males (24.0%). Fifty patients were in a relatively young age range (31 to 50 years), with an even more significant predominance of females, i. e., 83.3% *vs* 16.7% (Figure 1) .The remaining 175 patients were excluded from the study, either because the biopsy specimens of the antral or oxyntic mucosa were not fairly representative for histology or because they could be considered as cases of multifocal atrophic gastritis, regardless of the presence of *H. pylori* infection. Finally, the histological findings of the 196 patients with a diagnosis of atrophic body gastritis were correlated with the endoscopic reports (Table 2).

	Total of cases	%
All cases of chronic gastritis	2.564	100
Atrophic body gastritis	141	5,5
Unspecified atrophic gastritis	230	9,0
ABG after review of unspecified atrophic gastritis	55	2,2
Total of ABG diagnosed	196	7,6

Table 1. Main histological diagnosis of 6,005 gastroesophageal endoscopies carried out from 2007-2009 in a tertiary care unit of gastrointestinal endoscopy, Belo Horizonte, Brazil

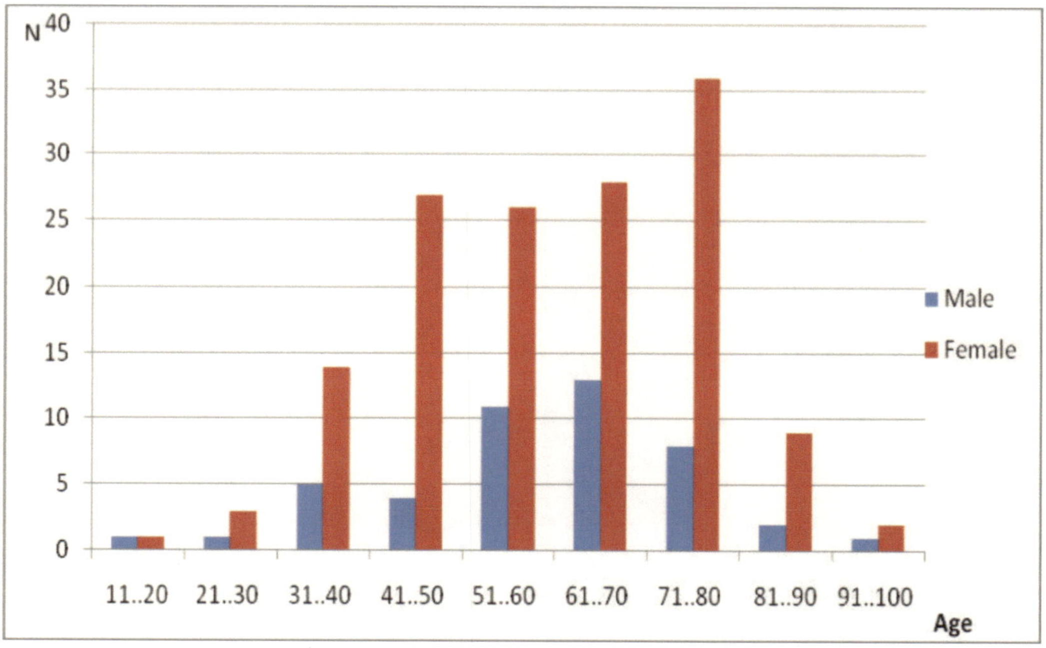

Fig. 1. Distribution of the 196 patients with the final diagnosis of ABG according to the age and gender

Among the 2,564 patients with chronic gastritis, 196 (7.6%) had a conclusive histologic diagnosis of atrophic body gastritis (type A chronic gastritis). Gastric mucosa samples of almost all of these patients showed well preserved antral mucosa, and severe glandular atrophy of the body mucosa (Figure 2 A, C, D). This atrophy was mainly represented by partial or complete replacement of oxyntopeptic glands with glands with intestinal metaplasia and antral-type mucous glands known as pseudoantral or pseudopyloric metaplasia (Figs. 2 D and 3). In several small fragments with poor representation of gastric mucosa, the pseudoantral metaplasia seemed to be a factor responsible for the failure to distinguish between antral and body atrophic mucosa. Small biopsy fragments of atrophic

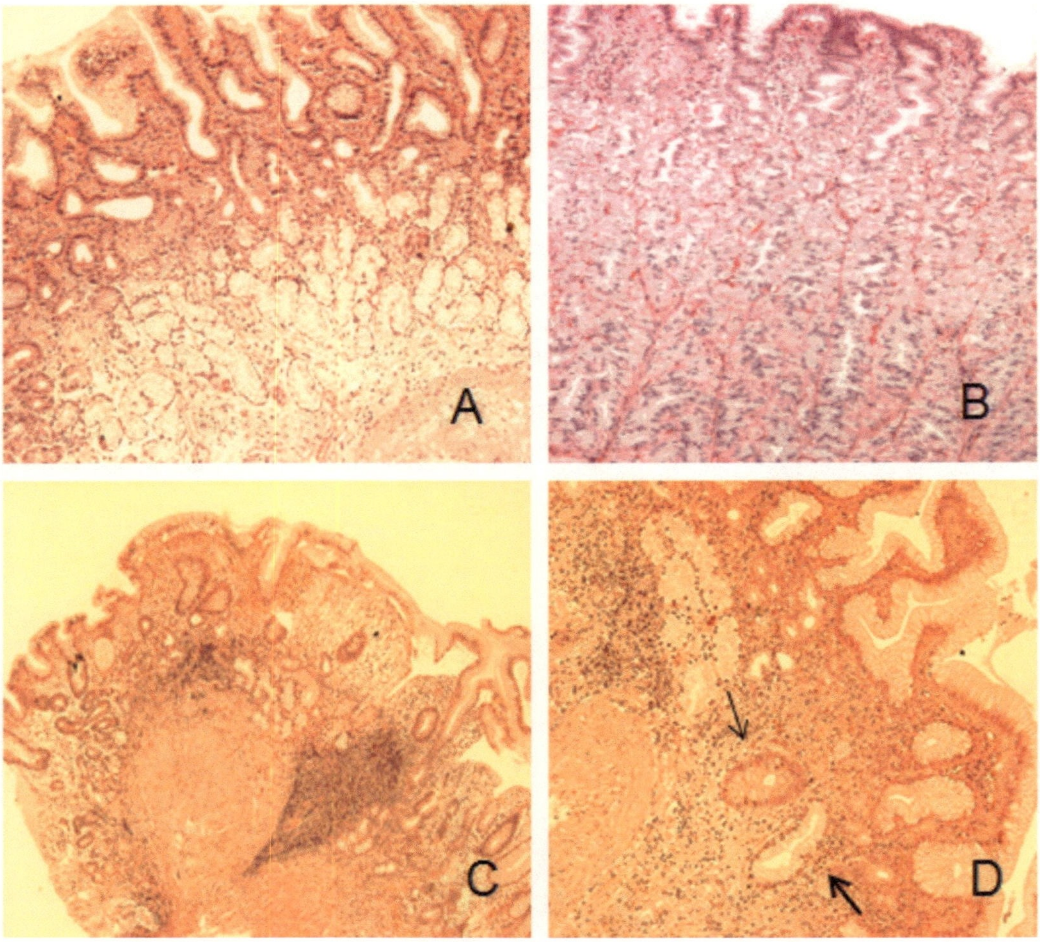

Fig. 2. Normal gastric mucosa of the antrum (A) and body (B) regions. Note that the foveolar region of the gastric antrum occupies approximately half the mucosa thickness while the mucus-secreting glands are distributed in the basal half of the mucosa. The connective tissue of the lamina propria is visible between the glands. Differently, the body mucosa (B) have short foveolas, and the oxintopeptic glands are numerous and justaposed occupy almost the entire space of conjunctive masking the lamina propria. C and D: body mucosa with severe glandular atrophy from a patients with ABG. Presence of glands with intestinal metaplasia (thin arrow) and pseudoantral metaplasia (thick arrow). The antral mucosa seen in A is from the same patient with ABG seen in C and D

body mucosa, or fragments that were cut tangentially, could present a morphological pattern similar to that of pyloric mucosa with chronic inflammation, thus leading to a diagnosis of multifocal gastritis instead of ABG (Figure 3). The boundaries between these two histological types of chronic gastritis become even more critical when *H. pylori* is present, which is an unusual occurrence. In the present series of ABG, *H. pylori* was found in only 9 (4.6%) cases.

The main endoscopic diagnosis of the 196 cases of atrophic body gastritis were as follows: (a) 76 (38.8%) cases of atrophic pangastritis, (b) 63 (32.1%) cases of pangastritis with apparent atrophy of the gastric body mucosa, (c) 42 (21.4%) cases of light enanthematous pangastritis, (d) 10 (5.1%) cases of pangastritis with gastric polyps, (e) 2 (1.0%) cases with endoscopically normal gastric mucosa, and 2 (1.0%) endoscopically unspecified cases (Table 2).

Main endoscopic reports	N	%
Atrophic pangastritis	76	38,8
Enantematous pangastritis/likely body mucosa atrophy	63	32,1
Light enantematous pangastritis	21	10,7
Antropyloric-predominant enantematous pangastritis	21	10,7
Body-predominant enentematous pangastritis	01	0,51
Gastric polyps	10	5,10
Normal gastric mucosa	02	1,02
Unspecified	02	1,02

Table 2. Main endoscopic report conclusions of the 196 patients with histologic ABG

3. Discussion

For many dyspeptic patients the diagnosis of ABG is the first step indicating the presence of autoimmune gastritis, associated or not with pernicious anemia. Since some of these patients should be monitored periodically from a clinical point of view and regarding the changes in their gastric mucosa, care should be taken not to overlook cases of gastritis with predominant or selective atrophy of the gastric fundus and body on the occasion of the first medical procedures they undergo. Knowing that the final diagnosis of this pathological entity usually depends on a close interaction between endoscopist and pathologist, an indication of the presence of these endoscopic changes to the pathologist directs more attention to the correct diagnosis. This correlation becomes even more necessary if we consider that the histologic processing artifacts, the absence of oxintopeptic glands in the histological sections plus the presence of extensive areas of intestinal and pseudoantral metaplasia, may complicate at first sight the differential diagnosis between ABG and atrophic multifocal gastritis.

Table 2 shows that standard endoscopic examination detected signs of gastric mucosa atrophy in 139 (70.9%) patients with ABG, although the affected gastric region was not specified. In the other 57 (29.1%) patients this change was not found although severe glandular atrophy of the body was found at histology. A more precise endoscopic report could direct the pathologist to a more conclusive histologic diagnosis. Most of the 55 patients confirmed as ABG cases among the 230 patients with varying degrees of mucosal atrophy at histology had an inaccurate endoscopy report.

3.1 Gastric mucosal atrophy: A problematic area of histopathology

The histologic diagnosis of gastric mucosa atrophy remains a difficult area to handle. In addition to the subjectivity of the histologic diagnosis, other factors contribute to blurring the histological interpretation, such as: (*a*) representativeness of the limited endoscopic biopsy. This bias occurs more often in cases in which a small number of biopsies are obtained for this purpose. It should be remembered here that both major types of chronic gastritis and glandular atrophy of the gastric mucosa occur with multifocal distribution. Therefore, the number of gastric biopsies, while important, need not exceed 2 to 4 fragments per region of the stomach, except for special conditions. Consensus among pathologists and endoscopists advocates, in routine cases, two biopsies from the antral region, two from the body and one from the *incisura angularis* (angular notch) (Dixon et al, 1999); (*b*) important for a more accurate diagnosis of glandular atrophy of the gastric mucosa is the good representativeness of the tissue sections. Slices containing the entire thickness of the mucosa, from the more superficial epithelial lining to the *muscularis mucosa*, favor a more reliable histopathological analysis for the interpretation of the presence of glandular atrophy (Fig. 2 A, C, D); (*c*) endoscopic biopsies showing histologic processing distortions arising from inappropriate tangential sections of the mucosa limit the observation of tissue components; (*d*) prominent inflammatory changes and exuberant lymphoid follicles can cause distortion or separation of glands, giving false impression of glandular rarefaction; (*e*) endoscopic biopsies from only one region of the stomach, for example, only from the antral region, leave the mucosa of the body without proper histological analysis. In these cases, selective glandular atrophy of the mucosa of the body may be missed in cases where the body mucosa presents a false endoscopic appearance of normality.

Although highly subjective and dependent on many factors inherent in sampling, the diagnosis and grading of glandular atrophy of the gastric mucosa rests on the final decision of the pathologist. Moreover, in cases of severe atrophy histopathological diagnosis consistently achieves high sensitivity and reproducibility when the endoscopic and histotechnical procedures prior to histological analysis run with relative normality.

It should be remembered that the oxyntic mucosa usually presents a much higher glandular density than that of the antral mucosa. At first, connective tissue and small vessels of the *lamina propria* are not so evident because they are masked by the large number of juxtaposed oxintopeptic glands (Fig. 2 B). This fact becomes more relevant because of tissue shrinkage caused by fixatives commonly used, such as formaldehyde. Tissue fixatives retract the mucosal structures, especially the loose connective tissue of the *lamina propria*. Thus, when examining a histological section of normal oxyntic mucosa the first impression one gets is that it appears to be constituted by almost only glandular epithelial tissue.

Therefore, the loss of oxyntic glands and their replacement with connective tissue tends to be clearly identified by histology. In these cases the degree of subjectivity for the diagnosis of atrophy can be considered small. In contrast, the antral mucosa usually presents less dense glandular tissue and the *lamina propria* is more apparent with a consequent more problematic histologic interpretation of moderate degrees of atrophy in this region (Fig. 2 A). The presence of areas of intestinal metaplasia that occur with relative frequency in the antral and body mucosa in *H. pylori* chronic gastritis is an objective histological sign indicating the replacement of specialized glands of the gastric mucosa with glands of the intestinal type. This fact strengthens the diagnosis of evolving or established glandular atrophy. What the presence of intestinal metaplasia may represent regarding the existence and grading of gastric atrophy is still a debatable issue (Genta, 1996, 1997). Whether in some cases of chronic gastritis the presence of few foci of intestinal metaplasia may correspond to the existence of established glandular atrophy is still an unresolved question. However, the presence of these foci in the gastric mucosa should be considered at least a signal of ongoing glandular loss, since in most cases intestinal metaplasia is associated with patent gastric atrophy. Some authors recommend that the histological diagnosis of moderate or severe atrophy of the gastric mucosa should be limited to cases of a glandular loss of at least 50%, replaced or not with metaplastic glands (Dixon et al, 1996).

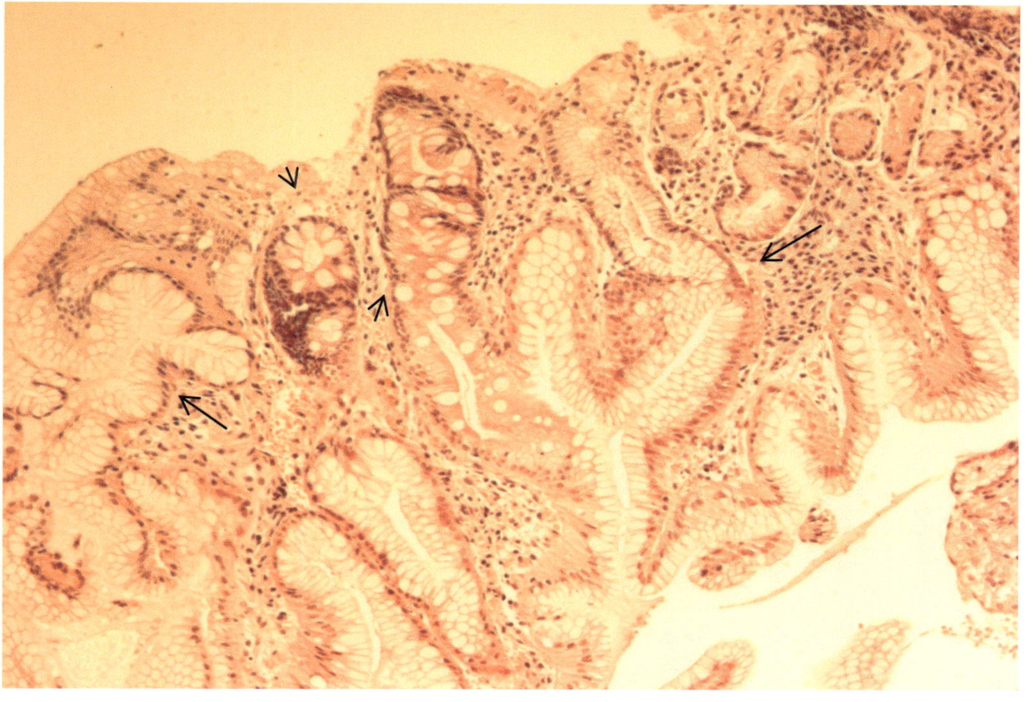

Fig. 3. Histological aspect of the body mucosa of a patient with ABG. Extensive areas of pseudoantral metaplasia (long arrows) and glands exhibiting intestinal metaplasia (short arrows). Oxyntopeptic glands are not observed. The picture may simulate atrophic antral mucosa and the diagnosis of multifocal gastritis, especially under conditions of limited interaction between endoscopists and pathologists and of inappropriate tissue processing

3.2 ABG: Waiting for a pathological definition

The designation of ABG has been extensively used without a specific definition of its limits. It is possible that the roots of this problem reside in the conceptual vagueness of what is called "atrophic gastritis" or even "gastric atrophy" (Genta, 1997). The criterion of ABG adopted for the present study involves only advanced cases of oxintopeptic mucosal atrophy with the antral mucosa showing no relevant histological changes. From a histological point of view, these patterns overlap those described for gastritis of autoimmune etiology. This definition of ABG is close to the one designated as "metaplastic autoimmune atrophic gastritis" (Park et al., 2010), and far from those defined by other authors (Vannella et al. 2011).

Therefore, when the atrophy of the gastric mucosa is clearly developed, with severe atrophy of the gastric body and fundus, the histological diagnosis of ABG can be relatively easy. Oxintopeptic glands are replaced entirely, or almost entirely, with intestinal glands (intestinal metaplasia), mucous glands (pseudoantral metaplasia) and other poorly differentiated glandular structures (Figs. 2 C, D, and 3). The endocrine cells of the oxyntic mucosa are spared from the process of atrophy, become hyperplastic what is commonly found in the ABG of autoimmune origin. Although these hyperplastic cells are considered to be enterochromaffin-like cells which are strongly reactive to the neuroendocrine marker chromogranin they can also express immunoreactivity to some peptide hormones such as ghrelin (Moreira et al. 2010).

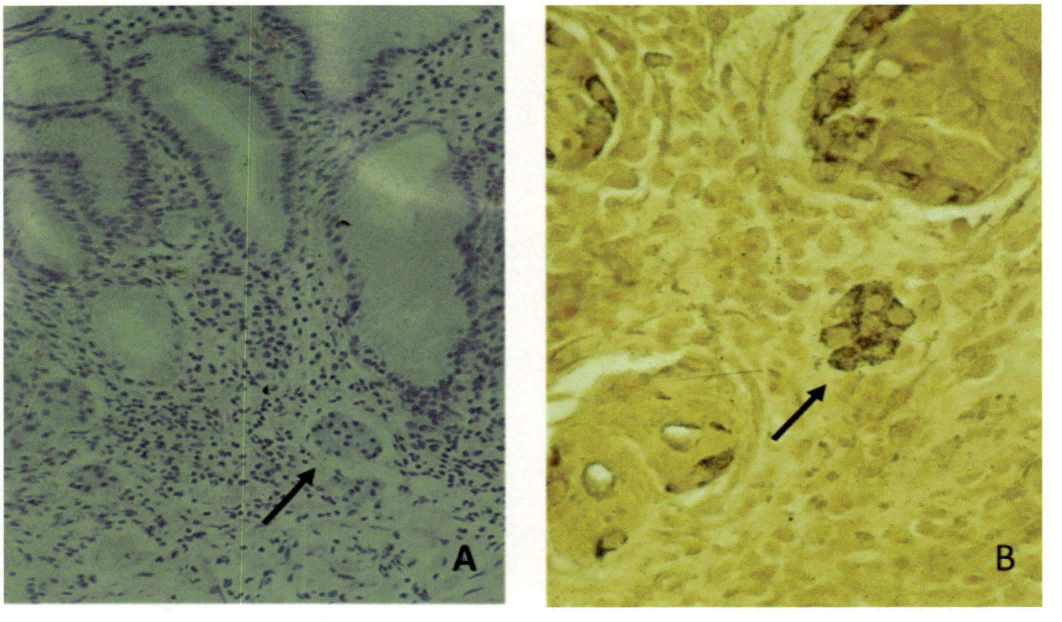

Fig. 4. Body gastric mucosa from a patient with autoimune ABG. A - Immersed in the *lamina propria* there is a nodule (arrow) composed of small cells, overlapping and even suggesting that it is related to endocrine cells (HE staining). B – Histological section of the same paraffin block stained by Grimelius technique showing hyperplasia of endocrine cells (argyrophilic cells) in the wall of the glands and hyperplastic nodules immersed in the *lamina propria* (arrow). These small nodules can be visualized in routine histological preparations, stained by HE and should raise the suspicion for the diagnosis of ABG. The presence of more intense inflammatory infiltrate in the *lamina propria* may mask the visualization of these endocrine nodules. For demonstrating the endocrine nature of these nodules, it is necessary special stainings as Grimelius technique for argyrophilic cells or immunohistochemistry using neuroendocrine markers, eg., chromogranin and neuron specific enolase

According to recent results from our laboratory regarding a large series of patients with ABG, we observed that most of the subjects presented an expressive number of ghrelin-immunoreactive cells in the different types of endocrine hyperplasia that occur in the atrophic body mucosa of these patients. Thus, ghrelin- expressing endocrine cells can be easily detected in both the hyperplastic endocrine nodules present in the *lamina propria* and diffusely in the walls of metaplastic glands (Fig. 5). Both intestinal metaplasia and pseudoantral metaplasia were frequent findings in these patients with ABG. Among 60 patients with a diagnosis of ABG, 51 presented areas of pseudoantral metaplasia in the body atrophic mucosa and most of them, i.e., 37 (72.5%) presented ghrelin-immunoreactive endocrine cells in the wall of pseudoantral metaplastic glands (Moreira & Barbosa, 2011). This fact may be of help in the differentiation between antral and body mucosa in cases of ABG. One of the methods currently used in this differentiation is the demonstration the absence of gastrin-producing cells (G cells) in the metaplastic glands of the body (pseudoantral metaplasia) since these cells are only present in the glands of the antral mucosa. In doubtful cases, this differential characteristic between the antral and pseudoantral mucosa has been used to characterize the mucosa of the body with pseudoantral metaplasia, which does not contain G cells, and to differentiate it from the true antral mucosa, which contains G cells (Park et al. 2010).Since this type of characterization of pseudoantral metaplasia is based on a negative fact (absence of G cells), the frequent presence of ghrelin-immunoreactive cells in pseudoantral metaplasia (a positive fact) could be a more reliable marker for this purpose, since these cells are rare in the glands of the normal antropyloric mucosa.

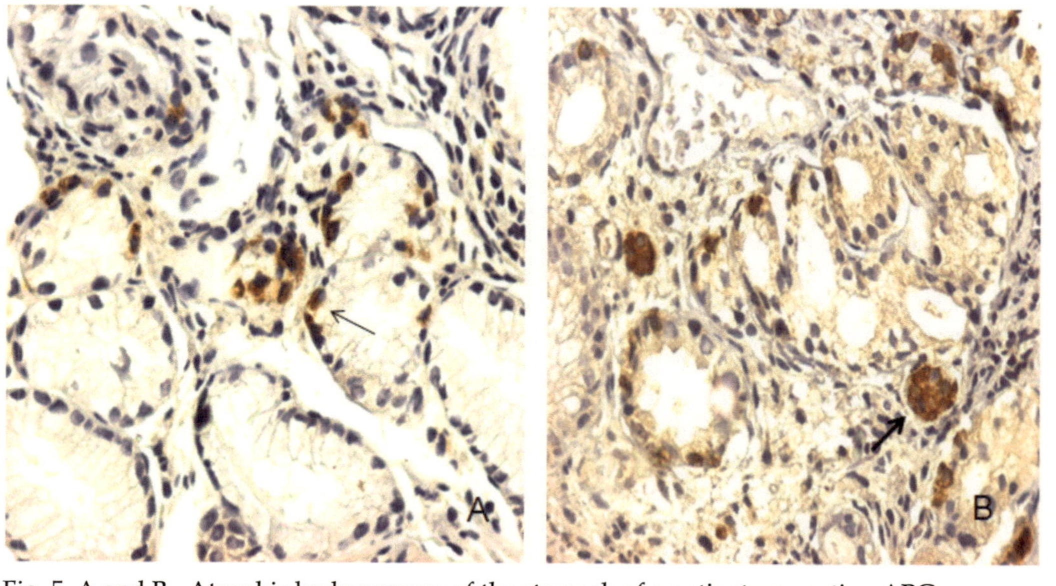

Fig. 5. A and B - Atrophic body mucosa of the stomach of a patient presenting ABG. Numerous glands exhibit pseudoantral metaplasia and most of them have endocrine cells immunoreactive to the peptide ghrelin (arrows). As ghrelin-immunoreactive cells are usually not present or are rare in antral mucosa this could be used as an reliable indication of pseudoantral metaplasia

This endocrine cell hyperplasia does not seem to occur in multifocal atrophic gastritis. Therefore, the presence of endocrine cell hyperplasia in the body mucosa of patients with ABG is a strong signal indicating the autoimmune etiology of the ABG. These florid changes of the body mucosa contrast with the discrete histological findings of the antral mucosa.

H. pylori is usually negative in these patients and, regardless of its presence, the atrophic gastritis with the morphological characteristics described above should preferably be regarded as autoimmune (Capella et al, 1999; Park et al, 2010). If necessary, serum anti-parietal cell and anti-intrinsic factor antibodies can be investigated to confirm this possibility. It should be noted that in a small percentage of patients with the pattern of morphological changes of the gastric mucosa typical of ABG, and clinically supposed to have autoimmune gastritis with pernicious anemia, the search for anti-parietal cells and/or anti-intrinsic factor antibodies may give negative results.

Some patients with pernicious anemia have been reported to have severe histological changes of the antral mucosa indistinguishable from those seen in the gastric body (Lewin et al, 1976). Recently, severe atrophic gastritis of the antrum and body mucosa has been reported in association with systemic autoimmune diseases. This pathological condition was not associated with *H. pylori* or endocrine cell hyperplasia and may affect a especific group of patients with a particular type of autoimmune gastritis. Hypothetically, these patients would develop the production of antibodies directed against multiple cell lines of the gastric mucosa (Jevremovic, 2006).

3.3 Gastric polyps and atrophic body gastritis

As seen in this series, the main endoscopic diagnosis of "gastric polyps" was relatively common among patients undergoing endoscopy who had a final diagnosis of ABG as the most important disease. We do not know how many of the 196 cases of ABG studied also had gastric polypoid lesions that were not described in the findings of endoscopic diagnostic by being considered irrelevant or by having been omitted. Likewise we are not aware of the frequency of cases of gastric polyps which, considered being the major and only injury, were removed by polypectomy without adequate sampling for histology of the mucosa of the gastric body and antrum. We believe that many pathologists face this reality in the laboratory routine, which may result in the omission of the diagnosis of the most important underlying gastric disease often responsible for the presence of polyps, such as ABG (Jain & R Chetty, R, 2009; Haruma et al, 1993).

Endoscopically, the term "gastric polyp" is applied to any bulge or swelling of the gastric mucosa, whether of epithelial origin or from underlying tissues. From a structural viewpoint, however, the term is being used by pathologists to designate lesions mainly consisting of epithelial proliferation that project into the lumen of the organ. However, the nomenclature of these lesions has not been fully defined. Moreover, the terminology used for polyps of the stomach and the description of their morphological structure are very similar to those used to describe polypoid lesions of the colon, although the biological behavior of gastric and colonic polyps does not always show the same evolutionary pattern. Gastric polyps can be divided into several types, many of which are still poorly understood in terms of their etiopathogenesis. The types for whose definition there is a more general consensus are: hyperplastic polyps, adenomatous polyps (adenomas), mixed polyps, fundic gland polyps, hamartomatous polyps, and retention polyps (juvenile). These different types of polyps may be associated with clinical syndromes (syndromic polyps) including the Peutz-Jeghers, Gardner, Cronkhite-Canada and Crowden syndromes. Among these various types of gastric polyps, the most common are hyperplastic non-syndromic polyps, which are also those most often associated with ABG. It should be added that the histological pattern of gastric hyperplastic polyps may be indistinguishable from that of polyps of syndromic origin (Lam-Himlinet al, 2010).

The gastric hyperplastic polyps are the result of reactive hyperplasia of the foveolar epithelium in response to injury or to primary disease of the gastric mucosa, including chronic gastritis with glandular atrophy, as previously mentioned (Abraham et al, 2001). Apparently, these types of polyps almost never occur in normal gastric mucosa (Fig. 6 A).

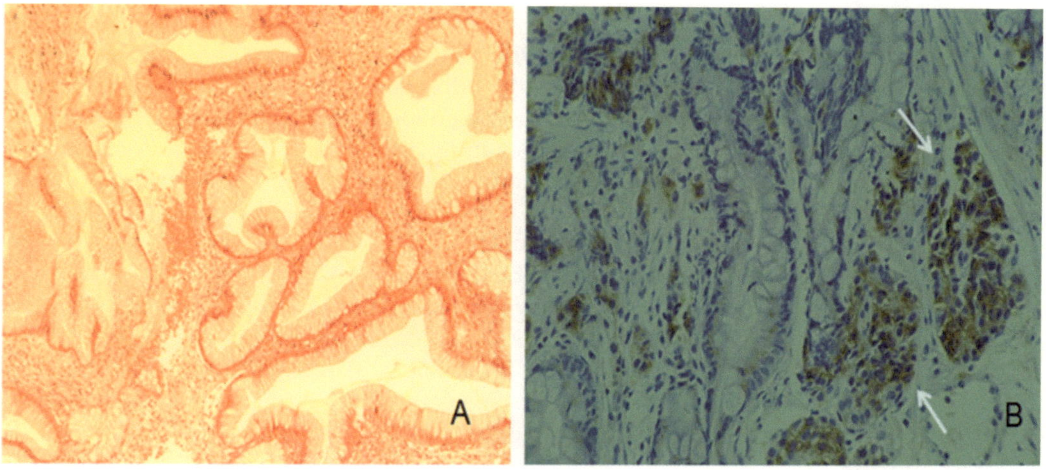

Fig. 6. Body gastric mucosa of a patient with the diagnosis of atrophic body gastritis. Intense hyperplasia of the foveolar epithelium (A), and of endocrine cells in the *lamina propria* (B) which could origin small gastric polyps. A - H.E. staining; B- Immunoperoxidase staining for chromogranin

Other endoscopic abnormalities often associated with ABG are the "gastric polyps" that occur in the body and fundus of the stomach and that derive from nodular proliferation of endocrine cells in the connective tissue of the *lamina propria* (Figure 6 B). They are usually multiple lesions located only in the body and fundus of the stomach and their presence should raise the suspicion of endoscopic ABG. Fusion of the endocrine hyperplastic nodules frequently occurs and the differential diagnosis of a neuroendocrine tumor should be considered. Since these nodules are usually multiple and not uniform, sampling of some of them does not always provide sufficient information for a final conclusion about the presence of endocrine neoplasia. In conclusion, there is a clinical and pathological significance of gastric polyps in relation to ABG because of its frequent association with both hyperplastic polyps and the polyps derived from endocrine cells proliferation (endocrine hyperplastic nodules or carcinoid tumors). However, the removal of these polyps must be accompanied by biopsies from the gastric antrum and body in order to characterize the primary process responsible for the appearance of polypoid lesions. The presence of these polyps may serve as a signal to the endoscopist of the presence of underlying disease or injury of the gastric mucosa, which is not always perceived by standard endoscopy.

3.4 Diagnosis of gastric mucosa atrophy: Endoscopic perspectives

The disagreement between endoscopic and histologic diagnosis for the presence of glandular atrophy of the gastric mucosa is not new and is relatively frequent (Torbenso et al, 2002). Standard endoscopy, although it can employ technical methods to study the thickness of the gastric mucosa such as stretching of the stomach wall by inflating air into the gastric cavity, continues to have a low accuracy index. The degree of distension of the stomach wall and visualization of the submucosal vascular network depends primarily on the professional skill and experience of the examiner, as well as on the availability of good quality equipment. Even at centers specialized in gastrointestinal endoscopy, the endoscopic-histologic correlation is weak, with sensitivity and specificity of about 40 to 60% (Eshmuratov, et al. 2010).

Therefore, since the histological method is also not reliable, at least for cases of mild or moderate atrophy, its use in combination with endoscopy continues to rest on quicksand. Opening good perspectives for the near future, the endoscopic method has progressed with the description of new visualization techniques to amplify the resolution and definition of gastrointestinal mucosa details. Thus, endoscopic techniques involving magnification with high resolution have been reported to be considerably more reliable than standard endoscopy to identify normal gastric mucosa, chronic gastritis and gastric atrophy (Anagnostopoulos et al. 2007). The progress of endoscopic techniques and the availability of high-resolution confocal laser endomicroscopy are now starting to gain firmer ground in the detection of minute lesions of the gastrointestinal mucosa, among them the different degrees of gastric mucosa atrophy (Li, CQ and Li, YQ, 2010; Goetz, M. and Kiesslich, R. 2010; Canto, 2010).

4. Conclusions

The term ABG was used in the present article to designate cases of chronic gastritis with selective glandular atrophy of the mucosa of the stomach body while the antral mucosa continued to show a normal aspect or only minimal inflammatory changes. Extensive areas of intestinal metaplasia, pseudoantral metaplasia and endocrine cell hyperplasia often occur in the atrophic mucosa of the body. Taken together, these changes of the gastric mucosa strongly suggest the presence of an inflammatory process of autoimmune etiology accompanied or not by pernicious anemia of subclinical or even clinical evolution. Thus, the major importance of the histologic diagnosis of ABG resides in the fact that, for many dyspeptic patients submitted to upper digestive endoscopy this may be the first opportunity they have to receive a correct diagnosis of their main disease.

The histologic diagnosis of glandular atrophy of the stomach of mild or moderate grade is highly subjective and depends on many factors linked to tissue collection and processing. From an endoscopic viewpoint, the diagnostic imprecision is even greater. However, the more extreme grades of atrophy of the gastric mucosa are easy to interpret histologically when tissue samples are collected, processed and interpreted in an appropriate manner. When this is not the case, the histologic diagnosis of ABG is frequently inconclusive or equivocal. In the present study, out of 230 cases with an inconclusive histological diagnosis reviewed by an expert pathologist in the gastrointestinal area, 55 (24%) were confirmed as ABG, many of them after new histologic sections were obtained from paraffin blocks. Although in the cases studied the degree of gastric atrophy was intense and circumscribed to the body, the standard endoscopic exam showed a very low correlation with the histological findings. This fact associated with problems regarding tissue collection and processing impairs a conclusive diagnosis of ABG in many cases, with a consequent delay in the diagnosis of the principal disease of a patient who seeks a service of digestive endoscopy due to nonspecific dyspeptic complaints. However, new endoscopic techniques show a clear progress that promises to reverse the current secondary role of endoscopy in combination with histology for the evaluation of patients with different degrees of gastric mucosa atrophy and consequently with chronic gastritis of autoimmune etiology.

5. Acknowledgment

This work was supported by grants from the Conselho Nacional de Desenvolvimento Científico e Tecnológico (CNPq), Brazil. The authors thank Ms. Luciene S. P. Faria for technical assistance.

6. References

Abraham, S.C., Singh, V.K., Yardley, J.K. & Wu, T.T. (2001). Hyperplastic polyps of the stomach: associations with histologic patterns of gastritis and gastric atrophy. *Am J Surg Pathol*, Vol.25, No.4, pp 500-507.

Anagnostoupoulos, G.K., Yao, K. et al. (2007). High-resolution magnification endoscopy can reliably identify normal gastric mucosa, Helicobacter pylori associated gastritis and gastric atrophy. Endoscopy, Vol.39, pp 202-207.

Canto, M.I. (2010). Endomicroscopy of Barrett´s Esophagus. Gastroenterol Clinic North Am, Vol.39, No.4, pp 759-769.

Capella, C., Fiocca, R., Cornaggia, M., Rindi, G., Moratti, R. & Solcia, E. (1999). Autoimmune gastritis, In: Gastritis, Graham, D.Y, Genta, R.M. & Dixon, M.F., pp 79-96, Lippincott Willians & Wilkins, ISBN 0-397-51675-4, Philadelphia, New York, London.

Carmel, R. (1996). Prevalence of undiagnosed pernicious anaemia in the elderly. Arch Intern Med, Vol.156. No.10, pp 1097-1100.

Correa, P. (1984). Chronic gastritis as a cancer precursor. Scand J Gastroenterol, Vol.19, pp 131-136.

Correa, P. (1992). Human gastric carcinogenesis: a multistep and multifactorial process – First American Society Award Lecture on Cancer Epidemiology and Prevention. Cancer Res, Vol.52, pp 6735-6740.

Dixon, M.F., Genta, R.M, Yardley, J.H. et al. (1996). Classification and grading of gastritis. The updated Sydney System. International Workshop on the Histopathology of Gastritis, Houston 1994. Am J Surg Pathol, Vol.20, pp 1161-1181.

Dixon, M.F., Genta, R.M., Yardley, J.H. & Correa, P. (1999). Classification and grading of gastritis. The updated Sydney System. In: Gastritis, Graham, D.Y, Genta, R.M. & Dixon, M.F., pp 35-49, Lippincott Willians & Wilkins, ISBN 0-397-51675-4, Philadelphia, New York, London.

Eshmuratov, A., Nah, J.C. et al. (2010). The correlation of endoscopic and histological diagnosis of gastric atrophy. Dig Dis Sci, Vol.55, pp 1364-1375.

Genta, R.M. (1996). Recognizing atrophy: another step toward a classification of gastritis. Am J Surg Pathol, Vol.20, No.1, pp 23-30.

Genta, R.M. (1997). Helicobacter pylori, inflammation, mucosal damage and apoptosis: pathogenesis and definition of gastric atrophy. Gastroenterology, Vol.113, No.6, pp 51-55.

Goetz, M. & Kiesslich, R. (2010). Advances of endomicroscopy for gastrointestinal physiology and diseases. Am J Physiol Gastrointest Liver Physiol, Vol.298, No.6, pp G797-806.

Haruma, K. et al. (1993). Gastric acid secretion, sérum pepsinogen I, and gastrin in Japanese with gastric hyperplastic polyps or polypoid-type early gastric carcinoma. *Scand J Gastroenterol*, Vol.28, No.7, pp 633-637.

Jain, R. & Chetty, R. (2009). Gastric hyperplastic polyps: a review. *Dig Dis Sci*, Vol.54, No.9, pp 1839-1846.

Jevremovic, D., Torbenson, M. et al. (2006). Atrophic autoimmune pangastritis: a distinctive form of antral and fundic gastritis associated with systemic autoimmune disease. Am J Surg Pathol, Vol. 30, No.11, pp 1412-1419.

Lam-Himlin, D., Park, J.Y., Cornish, T.C., Shi, C.& Montgomery, E. (2010). Morphologic characterization of syndromic gastric polyps. *Am J Surg Pathol*, Vol.34, No.11, pp 1656-1662.

Lewin, K.J., Dowling, F., Wright, J.P. & Taylor, K.B. (1976). Gastric morphology and serum gastrin levels in pernicious anaemia. Gut, Vol.17, No.7, pp 551-560.

Li, C.Q. & Li, Y.Q. (2010). Endomicroscopy of intestinal metaplasia and gastric cancer. Gastroenterol Clin North Am, Vol.39, No.4, pp 785-796.

Moreira, L.F.., Carvalho, M.R.N.V. & Barbosa, A.J.A. (2010). Ghrelin and pré-proghrelin immunoreactive cells in gastric neuroendocrine tumors associated with atrophic body gastritis. Jornal Brasileiro de Patologia e Medicina Laboratorial, Vol.46, pp 329-334.

Moreira, L.F. & Barbosa, A.J.A. (2011). Ghrelin and pré-proghrelin immunoreactive cells in atrophic body gastritis. Jornal Brasileiro de Patologia e Medicina Laboratorial. In press.

Park, J.Y., Cornish, T.C. et al. (2010). Gastric lesions in patients with autoimmune metaplasic atrophic gastritis (AMAG) in a tertiary care setting. Am J Surg Pathol, Vol.34, No.11, pp 1591-1598.

Solcia, E., Fiocca, R., Villani, L., Luinetti, O. & Capella, C. (1995). Hyperplasic, dysplasic, and neoplastic enterochromaffin-like-cell proliferations of the gastric mucosa: classification and histogenesis. Am J Surg Pathol, Vol.19, No.1, pp 51-57.

Tahara, T., Shibata, T. et al. (2009). Gastric mucosal pattern by using magnifying narrow-band imaging endoscopy clearly distinguishes histological and serological severity of chronic gastritis. Gastrointestinal Endoscopy, Vol.70, No.2, pp 246-253.

Torbenso, M., Abrham, S.C., Boitnott, J., Yardley, J.H. & Wu, T.T. (2002). Autoimmune gastritis: distinct histological and immunohistochemical findings before complete loss of oxyntic glands. Mod Pathol, Vol.15, No.2, pp 102-109.

Vannella, L., Lahner, E. et al. (2011). Reversal of atrophic body gastritis after H. pylori eradication at long-term follow-up. Digestive and Liver Disease, Vol.43, pp 295-299.

13

Evaluation of Duodenal Hypersensitivity to Acid Using Transnasal Endoscopy

Manabu Ishii et al.*
Division of Gastroenterology department of Internal Medicine,
Kawasaki Medical School, Kurashiki,
Japan

1. Introduction

According to the Rome III classification, functional gastroduodenal disorders (FGIDs) in adults are subdivided into six domains. Functional dyspepsia (FD) is a subcategory of the FGIDs. It is characterized by the presence of symptoms that are believed to be associated with gastroduodenal lesions, particularly epigastric pain or burning, postprandial fullness, or early satiation, without the evidence of organic disease to explain the onset of these symptoms at least 6 months before diagnosis (Tach J et al., 2006). Furthermore, FD is divided into 2 subtypes postprandial distress syndrome (PDS) and epigastric pain syndrome (EPS). The diagnostic criteria for PDS include the presence of 1 or both of the following symptoms several times in a week: bothersome postprandial fullness occurring after ordinary-sized meals, and early satiation that prevents finishing a regular meal. The diagnostic criteria for EPS include the presence of all of the following symptoms: moderately severe pain or burning localized to the epigastrium at least once per week, and intermittent pain, not generalized or localized to other abdominal or chest regions, not relieved by defecation or passage of flatus, and not fulfilling the criteria for gallbladder and sphincter of Oddi disorders.

FD is a functional disorder that affects 10-30% of the population worldwide. The results of an Itarian population-based study, indicated that the prevalence rates of FD were 11%. Of these, PDS, EPS, and PDS accompanied with EPS were 67.5%, 48.2%, and 15.8% respectively (Zagari RM et al.,2010).The results of a Swedish population-based study, indicated that the prevalence rates of FD, PDS, EPS, and PDS accompanied with EPS were 15.7%, 12.2%, 5.5%, and 1.7%, respectively (Aro P et al., 2009). The results of a Norwegian population-based study, showed that the lifetime prevalence rate of FD was 23% in men and 18% in women (Johnsen et al., 1988), and that in the United States, was 29% (Shaib Y et al., 2004).

---

* Hiroaki Kusunoki[2], Noriaki Manabe[3], Tomoari Kamada[1], Ken-ichi Tarumi[1], Hiroshi Matsumoto[1], Motonori Sato[1], Yoshiyuki Yamanaka[1], Takahisa Murao[1], Hideaki Tsutsui[1], Akiko Shiotani[1], Jiro Hata[3], and Ken Haruma[1]

[1]*Division of Gastroenterology department of Internal Medicine,* [2]*Division of General Medicine* [3]*Division of Endoscopy and Ultrasound Department of Clinical Pathology and Laboratory Medicine, Kawasaki Medical School, Kurashiki, Japan*

2. Pathogenesis and evaluation

Different factors such as delayed gastric emptying (Stanghellini V et al., 1996; Sarnelli G et al., 2003), hypersensitivity to gastric distension (Bradette M et al., 1991; Mearin F et al., 1991; Barbera R et al., 1995; Tack J et al., 2001), impaired gastric accommodation to a meal (Tach J et al., 1998), abnormal duodenojejunal motility (Holtmann G et al., 1996; Wilmer A et al., 1998), duodenal motor and sensory dysfunction (Samsom M et al., 1999; Schwarz MP et al., 2001), duodenal hypersensitivity (Schwartz MP et al., 2001), *Helicobacter pylori* infection, and psychosocial factors have been implicated in the pathogenesis of FD. Among these factors, acid is thought to be more important because proton pump inhibitors (PPIs) and histamine 2 (H2)-receptor antagonists have been proposed to be effective therapies for a subset of patients with FD.

2.1 Duodenal hypersensitivity to acid in patients with FD

Lee *et al.* (2004) reported that acid infusion into the duodenal bulb induced dyspepsia in healthy volunteers, and the symptoms of dyspepsia are more readily observed in patients with FD than in healthy subjects (Samsom *et al.*, 1999). Increased duodenal acid exposure plays a role in the onset of dyspeptic symptoms in patients with FD having prominent nausea (Lee *et al.*, 2004). A recent study indicated that acid infusion into the stomach predominantly induced dysmotility-like dyspeptic symptoms in healthy Japanese control subjects (Miwa *et al.*, 2007). PPIs and H2-receptor antagonists have been proposed as effective therapies for treating FD (Delaney *et al.*, 2005; Veldhuyzen van Zanten *et al.*, 2005; Kinoshita *et al.*, 2005; Seno *et al.* 2005). Guidelines for the management of dyspepsia suggest that PPI therapy is more effective than a placebo or H2-receptor antagonists in relieving the symptoms of patients with uninvestigated dyspepsia (Talley *et al.*, 2005).

2.2 Duodenal acid and gastroduodenal motility

Duodenal acidification suppresses antral contractions. Matsunaga *et al.* (1994) reported that intragastric acidification and intraduodenal acidification at pH 1.0 inhibited spontaneous phase III activity in dogs. Simrén *et al.* (2003) reported that after acid infusion in healthy volunteers, antral contractions were lesser and the number of contractions in the proximal duodenum was greater than those before the infusion. It has been shown that the greater the concentration of acid in the duodenum, the greater is the inhibition of gastric emptying (Hunt *et al.*, 1972). Duodenal pH influences interdigestive gastric motility in humans. Lowering of the duodenal pH prevents the occurrence of the gastric phase III (Woodtli *et al.*, 1995), and, in animals, duodenal acidification induces gastric relaxation by exerting an inhibitory effect on the stomach (Lu *et al.*, 1999). Duodenal acidification has an inhibitory effect on gastric emptying (Danzer *et al.*, 2004; Raybould *et al.*, 1993; Cooke, 1974; Mearadji *et al.*, 1999; Parkman *et al.*, 1998), and hydrochloric acid (HCl) may restrict gastric outflow by inducing tonic occlusion of the duodenum (Parkman *et al.*, 1998).

2.3 Pathophysiological mechanism of acid-sensing system

Visceral organs receive dual innervation from primary afferents commonly referred to as sympathetic afferents (splanchnic nerves) and parasympathetic afferents (vagus nerves). Lamb *et al.* (2003) reported that electromyographically recorded visceromotor responses increased after HCl administration in rats, but vagotomy and pretreatment with capsaicin abolished these responses. Their findings indicated that vagal pathways are involved in

mediating signals for the noxious stimulation of the stomach. Further, Scicho *et al.* (2005) reported that gastric acidification increased the expression of phosphorylated extracellular signal-regulated kinase-1 and -2 (p-ERK1/2) in the dorsal root ganglion neurons via *N*-methyl-D-aspartate receptors. They suggested that sympathetic pathways are involved in mediating signals for noxious stimulation of the stomach. Noxious mechanical stimulation showed that most of the increased p-ERK1/2 neurons coexpressed transient receptor potential vanilloid receptor 1 and acid-sensing ion channel 3 (Sakurai *et al.*, 2008).
Transient receptor potential vanilloid receptor 1 and the acid-sensing ion channel 3 are largely involved in the acid-induced nociception in mammals (Ugawa *et al.*, 2002), but it is still unknown which receptors of the peripheral sensory pathways encode and integrate an acidinduced nociceptive event in the gastric mucosa and the duodenal mucosa. Akiba *et al.* (2002) reported that the capsaicin pathway is an acid-sensing pathway that promotes hyperemia and mucus secretion in response to luminal acid in the duodenum.

2.4 Method for evaluating duodenal hypersensitivity to acid and gastric motility

Duodenal hypersensitivity to acid is one of the more important factors in the pathogenesis of FD. Although manometric methods, scintigraphic methods, electrogastrography and ultrasonography have been used to evaluate enterokinesis, a practical method for evaluating duodenal hypersensitivity to acid has not been reported. Transnasal endoscopy is a rescently developed, non-invasive and nondiscomforting method for examination of the upper gastrointestinal tract (Yagi *et al.*, 2005; Murata *et al.*, 2007). We developed a new method for evaluating duodenal hypersensitivity to acid and gastric motility by duodenal acidification using transnasal endoscopy (Ishii *et al.*, 2008).

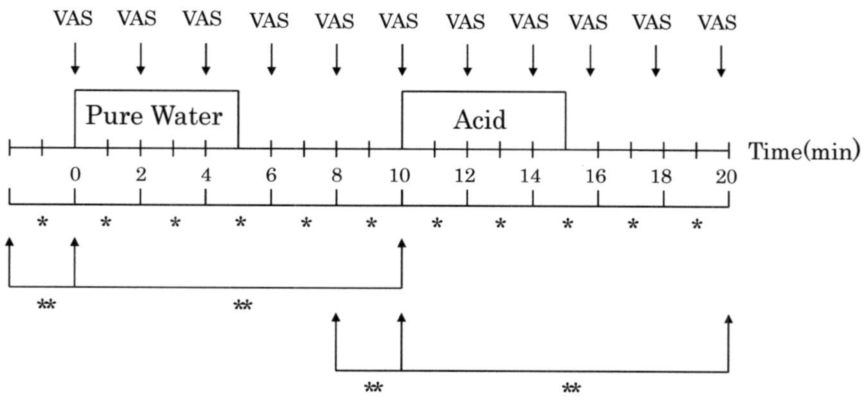

Fig. 1. *Number of antral contractions every two minutes; **Motility number; VAS: Visual Analogue Scale

The study protocol is shown in Fig. 1. All subjects underwent transnasal endoscopy as required in the left lateral decubitus position in the morning after overnight fasting. The infusion of air into their stomachs was minimized in order to observe their gastric motility. An infusion tube (outer diameter 1.5 mm) was then introduced by transnasal endoscopy until the tip was located in the duodenal bulb. The subjects changed their body position to the supine position, and their antral contractions and dyspeptic symptoms were evaluated before and after a duodenal infusion of pure water (36.5°C, 100 ml) and acid (36.5°C, 0.1 N

HCl, 100 ml). The images of transnasal endoscopy were recorded from the beginning until the end on a DVD and were analyzed after finishing the examination. We infused 100 ml of pure water and acid at a rate of 20 ml/min. The use of an electronic infusion pump, ensured

	2 min	4 min	6 min
Heavy feeling in the stomach			
Nausea or feeling sick			
Bloating			
Belching			
Cramping pain in the stomach			
Dull pain in the stomach			
Pricking pain in the stomach			
Tickling or tingling in the throat			
Sour or bitter taste			
Feeling that something is stuck in the throat			
Burning sensation in the chest			

Fig. 2.

Symptoms	Maximum severity scale (cm) (Mean±SEM)		
	0.1mol/L HCl	Pure Water	P-value
Heavy feeling in the stomach	4.76±0.74	0.54±0.24	0.0001
Nausea or feeling sick	4.65±1.1	0.19±0.16	0.001
Bloating	3.66±0.8	0.54±0.24	0.0006
Belching	1.61±0.61	0.76±1.1	0.2349
Cramping pain in the stomach	3.39±0.88	1.0±0.45	0.0016
Dull pain in the stomach	4.05±0.83	0.49±0.23	0.0005
Pricking pain in the stomach	1.58±0.72	0.51±0.75	0.125
Tickling or tingling in the throat	2.35±0.91	0.42±0.17	0.0539
Sour or bitter taste	1.1±0.16	0.55±0.09	0.0982
Feeling that something is stuck in the throat	1.6±0.64	0.45±0.25	0.0932
Burning sensation in the chest	2.67±0.75	0.16±0.1	0.0033

Maximum severity on the 10 cm visual analogue scale after infusion of 0.1 mol/L hydrochloric acid (HCl) or pure water (n=14)

Table 1.

that the subjects were blinded to the nature (acid or pure water) of the infusion. The acid infusion was started 5 min after the infusion of pure water was finished. The severity of each symptom was assessed by each subject using a 10-cm visual analogue scale every 2 min (Fig. 2). The symptoms assessed were as follows: a heavy feeling in the stomach, bloating, nausea or feeling sick, belching, a dull pain in the stomach, cramping pain in the stomach, a pricking pain in the stomach, tickling or tingling sensation in the throat, a sour or bitter taste, a feeling that something is stuck in the throat, and a burning sensation in the chest. The symptom severity scales were set at 0 cm before the duodenal infusion of water and acid. The maximum severity scale was calculated as the mean of the individual maximum values. We evaluated the differences between the maximum severity scales in the infusion of pure water and acid. Antral contractions beginning every 2 min before the duodenal infusion of water were counted every 2 min until the end of the examination. The macroscopic waves of gastric peristalsis propagating from the gastric body to the antrum were counted. The motility number was defined as the mean number of antral contractions in 1 min. We evaluated the differences between the motility numbers before and after the infusion of pure water and those before and after acid infusion. We compared the changes in the symptom severity scales, the maximum severity scales of each subject, the number of antral contractions, and the motility number between the acid and pure water infusion. Using this method, we showed that the maximum severity scale of a heavy feeling in the stomach, and other symptoms was significantly greater after the acid infusion than that the pure water infusion in healthy volunteers (Table 1). During pure water infusion, no changes were observed between the motility numbers. On the other hand, the motility number significantly decreased after duodenal acidification (before *vs.* after: 2.93 ± 0.12 times *vs.* 1.11 ± 0.23 times, $P<0.0001$) (Fig. 3).

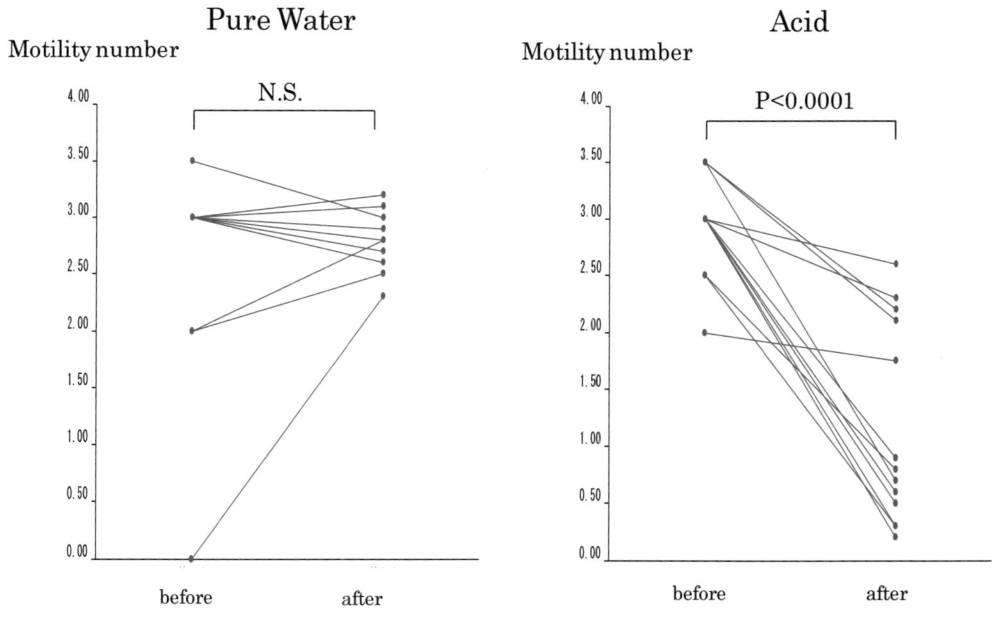

Fig. 3.

Furthermore, using this method we evaluated duodenal hypersensitivity to acid in healthy volunteers and patients with FD (Ishii *et al.*, 2010). The study protocol is shown in Fig. 4. In this study, we infused the patients with 20 ml of HCl at a rate of 20 ml/min. The severity of 12 symptoms was assessed by each subject using a 100-mm visual analogue scale (VAS) from the time acid infusion was started up to 30 min after the initiation of the infusion.

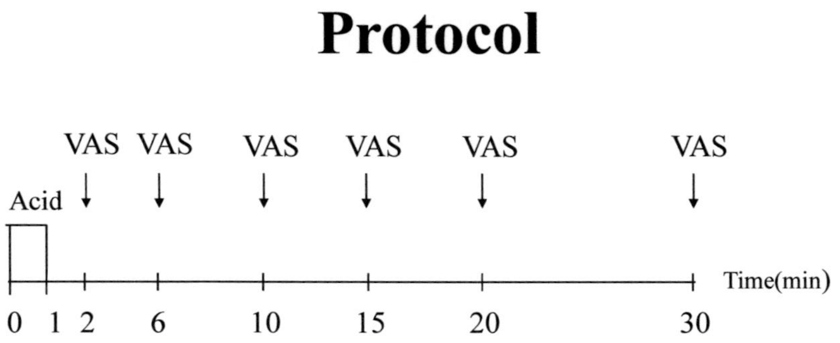

Fig. 4. Study protocols. This study consisted of monitoring of the assessment of symptoms using VAS

Symptoms	Maximum severity scale (mm) (Mean±SEM) Patients with FD	Healthy volunteers	P-value
Heavy feeling in the stomach	25.5±4.4	5.9±2.0	<0.001 *
Nausea or feeling sick	14.4±4.3	4.4±1.9	0.036 *
Bloating	39.1±5.1	14±3.5	<0.001 *
Belching	20.0±4.9	9.6±6.3	0.254
Cramping pain in the stomach	19.4±5.0	5.4±2.7	0.017 *
Dull pain in the stomach	21.8±5.0	4.5±2.3	0.003*
Prickling pain in the stomach	12.9±4.1	4.8±2.2	0.084
Tickling or tingling in the throat	9.7±3.2	0.6±0.6	0.008 *
Sour or bitter taste	8.9±3.1	0.6±0.6	0.011 *
Feeling that something is stuck in the throat	18.6±4.3	1.9±1.1	<0.001*
Burning sensation in the chest	10.6±3.6	3.1±2.0	0.073
Early satiety	35.6±5.3	9.0±3.9	<0.001*

Maximum severity on the 100-mm visual analogue scale after infusion of 0.1 mol/L hydrochloric acid (HCl) between healthy volunteers and patients with FD.
*P < 0.05, 2-sided non-paired *t* test

Table 2. Maximum severity scales between healthy volunteers and patients with FD

The maximum severity scale was defined as the maximum score of the symptom severity scale. The VAS was set at 0 mm just before the duodenal infusion of acid. The total score was defined as the aggregate score of the maximum severity scale for the 12 symptoms.

The differences in the rate of incidence of dyspeptic symptoms, maximum severity scales, and total scores between patients with FD and healthy volunteers were evaluated.
The rates of dyspeptic symptoms in patients with FD and healthy volunteers after acid infusion were 88.6% and 75%, respectively (P = not significant, using the X^2-test). The maximum severity scales of a heavy feeling in the stomach, nausea or feeling sick, bloating, cramping pain in the stomach, dull pain in the stomach, tickling or tingling in the throat, sour or bitter taste, feeling that something is stuck in the throat and early satiety significantly increased after acid infusion in patients with FD than in healthy volunteers ($P < 0.05$, using the two-sided non-paired t-test) (Table 2). There were significant differences in the total scores (patients with FD *vs* healthy volunteers: 233.8 ± 37.8 *vs* 63.9 ± 14.6; $P < 0.001$, using the two-sided nonpaired t-test) (Fig. 5). We found that duodenal acidification induced dyspeptic symptoms more significantly in patients with FD than in healthy volunteers.

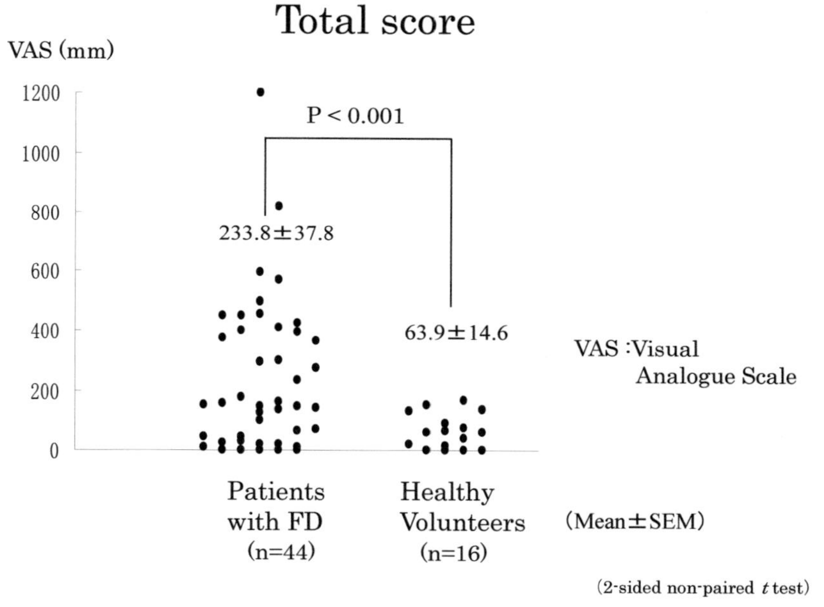

Fig. 5.

3. Conclusion

The effects of duodenal acidification by transnasal endoscopy significantly increased various dyspeptic symptoms not suppresses this symptoms. Further, this method enabled the evaluation of duodenal hypersensitivity to acid in healthy volunteers and in patients with FD. Using this method, we might be able to clarify a correlation between duodenal hypersensitivity to acid and the effectiveness of PPI therapy for the treatment of FD. A further examination is needed.

4. Acknowledgment

We thank nurses and officers at the Kawasaki Medical School for their kind help with the present survey.

5. References

[1] Tack, J.; Talley, N.J. & Camilleri, M. (2006). Functional gastroduodenal disorders. *Gastroenterol.* 130: 1466–1479.

[2] Zagari RM,; Law GR & Fuccio L. (2010). Epidemiology of functional dyspepsia and subgroups in the Italian general population: an endoscopic study. *Gastroenterol.* 138:1302-11.

[3] Aro, P.; Talley, N.J. & Ronkainen, J. (2009). Anxiety is associated with uninvestigated and functional dyspepsia (Rome III criteria) in a Swedish population-based study. *Gastroenterol.* 137: 94–100.

[4] Johnsen, R.; Straume, B. & Førde, O.H. (1988). Peptic ulcer and non-ulcer dyspepsia-a disease and a disorder. *Scand. J. Prim. Health Care* 6: 239–243.

[5] Shaib, Y.; & El-Serag, H.B. (2004). The prevalence and risk factors of functional dyspepsia in a multiethnic population in the United States. *Am. J. Gastroenterol.* 99: 2210–2216.

[6] Stanghellini, V.; Tosetti, C. & Pasternico, A. (1996). Risk indicators of delayed gastric emptying of solids in patients with functional dyspepsia. *Gastroenterol.* 110: 1036–1042.

[7] Sarnelli, G.; Caenepeel, P. & Geypens, B. (2003). Symptoms associated with impaired gastric emptying of solids and liquids in functional dyspepsia. *Am. J. Gastroenterol.* 98: 783–788.

[8] Bradette, M.; Pare, P. & Douville, P. (1991). Visceral perception in health and functional dyspepsia. Crossover study of gastric distension with placebo and domperidone. *Dig. Dis. Sci.* 36: 52–58.

[9] Mearin, F.; Cucala, M. & Azpiroz, F. (1991). The origin of symptoms on the brain-gut axis in functional dyspepsia. *Gastroenterol.* 101: 999–1006.

[10] Barbera, R.; Feinle, C. & Read, N.W. (1995). Nutrient-specific modulation of gastric mechanosensitivity in patients with functional dyspepsia. *Dig. Dis. Sci.* 40: 1636–1641.

[11] Tack, J.; Caenepeel, P. & Fischler, B. (2001). Symptoms associated with hypersensitivity to gastric distension in functional dyspepsia. *Gastroenterol.* 121: 526–535.

[12] Tack, J.; Piessevaux, H. & Coulie, B. (1998). Role of impaired gastric accommodation to a meal in functional dyspepsia. *Gastroenterol.* 115: 1346–1352.

[13] Holtmann, G.; Goebell, H. & Talley, J. (1996). Impaired small intestinal peristaltic reflexes and sensory thresholds are independent functional disturbances in patients with chronic unexplained dyspepsia. *Am. J. Gastroenterol.* 91: 485–491.

[14] Wilmer, A.; Van Cutsem, E. & Andrioli, A. (1998). Ambulatory gastrojejunal manometry in severe motility-like dyspepsia: lack of correlation between dysmotility, symptoms, and gastric emptying. *Gut* 42: 235–242.

[15] Samsom, M.; Verhagen, M.A. & van Berge Henegouwen, G.P. (1999). Abnormal clearance of exogenous acid and increased acid sensitivity of proximal duodenum in dyspeptic patients. *Gastroenterol.* 116: 515–520.

[16] Schwartz, M.P.; Samsom, M. & van Berge Henegouwen, G.P. (2001). Effect of inhibition of gastric acid secretion on antropyloroduodenal motor activity and duodenal acid hypersensitivity in functional dyspepsia. *Aliment. Pharmacol. Ther.* 15: 1921–1928.

[17] Schwarz, M.P.; Samsom, M. & Smout, A.J. (2001). Chemospecific alterations in duodenal perception and motor response in functional dyspepsia. *Am. J. Gastroenterol.* 96: 2596–2602.

[18] Lee, K.J.; Demarchi, B. & Demedts, I. (2004). A pilot study on duodenal acid exposure and its relationship to symptoms in functional dyspepsia with prominent nausea. *Am. J. Gastroenterol.* 99: 1765–1773.

[19] Samsom, M.; Verhagen, M.A. & van Berge Henegouwen, G.P. (1999). Abnormal clearance of exogenous acid and increased acid sensitivity of proximal duodenum in dyspeptic patients. *Gastroenterol.* 116: 515–520.

[20] Lee, K.J.; Vos, R. & Janssens, J. (2004). Influence of duodenal acidification on the sensorimotor function of the proximal stomach in humans. *Am. J. Physiol.* 286: G278- G284.

[21] Miwa, H.; Nakajima, K. & Yamaguchi, K. (2007). Generation of dyspeptic symptoms by direct acid infusion into the stomach of healthy Japanese subjects. *Aliment. Pharmacol. Ther.* 26: 257- 264.

[22] Delaney, B.; Ford, A.C. & Forman, D. (2005). Initial management strategies for dyspepsia. *Cochrane Database Syst. Rev.* 4: CD001961.

[23] Veldhuyzen,; van Zanten S.J. & Chiba, N. (2005). A randomized trial comparing omeprazole, ranitidine, cisapride, or placebo in helicobacter pylori negative, primary care patients with dyspepsia: the CADET-HN Study. *Am. J. Gastroenterol.* 100: 1477–1488.

[24] Kinoshita, Y.; Hashimoto, T. & Kawamura, A. (2005). Effects of famotidine, mosapride and tandospirone for treatment of functional dyspepsia. *Aliment. Pharmacol. Ther.* 21 (Suppl. 2): 37–41.

[25] Seno, H.; Nakase, H. & Chiba, T. (2005). Usefulness of famotidine in functional dyspepsia patient treatment: comparison among prokinetic, acid suppression and anxiety therapies. *Aliment. Pharmacol. Ther.* 21 (Suppl. 2): 32–36.

[26] Talley, N.J.; Vakil, N.B. & Moayyedi, P. (2005). American gastroenterological association technical review on the evaluation of dyspepsia. *Gastroenterol.* 129: 1756–1780.

[27] Matsunaga, Y.; Yamamoto, O. & Ueki, S. (1994). Inhibition of phase III activity by acid in canine stomach. *Regul. Pept.* 52: 61–72.

[28] Simrén, M.; Vos, R. & Janssens, J. (2003). Acid infusion enhances duodenal mechanosensitivity in healthy subjects. *Am. J. Physiol.* 285: G309–G315.

[29] Hunt, J.N. & Knox, M.T. (1972). The slowing of gastric emptying by four strong acids and three weak acids. *J. Physiol. (Lond.)* 222: 187–208.

[30] Woodtli, W. & Owyang, C. (1995). Duodenal pH governs interdigestive motility in humans. *Am. J. Physiol.* 268: G146–G152.

[31] Lu, Y.X. & Owyang, C. (1999). Duodenal acid-induced gastric relaxation is mediated by multiple pathways. *Am. J. Physiol.* 276: G1501–G1506.

[32] Danzer, M.; Jocic, M. & Samberger, C. (2004). Stomach-brain communication by vagal afferents in response to luminal acid backdiffusion, gastrin, and gastric acid secretion. *Am. J. Physiol.* 286: G403–G411.

[33] Raybould, H.E. & Hölzer, H.H. (1993). Duodenal acid-induced inhibition of gastric motility and emptying in rats. *Am. J. Physiol.* 265: G540–G546. Cooke, 1974;

[34] Mearadji, B.; Straathof, J.W. & Lamers, C.B. (1999). Effect of gastrin on proximal gastric motor function in humans. *Neurogastroenterol. Motil.* 11: 449–455.

[35] Parkman, H.P.; Urbain, J.L. & Knight, L.C. (1998). Effect of gastric acid suppressants on human gastric motility. *Gut* 42: 243–250.

[36] Lamb, K.; Kang, Y.M. & Gebhart, G.F. (2003). Gastric inflammation triggers hypersensitivity to acid in awake rats. *Gastroenterol.* 125: 1410–1418.

[37] Scicho, R.; Liebmann, I. & Lippe, I.T. (2005). Extracellular signal-regulated kinase-1 and -2 are activated by gastric luminal injury in dorsal root ganglion neurons via N-methyl- D-aspartate receptors. *Neuroscience* 134: 505–514.

[38] Sakurai, J.; Obata, K. & Ozaki, N. (2008). Activation of extracellular signal-regulated protein kinase in sensory neurons after noxious gastric distention and its involvement in acute visceral pain in rats. *Gastroenterol.* 134: 1094–1103.

[39] Ugawa, S.; Ueda, T. & Ishida, Y. (2002). Amiloride-blockable acid-sensing ion channels are leading acid sensors expressed in human nociceptors. *J. Clin. Invest.* 110: 1185–1190.

[40] Akiba, Y.; Nakamura, M. & Nagata, H. (2002). Acid-sensing pathway in rat gastrointestinal mucosa. *J. Gastroenterol.* 37: 133–138.

[41] Yagi, J.; Adachi, K. & Arima, N. (2005). A prospective randomized comparative study on the safety and tolerability of transnasal esophagogastroduodenoscopy. *Endoscopy* 37: 1226–1231.

[42] Ishii, M.; Manabe, N. & Kusunoki, H. (2008). Real-time evaluation of dyspeptic symptoms and gastric motility induced by duodenal acidification using noninvasive transnasal endoscopy. *J. Gastroenterol.* 43: 935–941.

[43] Ishii, M.; Kusunoki, H. & Manabe, N. (2010). Evaluation of duodenal hypersensitivity induced by duodenal acidification using transnasal endoscopy. *J. Gastroenterol. Hepatol.* 25: 913-918.

Part 4

The Colon

14

The Role of Colonoscopy in the Prevention of Colon and Rectal Cancer

David Martínez Ares and Pamela Estévez Boullosa
Gastroenterology Unit. Complejo Hospitalario Universitario de Vigo, Vigo-Pontevedra
Spain

1. Introduction

Colorectal cancer (CRC) is one of the most common tumors in our society. It is the most common gastrointestinal tumor and it is also estimated that between 5 and 6% of the population will suffer this tumor along their lives. Colorectal cancer is a tumor in which it is possible to perform primary and secondary prevention. It ranks second in frequency in both men and women, and it represents the second leading cause of cancer-related deaths in both men (after lung cancer) and women (after breast cancer). Indeed, CRC is responsible for 12% of cancer-related deaths in men and for 15% in women. It represents, therefore, a public health problem of first magnitude, causing over 10,500 annual deaths in Spain; so it is well established and cost effectiveness to use a program for early detection and prevention of this disease. CRC mortality in 2006 was almost double that the one recorded in Spain in 1975 in both sexes, considering them separately, and in the entire population as a whole. In relation to the rest of the Europe, Spain has an intermediate CRC mortality, lower than that recorded in Czech Republic or Slovakia, and well above from CRC mortality in Finland or Cyprus. In Spain, cancer mortality is higher in the north than in the south, and this difference is more significant in males. Furthermore, cancer mortality in the whole country is quite stable since the beginning of this century, observing a slight increase in northern regions.

The survival of patients diagnosed with CRC is approximately 54% at 5 years after diagnosis. However, survival is significantly lower in the group of patients in advanced stages, and much higher, with a survival rate around 90%, when it comes to patients in early stages. Therefore, an early diagnosis of colorectal cancer can lead to a significant reduction in cancer mortality. Consequently, a program of screening or early detection could considerably improve the prognosis of this disease.

Colorectal cancer is a health problem that fulfills all the requirements that the World Health Organization requires to consider a cost-effective screening program for early detection of neoplasia: first it is a very common disease, representing a major public health problem; second it is a disease with a well-known natural history, fulfilling in most cases the adenoma-carcinoma sequence (Figure 1), and this natural history is long enough so it can be interrupted by various diagnostic and therapeutic strategies; thirdly, we have diagnostic methods with enough diagnostic accuracy and at reasonable cost; fourthly, there is an effective treatment and, finally, this approach seems to be cost-effective. However, these screening programs have been implemented in very few sites in the world, having to be reduced in many cases to opportunistic screening or, at best, reduced to population at

highest risk of developing the disease, such as those suffering from predisposing diseases such as ulcerative colitis, or individuals with high familial risk of developing the disease.
There is little doubt about the beneficial of a program for early detection of colon cancer: the diagnosis of the disease in an early stage practically ensures its cure, and even in many cases, we will be able to diagnose precancerous lesions and removing them we can avoid the appearance of cancer. The best prevention strategy is subject of discussion, especially in lower-risk patients.
As expected, before proposing an individual for inclusion in a screening program it is essential to establish their individual risk of developing colon cancer. Routinely, the population is divided into three groups according to their risk of developing colorectal cancer (CRC):

- Low-risk population: includes individuals younger than 50 years, without personal or family risk factors for developing CRC. In this population is not recommended CRC screening.
- Average-risk population: they are people whose only risk factor for the condition of the disease is having an age over 50 years. Given the high incidence of the disease after this age, it is justified to perform an early diagnosis.
- High-risk population: includes all individuals with personal risk factors (history of polyps or colorectal cancer or predisposing conditions such as inflammatory bowel disease) or family risk factors for cancer development. It is well known that the existence of first-degree relatives of colon cancer increases the risk for the disease; in addition, there are familial forms of cancer or hereditary syndromes (familial adenomatous polyposis and hereditary non-polyposis colorectal cancer are the most common).

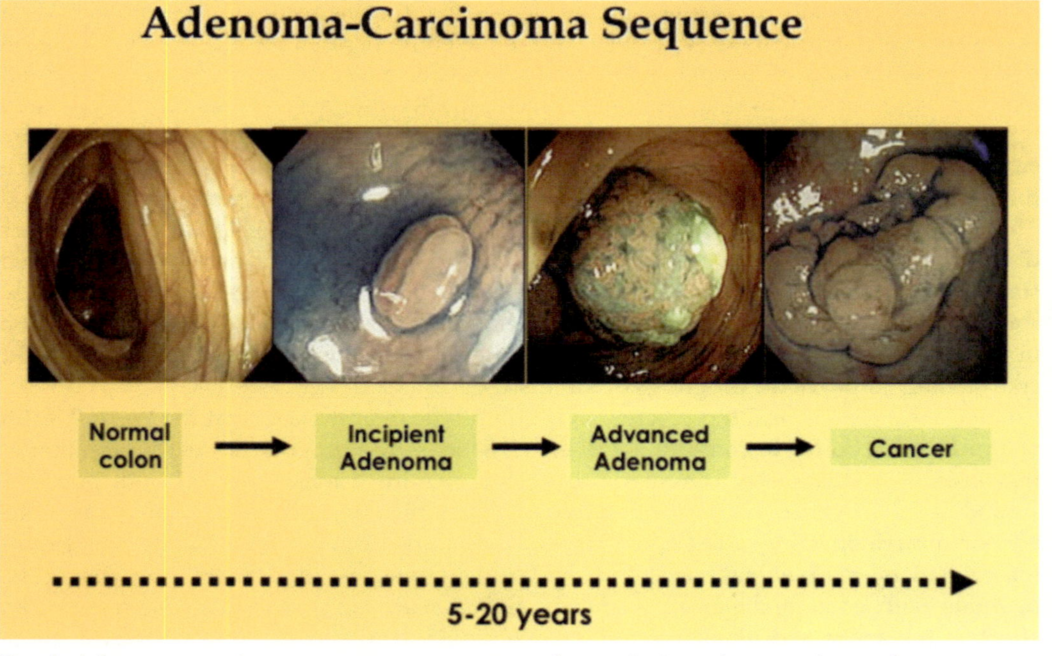

Fig. 1. Adenoma-carcinoma sequence represents the evolution of most colorectal carcinomas, from a normal colon to the development of an invasive carcinoma

2. The role of colonoscopy in preventing colorectal cancer

Colonoscopy plays a dual role in preventing colorectal cancer. First, endoscopic examination of the colon and rectum is the gold standard in the diagnosis of neoplastic and preneoplastic lesions in the large intestine. On the other hand, the development of therapeutic techniques such as polypectomy or more complex techniques like endoscopic mucosal resection or endoscopic submucosal dissection, allows the removal of some of these lesions. Indeed, endoscopic resection is curative in almost all preneoplastic lesions (benign lesions) and may be curative in early malignant lesions, which are those that only affect the mucosa and submucosa.

Colonoscopy is useful for the diagnosis of cancer and precancerous lesions. Unquestionably, despite radiological techniques are useful for diagnosis, the role of colonoscopy is essential firstly to confirm the radiological findings and also to obtain biopsy specimens for histological diagnosis. Colorectal cancer is frequently presented as proliferative lesions that produce some stenosis of the intestinal lumen, with ulcerated surface and even with hemorrhagic necrotic areas (Figure 2); sometimes they are polypoid lesions that can also have ulcerated areas (Figure 3), or just be circumscribed ulcerations (Figure 4).

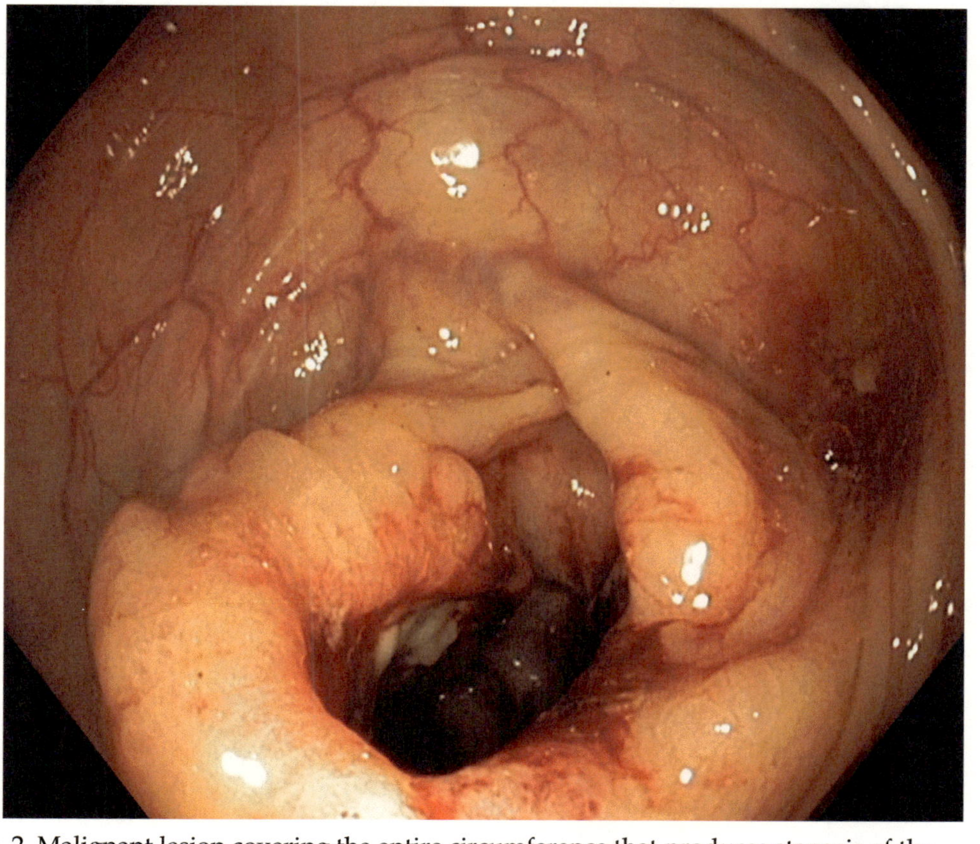

Fig. 2. Malignant lesion covering the entire circumference that produces stenosis of the intestinal lumen, with ulcerated surface, hemorrhagic necrotic areas and bleeding easily at the touch of endoscope

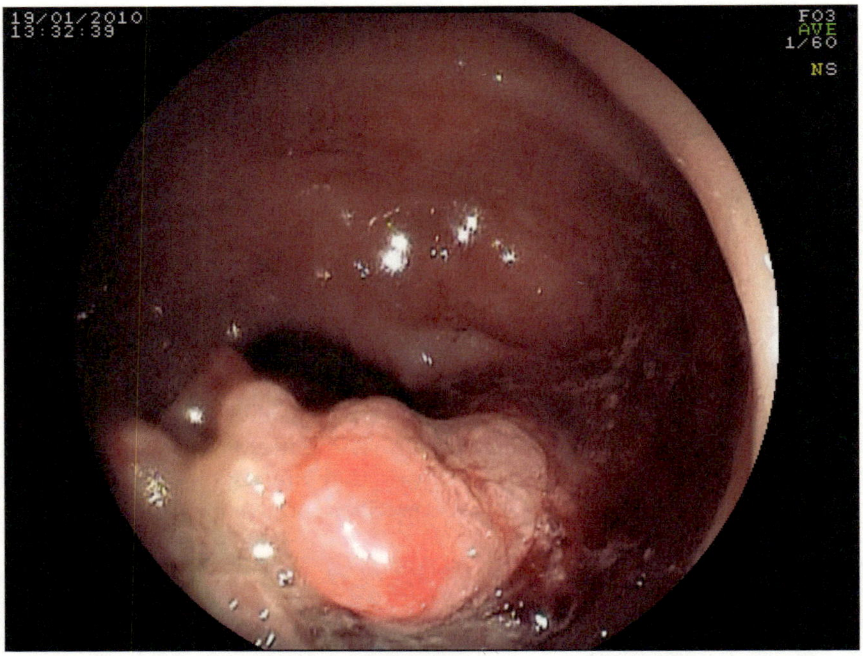

Fig. 3. Sessile polyp, with wide-based attachment, embossed surface, with ulcerated areas and a friable mucosa. Biopsies from the lesion suggest adenocarcinoma arising in a villous adenoma

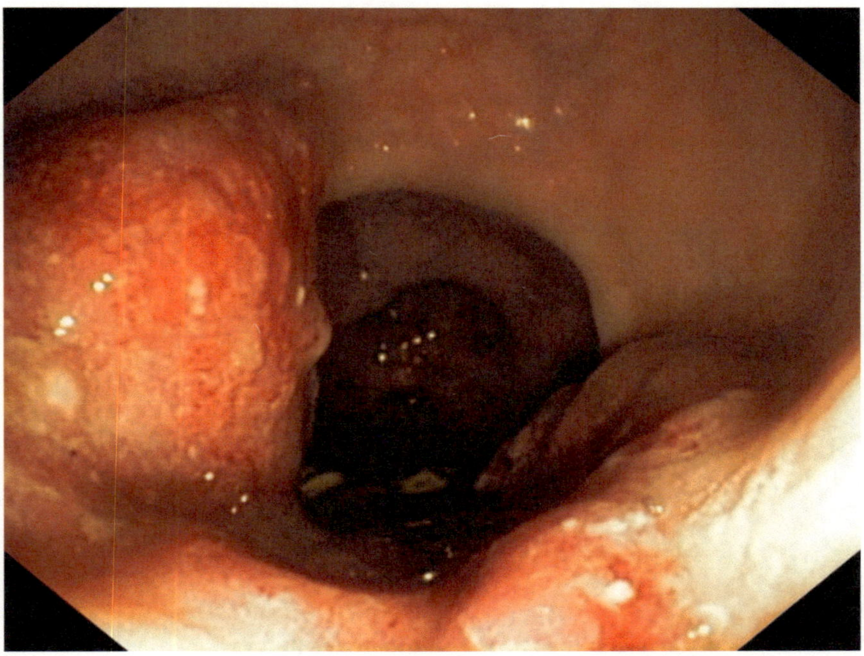

Fig. 4. Ulcer that affects 2 / 5 parts of the circumference of intestinal lumen, with raised and indurated edges. Biopsies suggested undifferentiated adenocarcinoma

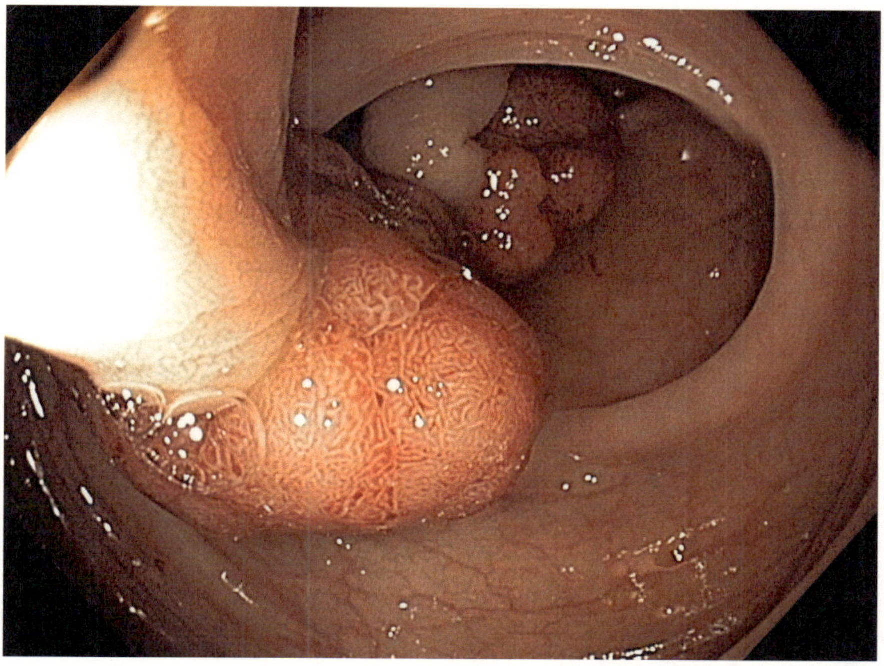

Fig. 5. The picture shows two large pedunculated polyps. Adenomatous tissue is easily differentiated from the pedicle, consisting of normal mucosa, non-neoplastic

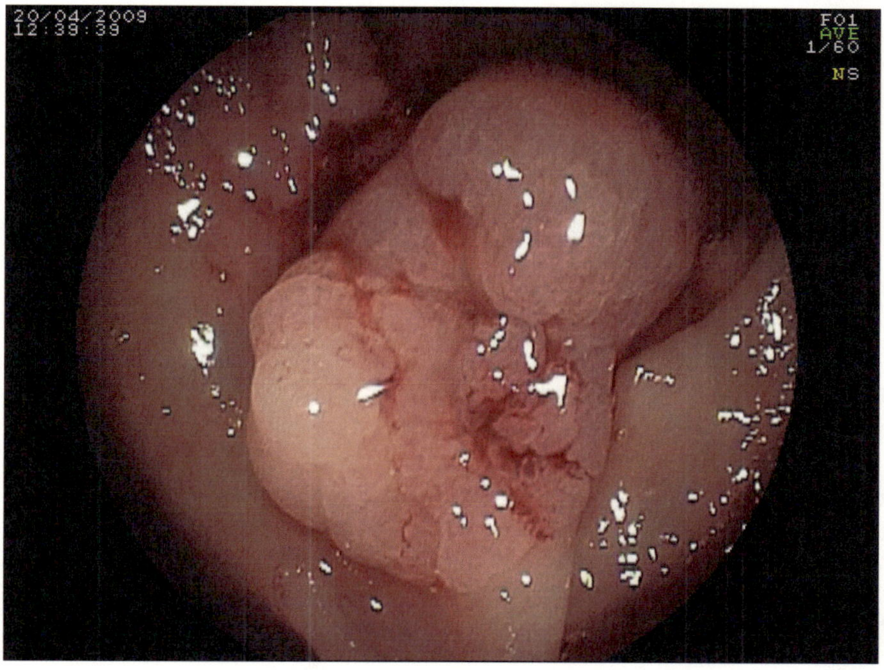

Fig. 6. Sessile polyp, with wide-based attachment, in which it does not recognize any pedicle

The diagnosis of polyps is also quite distinctive, as outgrowths on the colonic mucosa with variable size and morphology. They can present as pedunculated lesions (Figure 5), sessile lesions (Figure 6), or as flat or very slightly raised lesions (Figure 7). Occasionally, lesions can be almost undetectable during a conventional colonoscopy, so some special techniques such as chromoendoscopy or modern techniques of Narrow Band Imaging and Computed Virtual Chromoendoscopy can be helpful to identify and study the lesions more accurately (Figure 8). After these lesions have been located and characterized, we should think in the possibility to perform the resection of the lesion by polypectomy (Figure 9) or endoscopic mucosal resection (Figure 10).

Although, in general, the role of colonoscopy in preventing CRC can be summarized in the above, there are some differences in the groups of patients that have been differentiated according to their risk of developing the disease. For this reason, then we will discuss in greater detail, the place of colonoscopy in the screening strategies proposed for each of these patients.

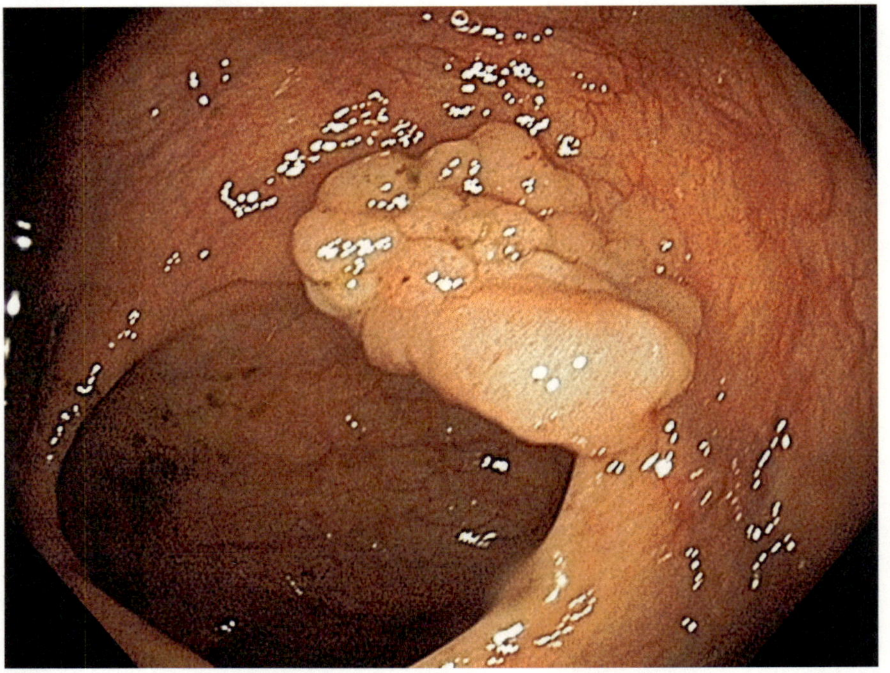

Fig. 7. Flat polyp, located in right colon close to the ileocecal valve. The lesion has a thickness of a few millimeters and a granular surface

2.1 Usefulness of colonoscopy in preventing CRC in average risk population

This is the largest group of individuals who would be subsidiaries of CRC prevention programs, so the group would consume a greater amount of resources. In fact, most colorectal carcinomas are sporadic, appearing in patients who have neither family history of disease or conditions predisposing to disease.

The prevention strategy that arises in this population is, once assumed the failure of primary prevention, it takes place secondary prevention. That is, it is an early diagnosis of cancer or

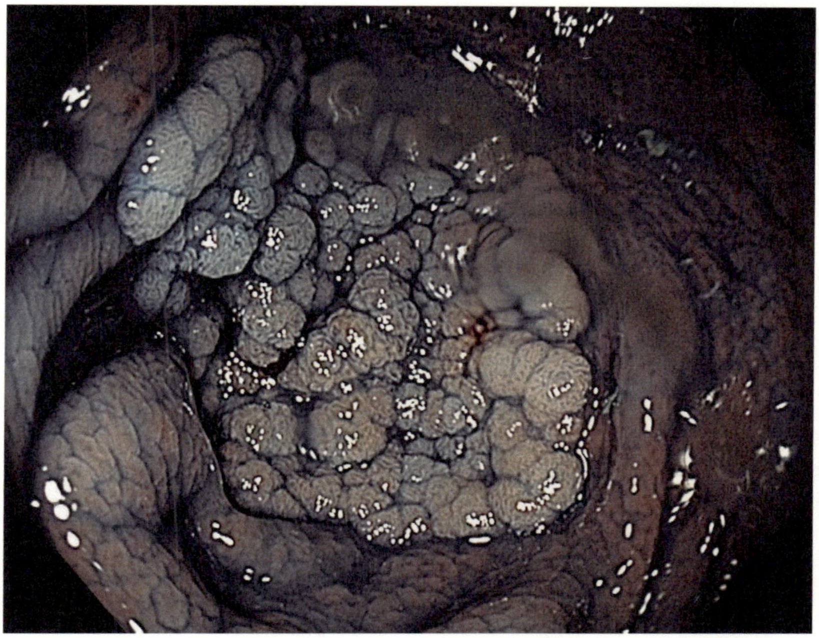

Fig. 8. Laterally spreading tumor with granular surface, with sharply demarcated edges after performing vital staining with indigo carmine 2%

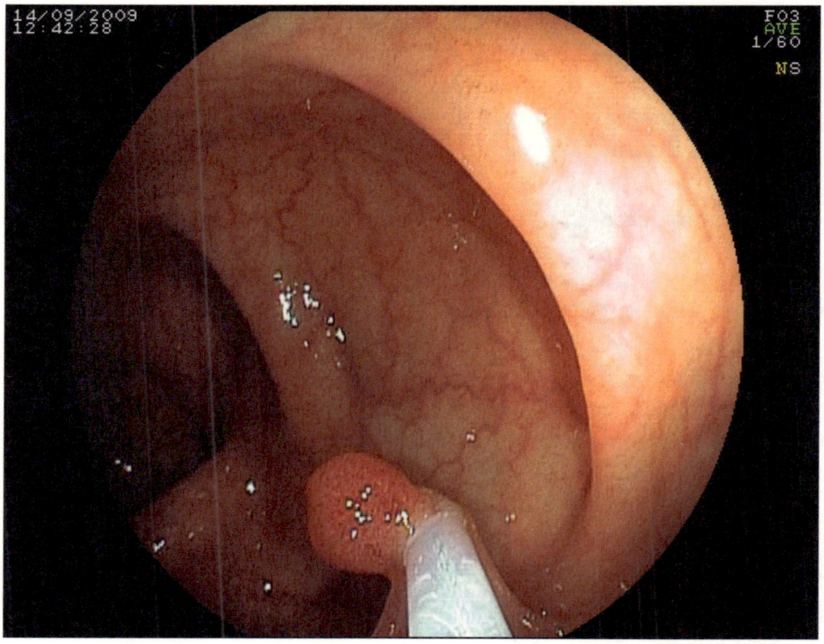

Fig. 9. Endoscopic polypectomy by polypectomy snare of a pedunculated lesion of about 7 mm in diameter, located in proximal transverse colon. The pathological study revealed the presence of a tubular adenoma with low grade dysplasia

precancerous lesions, in order to ensure a treatment with the best outlook for cure. In the case of diagnosis of polyps, colonoscopy and polypectomy allow the resection of the lesions and, thus, to prevent the occurrence of CRC.
In this group the screening strategies accepted and recommended by different international and Spanish scientific societies are:

- Fecal occult blood, immune test preferably (FOBT), on an annual or biennial periodicity.
- Barium enema, replaced in most developed countries by the CT-colonography, every 5 years.
- flexible sigmoidoscopy every 5 years
- total colonoscopy, every 10 years

No comparative studies are available that allow us to establish which is the most cost effective strategy. Taking into account that the most questionable option is represented by radiological tests, it seems that the discussion focuses on the choice of test FOBT or colonoscopy. If we accept the numbers described in several studies, stating that, in patients at average risk, adenomas should be detected in at least 25% of screening colonoscopies, there are doubts about the profitability of the radiological techniques. However, at present, we do not have enough scientific evidence to choose any strategy, although there is an American study which points in this direction. In Spain it is estimated that the cost per year of life saved using immunological fecal occult blood annually is around € 1,200, and it is € 2,300 for sigmoidoscopy every 5 years or colonoscopy every ten years. Both cases demonstrate the low cost of these screening programs when we compared them with other established screening systems for other malignancies such as cervical or breast cancer, whose cost is approximately 5-6 times higher.
The screening of colorrectal cancer in average risk population implies a significant increase in the number of colonoscopies that we must perform in our units. There are some concers about this situation. Perharps, there are no enough endoscopists in our health system to answer this raising demand of colonoscopies. The spanish health system should consider this limitations before the implementation of a screening program.

2.2 Prevention of colorrectal cancer in patients with personal history of polypectomy or CRC

Patients in which colonic polyps were removed or that have been treated for colon cancer should be included in specific monitoring systems. So this is tertiary prevention, and the aim is to detect metachronous lesions that appear in the months or years after the onset of the initial lesion. This disclosure is based on the possibility that the patient could have synchronic small lesions that could have not been detected in the initial colonoscopy. When performing a new examination in a reasonable period of time, these lesions would be detected in early stages yet. On the other hand, it is also known that these patients have an increased risk of presenting new lesions in the future. The only test accepted by all societies for these patients is colonoscopy.
The frequency of follow-up colonoscopies will be determined by the type of lesions presented by the patients. Naturally, any recommendation is based on the fundamental principle that colonoscopies performed meet all the standards of quality: good bowel preparation, full colon examination and mean colonoscopic withdrawal times of at least 6 minutes. In fact, all the factors mentioned above, especially the last one, are significantly correlated with the rate of polyps detected at screening colonoscopy.

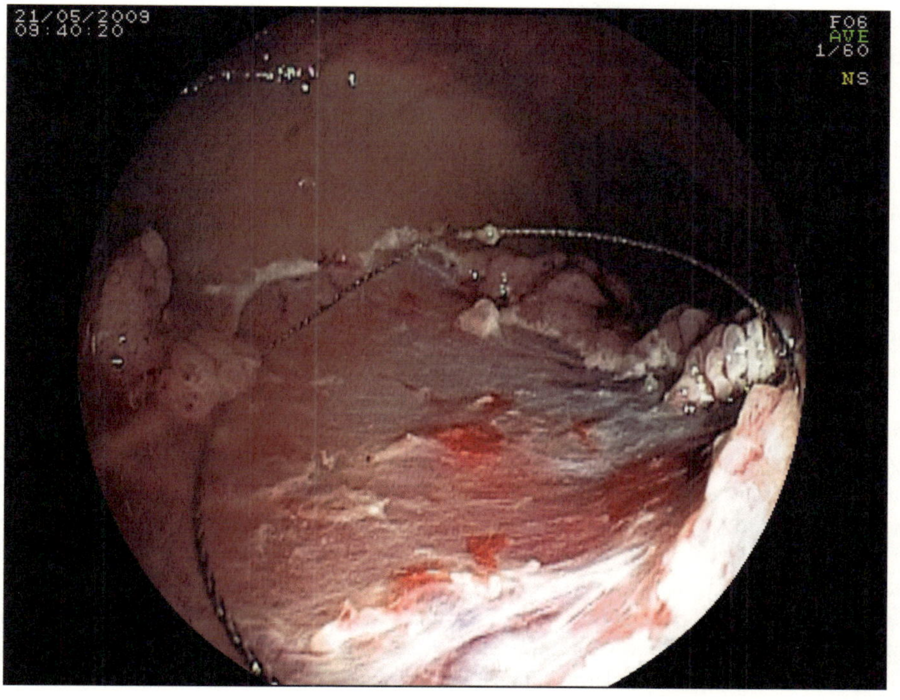

Fig. 10. Picture showing endoscopic mucosal resection of a large flat polyp placed in rectum. The size of the polypectomy snare allows us to approximate the size of the lesion, which is about twice the size of it, so about 6 cms. The resection is performed gradually, in several fragments (piecemeal resection). By this way large lesions can be removed

The number and characteristics of the resected polyps are, therefore, the key factors to establish the date of the next examination. The existence of multiple adenomas (more than three) or a polyp that has a size greater than 10 mm or, regardless of size, the polyp has a villous component or high grade dysplasia (advanced adenoma); leads to set the following colonoscopy within three to five years. If the number of adenomas removed is larger than 10, we recommend surveillance colonoscopy within less than 3 years. When these conditions are not are satisfied (less than three adenomas, without advanced adenoma characteristics), the next examination should be done within five to ten years. In case of a first surveillance examination without evidence of new adenomas, subsequent colonoscopies should be performed every 5 years.

In patients who have been treated for colorectal cancer, as well as in patients with adenomas, we should have a complete study of the colon before surgery or at least within 6 months. In case of obstructive tumors in which it is impossible to complete a study by colonoscopy, we can complete the examination of the colon with a CT-colonography. Most clinical practice guidelines recommend a review of the surgical anastomosis within one year after the intervention, to rule out a possible anastomotic recurrence and then, the recommendations are the same as those for patients undergoing endoscopic polypectomy: the first examination after three years and the following ones, if not metachronous lesions were detected, should be performed at intervals of 5 years. In case of detecting lesions during follow-up, its features will condition the surveillance.

2.3 CRC screening in patients with inflammatory bowel disease

People suffering from inflammatory bowel disease, especially ulcerative colitis have an increased risk of colon cancer. The risk is only increased in patients with extensive disease, thus it is not indicated endoscopic surveillance in patients with ulcerative colitis that only affects the rectosigmoid region. However there are a number of factors that are associated with a significant rise in the incidence of colon cancer. Indeed, the risk increases significantly if there are family history of colon cancer, if primary sclerosing cholangitis is associated with ulcerative colitis and, undoubtedly, if it is a disease with difficult control with persistent inflammation and presence of inflammatory pseudopolyps. Patients with Crohn's disease with extensive colonic involvement may also have an increased risk of developing colon cancer, so surveillance should also be extended to this group of patients.

The risk increases significantly after 8-10 years of development, being that the moment in which it is recommended to start the monitoring programs. Naturally, and taking into consideration that what we are looking for is the presence of dysplasia, colonoscopy with biopsy of colorectal mucosa is the only valid screening strategy. However, the evidence supporting this colorectal cancer screening is poor. Several studies suggest that the inclusion of patients in screening programs improves the prognosis of the disease because many cases would be diagnosed in early stages. In contrast, other studies doubt about the utility of specific screening programs, since most malignancies would be diagnosed as interval cancers.

Although scientific evidence is little and poor, the majority of international clinical practice guidelines, and also guidelines available in Spain, recommend to start with screening from 8-10 years after development of the disease in extensive colitis, and from 15 years in colitis that just involve the left colon. As explained before, it is not justified to perform any kind of endoscopic screening in patients with only rectal involvement. Initially it would be recommended to perform colonoscopy every 2-3 years, and then to increase in frequency because the incidence of colon cancer increases with duration of disease. It has been suggested to perform colonoscopies every two years after 20 years since the diagnosis of the disease and annually after 30 years of development of ulcerative colitis. It is also included in most guidelines the recommendation to intensify surveillance in patients with sclerosing cholangitis due to its association with an increased risk of CRC, indicating to perform an annual colonoscopy at the time of diagnosis of primary sclerosing cholangitis.

The best way to prevent the appearance of colon cancer is an early detection of dysplasia. Therefore, we should carefully explore all of the colon mucosa, trying to detect any mucosal lesion (minimum mucosal elevation, polyp, mass ...) and if so, we should take biopsies. Additionally, biopsies from the entire colonic mucosa should be systematically taken and the most widely recommendation accepted is taking 4 biopsy specimens every 10 cm of intestine. As expected, the examinations are hardworking and, with the available evidence, we can not ensure its cost effectiveness. In order to make these examinations less time-consuming and possibly more cost effective, several studies propose to take biopsies in a targeted way, using magnification endoscopy and chromoendoscopy. Thus, these techniques help us to choose the areas that we need to biopsy, and this could probably improve the detection of dysplasia and also they can help us in reducing the number of biopsies that should be taken. At the present time confocal endomicroscopy is under study. This technique allows subsurface histological diagnosis in situ, without taking biopsies, and it could probably be more helpful detecting dysplasia. However, these are very long examinations, and this technique requires an expensive technology and a specialized training by the endoscopist, so it becomes a technique restricted to highly specialized centers.

There is some agreement on the way to approach after detecting dysplasia. Due to the high incidence of synchronous adenocarcinoma with high-grade dysplastic foci, it is usually recommended to perform a total proctocolectomy after detecting high-grade dysplasia. In case a low-grade dysplasia, the decision is more controversial. If multiple foci of dysplasia on flat mucosa are detected, it is recommended to perform a proctocolectomy. On the other hand, if isolated foci of dysplasia are detected the recommendation should be to perform a new colonoscopy within approximately 3-6 months. Subsequently, following colonoscopies should be performed every 6 months.

Elevated lesions or masses can appear in patients with ulcerative colitis, and in many cases they are similar to adenomas. The presence of dysplasia on these raised lesions causes a difficult differential diagnosis with sporadic adenomas that are defined by the presence of dysplasia and whose treatment could be endoscopic polypectomy. Generally, we consider dysplasia-associated lesion or mass (DALM) if the lesion is located on "colitic" mucosa (even in quiescent ulcerative colitis), while if it appears on normal mucosa, it is probably sporadic adenoma. Sporadic adenoma should be treated as in the general population and DALM could also be endoscopically removed after ruling out the presence of dysplastic lesions in the surrounding mucosa. If this is not technically possible or perilesional mucosal biopsies present dysplastic foci, we should perform a total colectomy. If we have performed endoscopic resection of the lesion, we should take biopsies of the mucosa around the lesion in 3-6 months, and also the following colonoscopies should be performed every six months.

The work for pathologist is not always easy and he can find cases in which, mainly due to the persistence of inflammatory activity, the findings are not definitive to confirm or exclude dysplasia. In these cases, endoscopy should be repeated within 3-6 months after an appropriate control of mucosa inflammation under a specific treatment.

As presented, colonoscopy is essential in monitoring these patients, being the only tool that allows taking biopsies to detect dysplasia. However, there is a long way to walk until we find the ideal strategy to make examinations less time-consuming and more cost effective. Everything suggests that modern endoscopic techniques (magnification endoscopy and chromoendoscopy) can be the key, but there is little scientific evidence by now. Secondly, the steps to follow in case of dysplasia seem to be more established. Finally, colonoscopy may have a therapeutic role if we detect low-grade dysplastic foci on lesions and masses similar to adenomas.

2.4 Colorectal cancer screening strategies in patients with family history of CRC

The risk of colorectal cancer is higher in those people who belong to families where cases of CRC have been recorded, even after having ruled out the possibility of polyposis syndromes and hereditary colorectal cancer. However, the risk depends on several factors: the number of relatives affected, the degree of kinship and age at which the neoplasm is detected. In second-degree relatives, excepting they were multiple family members affected, it is not justified any special CRC screening, and the recommendations are the same as for medium-risk population. In case of multiple second-degree relatives affected, the different scientific societies recommend the same screening strategy as for people at average risk, but starting the screening program at age 40 years. In case of several first-degree relatives or a single family member younger than 60 years at the time of diagnosis, the only recommendation accepted is to perform colonoscopy every five years. The age to start the screening will be at 40 years of age or at age 10 years younger than the youngest case diagnosed in the family. The presence of a single first-degree relative older than 60 years increases the risk of developing the disease but in a lesser way, so the recommendations are the same as if there were second-degree relatives affected.

In summary, if there is a family history of colorectal cancer, the risk is increased respecting to the average risk population. If there is a low risk family history, as well as medium-risk population, the acceptable screening tests include fecal occult blood testing, colonoscopy and radiological tests. By contrast, if there is a high risk family history the only accepted screening test is colonoscopy because there are higher possibilities of detecting cancer or polyps.

2.5 Hereditary CRC syndromes: non-polyposis colorectal cancer and familial adenomatous polyposis

2.5.1 Hereditary non-polyposis colorrectal cancer or Lynch syndrome

Hereditary non-polyposis colorectal cancer (HNPCC) or Lynch syndrome is an autosomal dominant disease which represents less than 2% of total CRC. It is mostly due to mutations in DNA repair genes and, clinically, it is characterized by the development of neoplasia in young people (under 50 years) with high preference for right colon, with great tendency to develop synchronous and metachronous neoplasms as well as in other organs (urinary tract, biliary tract, endometrium, pancreas, stomach, small intestine and ovary). It is more uncommon to find development of osteomas, skin or brain tumors. Pathologically it is characterized by a strong tendency to present a mucinous histology.

The diagnosis is based on the Amsterdam criteria: at least three relatives affected, one of whom is a first degree relative of the other, at least two successive generations involved and at least one case diagnosed of cancer before age 50. Then, these criteria were found to be too strict and were expanded to include the associated non-colorectal cancers (Amsterdam II). In any case, these criteria have poor sensitivity for the diagnosis of the disease, although its specificity is very high. Therefore, the Bethesda criteria were established, suspecting the disease by demonstrating on the resected tumor the presence microsatellite instabilty (expression of mutations in repair genes). It is mandatory to perform a genetic analysis whether if diagnosis is based on the Amsterdam criteria or on the analysis of microsatellite instability. If the mutation responsible for the disease is detected in a patient, the family members should be studied, and only those who file such mutations will be subsidiary to perform the screening program.

The aim of endoscopic surveillance of people belonging to families with Lynch syndrome is the early detection of cancer or polyps and their removal when it is possible. In many cases, precancerous lesions are flat lesions, and may not be detected by non-endoscopic techniques, so the only acceptable diagnostic technique for monitoring is the colonoscopy. Even these lesions are difficult to detect with conventional endoscopy, which may explain the high frequency of interval cancers. For this reason it was suggested to use more sophisticated endoscopic techniques (Narrow Band Imaging and chromoendoscopy) to facilitate the detection of these lesions. In our experience, chromoendoscopy seems to be easier to perform and to interpret. To do it, it is essential a correct colon cleansing and staining of the colonic mucosa with a solution of Indigo Carmine 0.2%. This will significantly improve the detection of flat lesions, almost imperceptible by conventional colonoscopy. The use of magnification endoscopy can further improve diagnostic accuracy. Computed virtual chromoendoscopy (CVC or FICE, Fujinon) (Figure 11) can be an alternative to conventional chromoendoscopy (Figure 12), avoiding the use of colorants and making even shorter examinations, but of course, it depends on the availability of this technology. The use of NBI (Figure 13) may be helpful for the characterization of lesions, but this technique may be more complicated than chromoendoscopy.

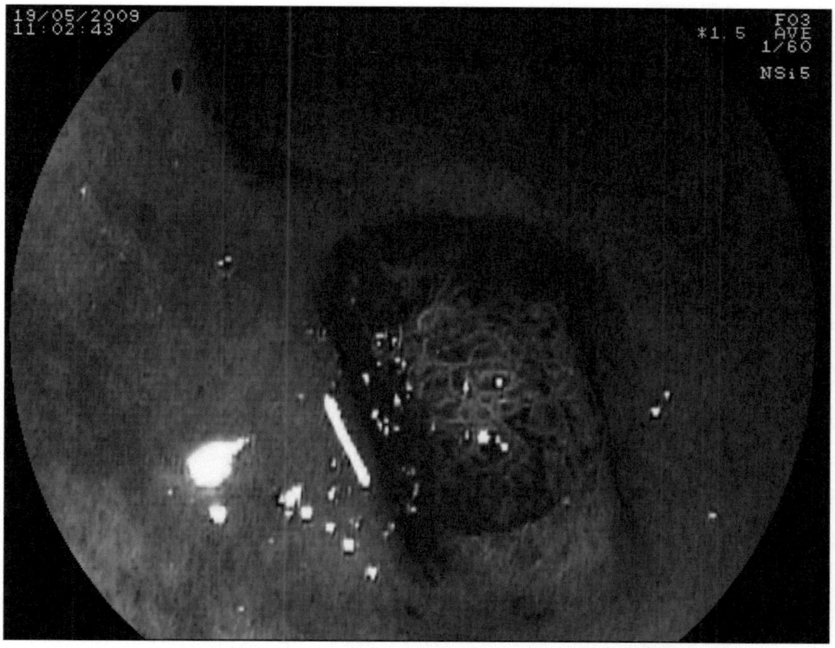

Fig. 11. Flat lesion in the right colon in a patient with quiescent ulcerative colitis, studied by CVC, Set 4

The interval between examinations in these cases is determined by finding the adenoma-dysplasia-carcinoma progression significantly shortened or even that it does not exist. It has been shown that performing examinations every 3 years had managed to reduce the incidence and the CRC mortality in more than 60%. However, widespread recommendations propose to perform colonoscopies every 1 or 2 years. Patients operated on for CRC in the context of Lynch syndrome have a high possibility of metachronous lesions, so post-resection surveillance recommendation is the same as the screening strategy for relatives at risk. The age at onset of endoscopic surveillance is usually established around 20-25 years of age or 10 years younger than the youngest case in the family, choosing the option that happens before.
In conclusion, in people from families with Lynch syndrome it is justified to perform surveillance programs. The only acceptable alternative is to conduct endoscopic surveillance and, based on current evidence, conventional endoscopy may not be sufficient. The use of chromoendoscopy and magnification endoscopy may be useful, so monitoring of these patients should be performed in specialized endoscopy units with endoscopists trained in these techniques.

2.5.2 Familial adenomatous polyposis

The classic form of familial adenomatous polyposis (FAP) is characterized by the development of hundreds of polyps in the colon, usually after puberty. Its pattern of inheritance is autosomal dominant and in the absence of surgical treatment, 100% of patients would develop cancer. An attenuated form of familial adenomatous polyposis has been identified. Individuals with attenuated FAP develop 20-100 adenomatous polyps and the average age of diagnosis is ten years later than in the classic form. There is the possibility of developing polyps at other gastrointestinal levels or tumors in other locations.

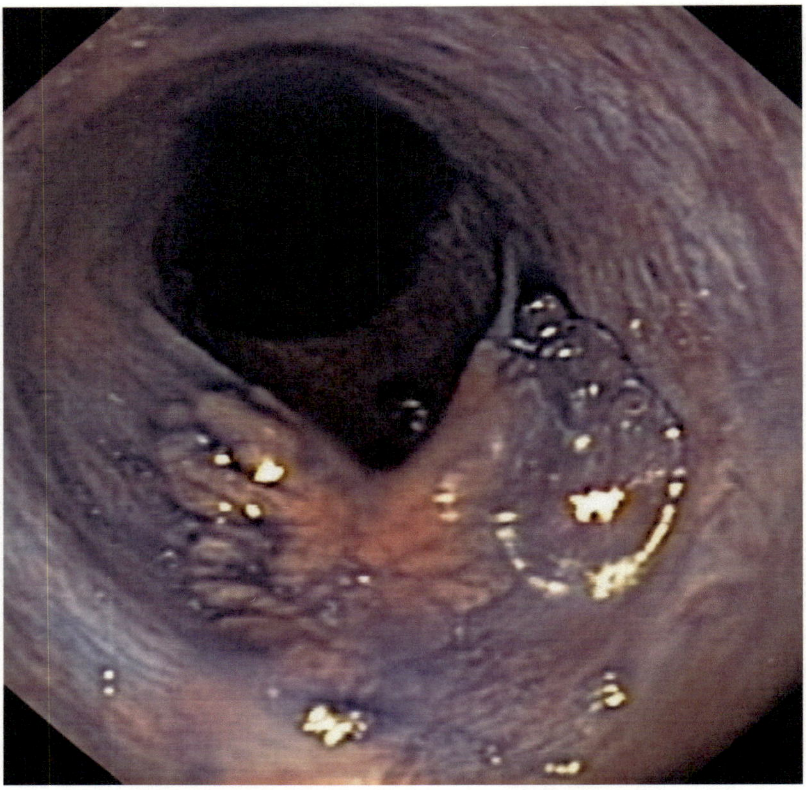

Fig. 12. Flat lesion, almost imperceptible to conventional endoscopy, which clearly demarcates with 0.2% indigo carmine. This is a patient who performed a colonoscopy as colorectal cancer screening method because he belonged to a family that fulfilled the Amsterdam criteria for diagnosing HNPCC. This is a lesion that, according to the Paris classification of superficial gastrointestinal neoplasia, can be a category IIc (excavated or depressed). According to its size (about 25 mm) endoscopic resection can not be considered. Indeed, the study of the surgical specimen showed the presence of adenocarcinoma with infiltration of the muscularis propria (pT2)

The diagnosis is based on detection of polyps by endoscopy and histologic confirmation of the presence of adenomas. Then, genetic testing should be performed to identy APC gene mutations. However, mutations are not identified up to 30% of cases. Most diagnoses occur in relatives of patients affected, who are included on endoscopic surveillance programs. The recommended strategy in most guidelines is performing sigmoidoscopy every 1-2 years from 13-15 years of age and up to 40. From this age, they are recommended every 5 years until 60 years. In attenuated FAP, screening begins at age 10 years older than in classical FAP, and as polyps are more likely to appear on the right colon, colonoscopy should be complete. Also, chromoendoscopy may improve the detection rate of polyps on these patients.

When individuals are diagnosed, prophylactic colectomy should be considered. The standard surgery is proctocolectomy with ileo-anal reservoir. In patients with reservoir, endoscopic examinations should be performed every 3 years. In patients who have preserved the rectum (for example in attenuated FAP it is a good option, if there are few polyps in rectum), endoscopic examination should be performed every 6-12 months.

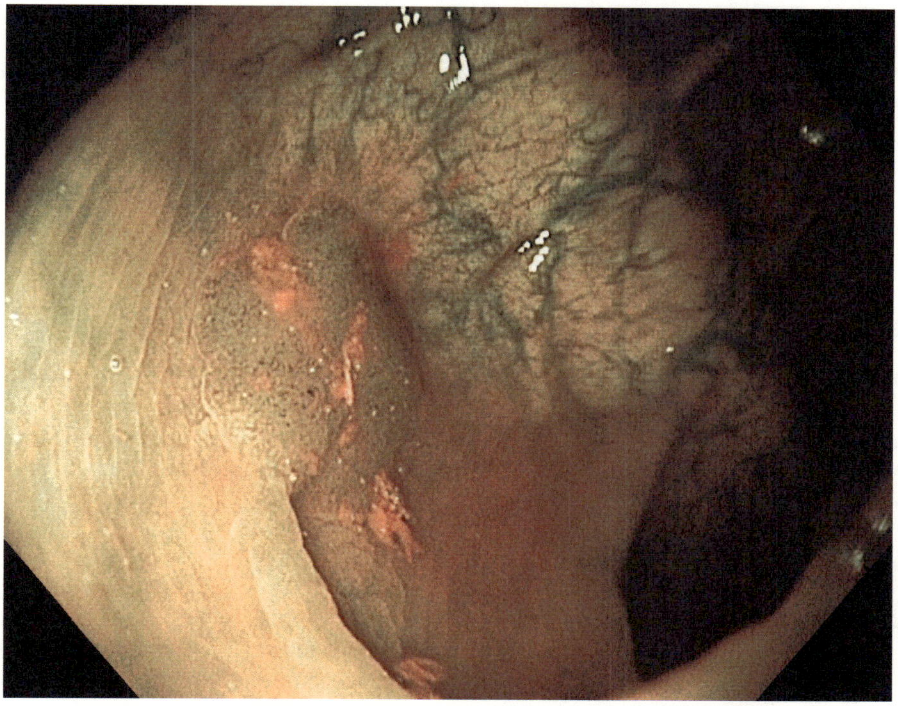

Fig. 13. Flat lesion, about 10 mm, located in the hepatic flexure of colon, visualized with NBI. This is a IIa lesion according to the Paris classification. Endoscopic resection and histological study of it showed a villous adenoma with high grade dysplasia

Due to these patients may have adenomas in other locations of the upper gastrointestinal tract, other endoscopic procedures should be performed. It is recommended to perform a gastroscopy every 4-5 years starting from age 25. If no adenomas are detected, another possibility is to take random biopsies on the duodenal folds. Additionally, it is recommended using side vision duodenoscope for further examination of the papillary area to detect ampulomas. Treatment of duodenal adenomas is controversial. Endoscopic resection of them seems to be not very effective, especially if they are many, and it is a technique that is not exempt of complications. The severity of the lesions is established by Spiegelman classification, which takes into account the number of adenomas, size, histological type and presence of dysplasia. In patients with duodenal adenomas Spiegelman stage I-II disease, endoscopic surveillance could be performed every 2-3 years, but in patients with more complex cases, monitoring should be stricter, like performing endoscopy every 6-12 months, but probably surgical treatment should be the best option in these cases. On the other hand, endoscopic removal of the most significant adenomas could delay surgical decision.

There are some other forms of polyposis, like MYH-associated polyposis (MAP) which appears to be similar to other hereditary conditions as attenuated familial adenomatous polyposis, so screening strategies in people with MAP should be similar to screening in people with attenuated FAP.

3. Conclusions

As we have explained, colonoscopy plays an important role in preventing colorectal carcinoma. In average risk populations for developing of cancer, it is one of the recommended screening strategies. In this population it has not yet been demonstrated which one is the most cost-effective strategy. What is unquestionable is the role of colonoscopy because of its therapeutic approach on the removal of lesions detected by other techniques or by its own. In high-risk populations, the only acceptable strategy is screening colonoscopy. The frequency of examinations is determined in each case by the particular risk of developing CRC. In some cases, such as patients with long-standing ulcerative colitis or individuals from families with Lynch syndrome, conventional colonoscopy is not enough, requiring using special techniques for endoscopic diagnosis, such as chromoendoscopy and magnification endoscopy.

4. Acknowledgment

Our thanks to Dr. Vincent Hernandez Ramirez for providing us the latest data on colorectal cancer epidemiology in our country, and to Dr. Maria Luisa de Castro Parga to transfer us some of her images. In addition, we would like to thank the whole team and staff of the Endoscopy Unit in our hospital. Without their knowledge and dedication, our work would be less productive.

5. References

Castells A, Marzo-Castillejo M, Mascort JJ, Amador FJ, Andreu M, Bellas B, Fernandez A, Ferrandiz J, Giraldez M, Gonzalo V, Jover R, Quintero E, Alonso-Coello P, Bonfill X, Lanas A, Piñol V, Piqué J. [Clinical practice guideline. Prevention of colorectal cancer. 2009 update. Asociación Española de Gastroenterología. Gastroenterol Hepatol. 2009; 32:717.e1-58.

Winawer SJ, Zauber AG, Fletcher RH, Stillman JS, O'Brien MJ, Levin B, Smith RA, Lieberman DA, Burt RW, Levin TR, Bond JH, Brooks D, Byers T, Hyman N, Kirk L, Thorson A, Simmang C, Johnson D, Rex DK; US Multi-Society Task Force on Colorectal Cancer; American Cancer Society. Guidelines for colonoscopy surveillance after polypectomy: a consensus update by the US Multi-Society Task Force on Colorectal Cancer and the American Cancer Society. Gastroenterology 2006;130:1872-85.

Rex DK, Johnson DA, Anderson JC, Schoenfeld PS, Burke CA, Inadomi JM; American College of Gastroenterology. American College of Gastroenterology guidelines for colorectal cancer screening 2009 [corrected]. Am J Gastroenterol. 2009; 104:739-50.

Levin B, Lieberman DA, McFarland B, Andrews KS, Brooks D, Bond J, Dash C, Giardiello FM, Glick S, Johnson D, Johnson CD, Levin TR, Pickhardt PJ, Rex DK, Smith RA, Thorson A, Winawer SJ; American Cancer Society Colorectal Cancer Advisory Group; US Multi-Society Task Force; American College of Radiology Colon Cancer Committee. Screening and surveillance for the early detection of colorectal cancer and adenomatous polyps, 2008: a joint guideline from the American Cancer Society, the US Multi-Society Task Force on Colorectal Cancer, and the American College of Radiology. Gastroenterology. 2008; 34 :1570-95.

Zauber AG. Cost-effectiveness of colonoscopy. Gastrointest Endosc Clin N Am. 2010; 20: 751-70.

15

Recent Advances in Diagnostic Endoscopy for Colorectal Neoplasm

Yoji Takeuchi, Noboru Hanaoka and Masao Hanafusa
Department of Gastrointestinal Oncology, Osaka Medical Center for Cancer and Cardiovascular Diseases
Japan

1. Introduction

Colorectal cancer is one of the most common causes of cancer-related death in the western world (Jemal et al., 2009). Most non-hereditary colorectal cancers arise from benign adenomas (Morison et al., 1974). It has been reported that removal of adenomatous polyps reduces the risk of subsequent colorectal cancer by as much as 80% (Winawer et al., 1993). Therefore, detection and removal of colorectal adenomas, as well as of cancer in the early stages, is utmost importance in improving the prognosis of patients with colorectal cancer. Although colonoscopy is one of the most reliable methods for diagnosis of colorectal neoplasms, conventional colonoscopy could be improved by addressing some of its shortcomings.

In this article, the new and promising technologies that comprise image-enhanced endoscopy (IEE) are reviewed, and a new colonoscopic strategy that incorporates some of these techniques is proposed.

2. Detection of colorectal neoplasms using colonoscopy

It is generally known that conventional colonoscopy fails to detect some colorectal neoplasms (Rex, et al., 1997) and that such failure may lead to interval cancers between successive colonoscopies. To date, many attempts have been made to improve screening and surveillance colonoscopy. Mounting a transparent hood (TH) on the tip of the colonoscope helps in the detection of colorectal neoplasms by pressing and flattening the colonic folds, thus improving the endoscopic view (Hewett & Rex, 2010). On the other hand IEE, including the total colonic dye-spray method, narrow-band imaging (NBI), flexible spectral imaging color enhancement (FICE) and autofluorescence imaging (AFI) offers the possibility of increasing the detection rate of colorectal neoplasms by increasing the visibility of colorectal neoplasms.

Although the reasons for overlooking colorectal neoplasms are unknown, there are two major possibilities (Fig. 1). One is that the overlooked lesions are small and hidden behind colonic folds. Endoscopists should check possible blind spots by using 'mechanical' devices which allow them to look behind colonic folds. The other possible reason is that the overlooked lesions are flat and similar in color to the surrounding mucosa, which makes them difficult to recognize using conventional white light endoscopy. Some type of 'optical' image enhancing device should be used for detection of this type of lesion. Therefore, endoscopists should utilize both 'mechanical' and 'optical' devices to minimize the overlooking of colorectal neoplasms.

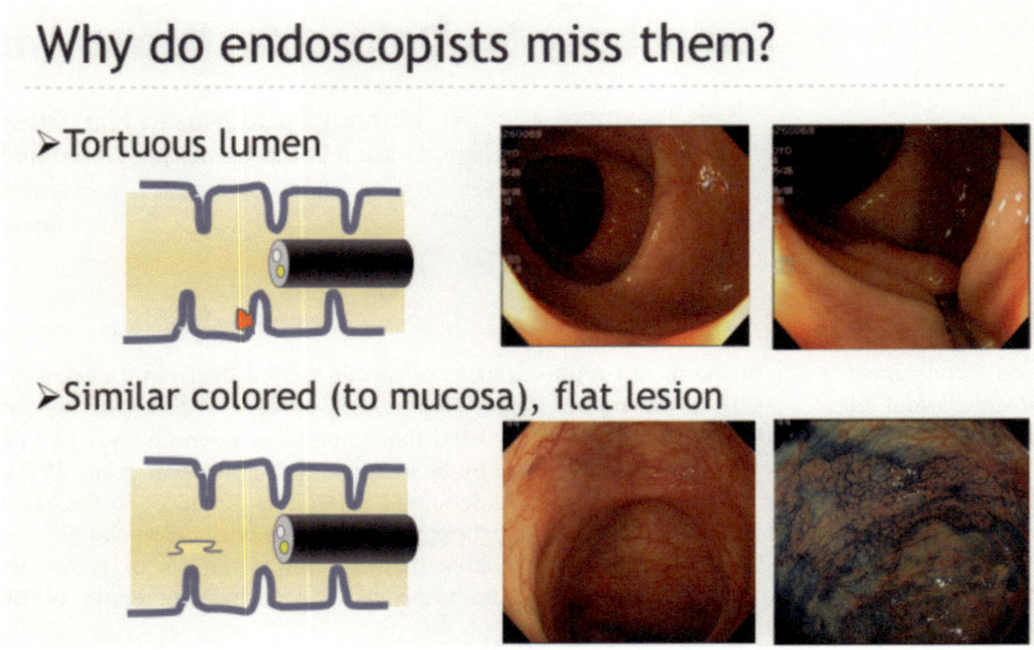

Fig. 1. Possible reasons for overlooking colorectal lesions. A tortuous lumen with colonic folds can result in the overlooking of small lesion behind the folds. Flat lesions of a similar color to the surrounding mucosa can also be easily overlooked

2.1 Mechanical methods for minimizing the overlooking of colorectal neoplasm

Some mechanical methods for minimizing the overlooking of colorectal neoplasms have been proposed. One of them is the Third Eye Retroscope, which is passed through the working channel of a standard colonoscope and provides retrograde visualization of the colon (Triadafilopoulos, et al., 2007). In a multicenter randomized controlled trial, it resulted in the diagnosis of about 50% additional adenomas (Leufkens, et al., 2011). The other is the Aer-O-Scope, which provides simultaneous 360° viewing of the mucosal surface of the colon. The use of this device was reported in a preliminary pilot feasibility study (Vucelic, et al., 2006). Although both are promising devices that allow direct visualization of the back of colonic folds, they require an additional endoscope or endoscopic system and are much too complicated technically. Therefore, they have not become standard methods for screening colonoscopy.

Cap-fitted colonoscopy uses a TH affixed to the colonoscope tip (Fig. 2). It flattens the colorectal folds and improves mucosal exposure. The method is very simple and requires only a TH, which costs about $20. The efficacy of THs has been reported previously (Matsushita et al., 1998). They performed tandem colonoscopy on 24 patients and proved that the TH reduced the miss rate for polyps from 15% to 0%. In their randomized tandem colonoscopy study, Hewett & Rex also reported that cap-fitted colonoscopy reduced the miss rates for all adenomas, and specifically for small adenomas (Hewett & Rex, 2010).

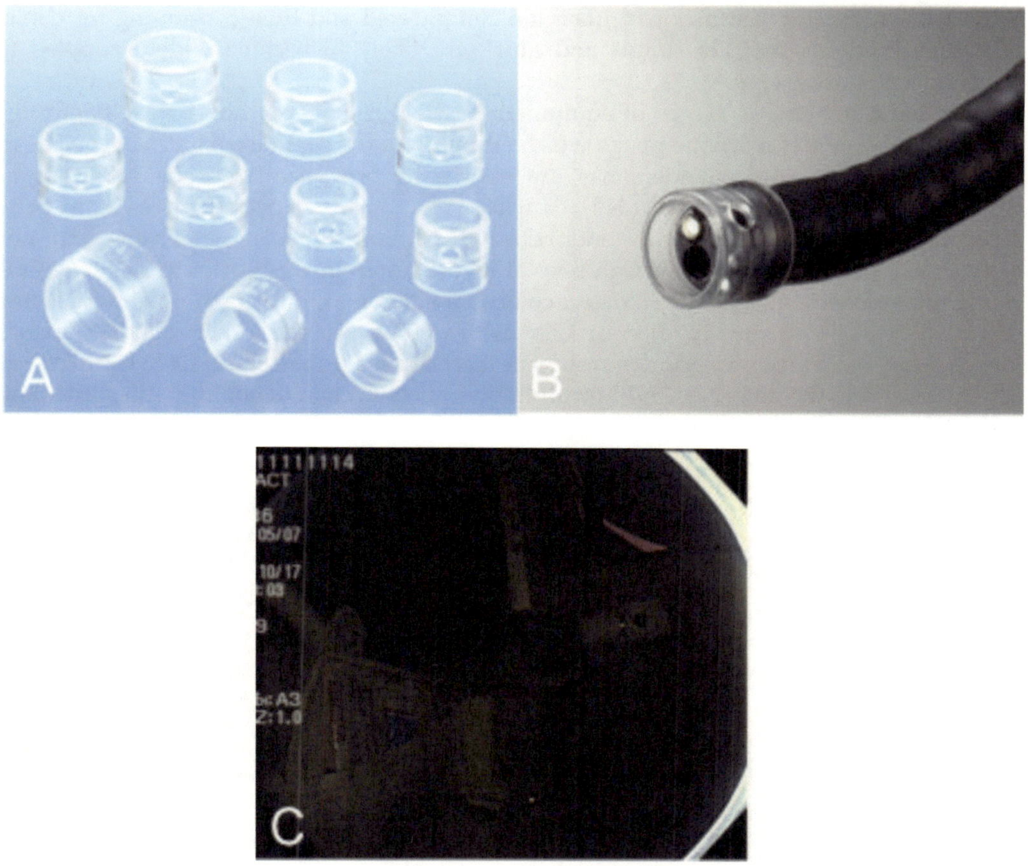

Fig. 2. (A) Transparent hood (TH, D-201 series; Olympus Medical Systems, Tokyo, Japan). (B) The TH attached to the tip of the colonoscope. (C) The endoscopic view of the cap-fitted colonoscope. The tip of TH is seen on the right edge of the endoscopic view

2.2 Optical methods for minimizing the overlooking of colorectal neoplasms

Image-enhanced endoscopy is expected to be better at detecting adenomas than conventional white light imaging (WLI). There are two types of IEE: dye-based and equipment-based (Kaltenbach, et al., 2008). In dye-based IEE, absorptive or contrast dye is used to enhance the features of the lesion. The typical absorptive dye for colonoscopy is crystal violet and the typical contrast dye indigo carmine. Indigo carmine, which can provide enhancement of the details of lesions by highlighting subtle changes in mucosal topography, is usually used to minimize the overlooking of colorectal neoplasms. On the other hand, there are a number of categories of equipment-based IEE. These include optical method such as NBI, electronic methods such as FICE, and optical-digital methods such as AFI.

Brooker et al. reported that total colonic dye-spray increases the detection of diminutive adenomas (Brooker et al., 2002). In their trial, they detected 89 diminutive adenomas using total dye-spray colonoscopy and 37 using conventional colonoscopy. Certainly, total colonic dye-spray might improve the adenoma detection rate, but it has not become a standard method for screening because it is much too complicated and time consuming for clinical use. Only methods that are simple and quick are likely to become widely adopted for screening colonoscopy.

Narrow band imaging is a type of equipment-based IEE that uses short-wavelength light (Fig. 3). NBI provides a unique image which emphasizes the capillary pattern as well as the surface pattern. Colorectal adenomas are shown as brownish areas by NBI and are significantly better visualized by NBI than by WLI. NBI is expected to result in better detection of colorectal adenomas and better distinction between neoplasms and non-neoplastic lesions. Recently, although several investigators in western countries have been trying to demonstrate its ability to detect colorectal adenomas, most randomized trials have reported negative results (Adler et al., 2008, 2009). On the other hands, Japanese investigators have reported positive results in their articles (Inoue et al., 2008; Uraoka et al., 2008). Therefore, the efficacy of NBI for detection of colorectal adenoma is still contentious and further investigation is needed.

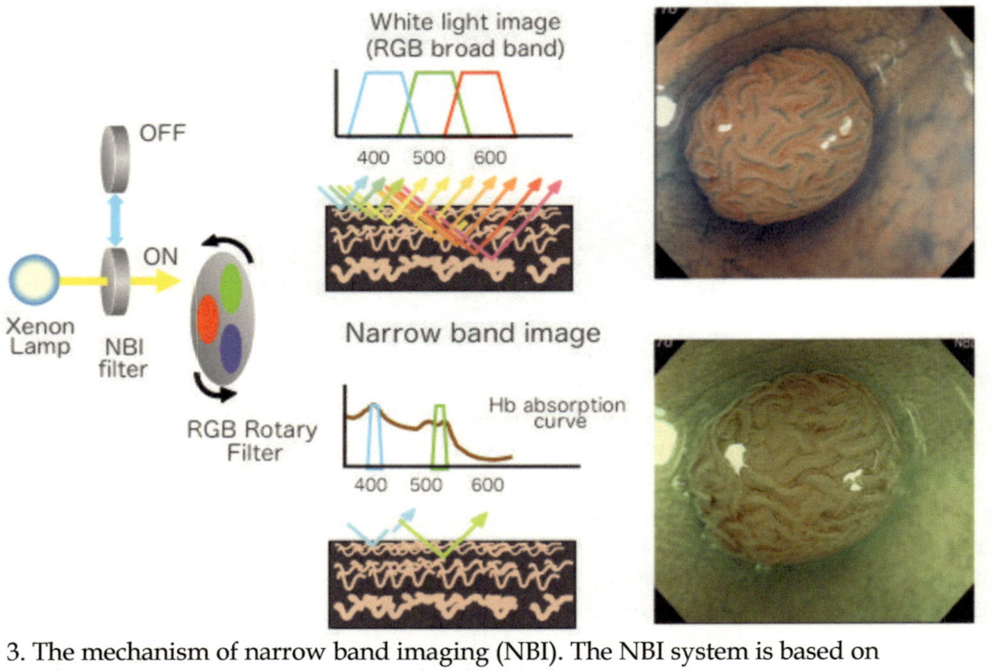

Fig. 3. The mechanism of narrow band imaging (NBI). The NBI system is based on modification of spectral features with each optical filter narrowing a bandwidth of spectral transmittance. (RGB; Red, Green, Blue)

Flexible spectral imaging color enhancement modifies spectral transmittance arithmetically by using a computing processor; therefore, it does not require optical filters. Furthermore, because of its variable setting functions (up to 10), the operator has flexibility in selection of the most suitable wavelengths for each examination. Although some randomized controlled trials have been conducted (Aminalai et al., 2010 Chung et al., 2010), no one has yet demonstrated improvement in adenoma miss or detection rates compared with WLI.

Autofluorescence imaging is an endoscopic technique for visualizing with reflected autofluorescence, which is emitted from an endogeneous fluorophore by exposing it to short wavelength excitation light (Fig. 4). The latest model of AFI system can switch between observation modes in a few seconds. Because colonic adenomas are shown as distinct purple areas in the surrounding green mucosa using AFI, this technique is expected to improve the detection rate of colonic tumors during screening colonoscopy, especially in regard to flat lesions, which are difficult to detect using WLI (Fig. 5). Matsuda et al. reported that AFI is better than WLI at detecting polyps in the right-sided colon. The miss rate for all polyps with AFI (30%) was significantly less than that with WLI (49%, P=0.01) (Matsuda et al., 2008).

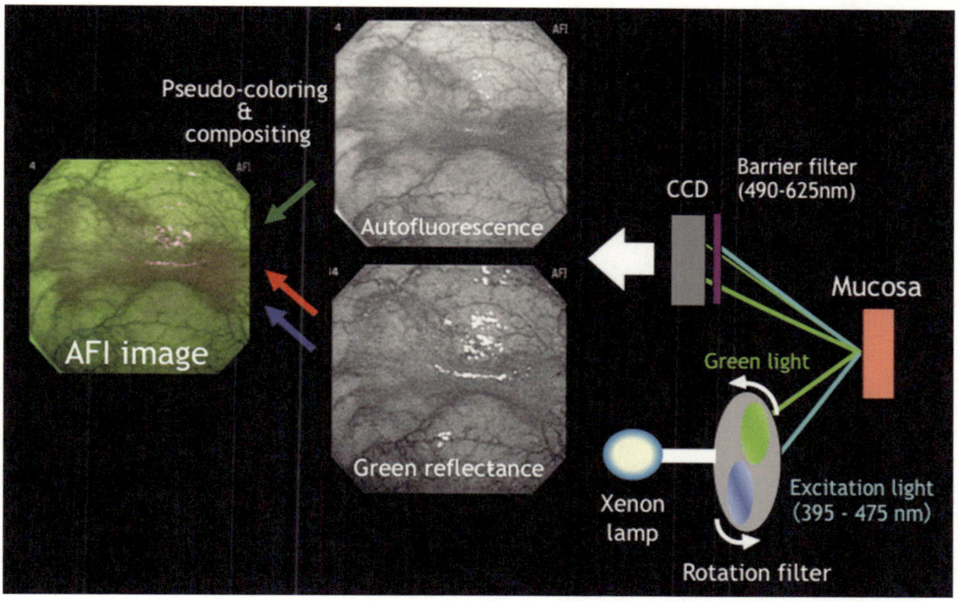

Fig. 4. The mechanism of autofluorescence imaging (AFI). AFI images are produced by illuminating the mucosa by light that has passed through a rotation filter. The image processor artificially colors the autofluorescence images green, and the green reflection images red and blue, then composite images are displayed on the video screen

2.3 Combination of mechanical and optical methods for minimizing the overlooking of colorectal neoplasms

To determine whether a combination of the different complementary mechanisms of AFI and a TH would be better at detecting colorectal neoplasms than conventional WLI without a TH, a prospective, randomized controlled trial was conducted.

In this trial, both patients undergoing colonoscopy for investigation of a positive screening fecal occult blood testing (FOBT) and those who had been referred for surveillance colonoscopy after endoscopic resection of colorectal neoplasms were enrolled. A 2 × 2 factorial design was adopted to investigate the impact of simultaneous AFI and a TH. The

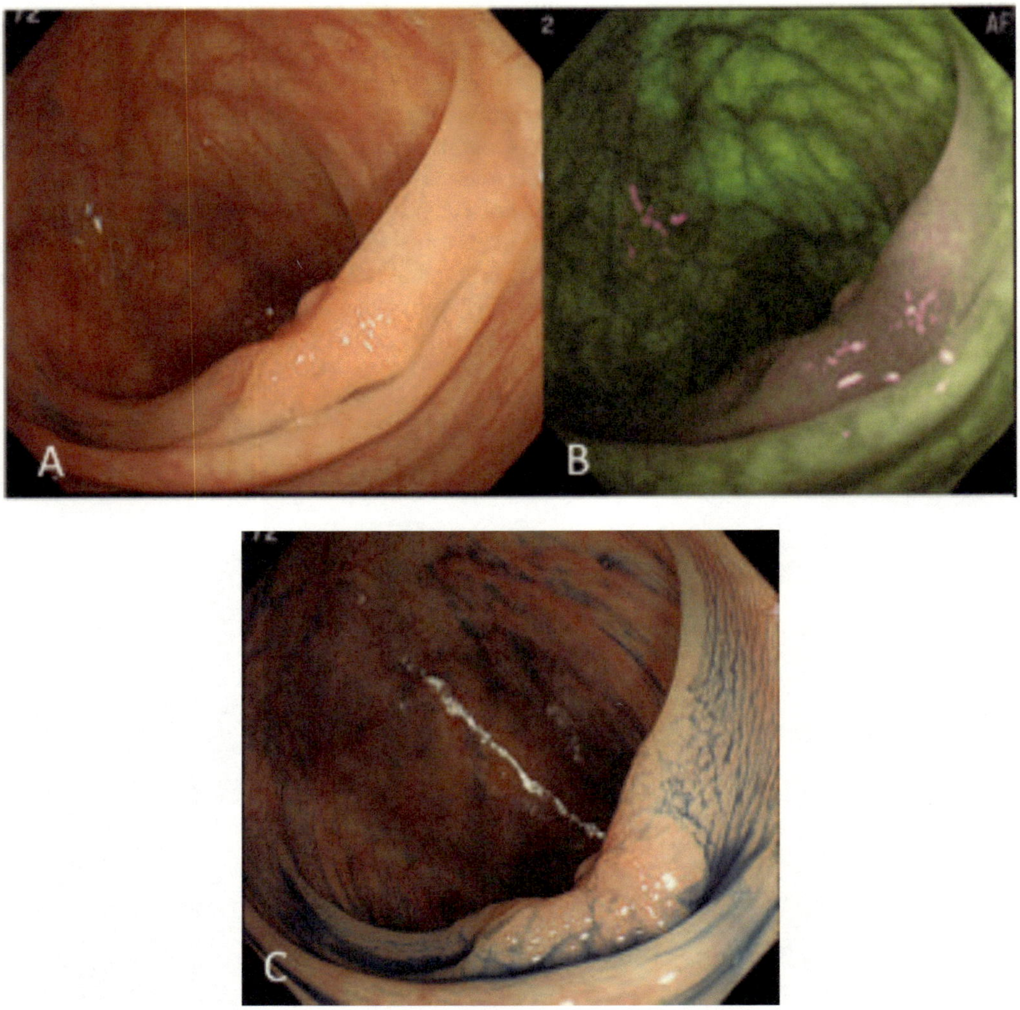

Fig. 5. Images of colonic tumor using autofluorescence imaging (AFI). (A) Conventional endoscopic image of colon cancer in the transverse colon. The lesion is flat and similar in color to the surrounding mucosa. (B) AFI image of the lesion. The lesion shows as a distinct purple area surrounded by green mucosa. (C) Chromo-endoscopic image of the lesion. The features of the lesion are enhanced by indigo carmine

participants were assigned randomly to the following four groups: (1) WLI: colonoscopy using WLI without a TH; (2) WLI + TH: colonoscopy using WLI with a TH; (3) AFI: colonoscopy using AFI without a TH; and (4) AFI + TH: colonoscopy using AFI with a TH (Fig. 6). All patients gave written informed consent to participate in this study and the study protocol was approved by the Research Ethics Committee of our center.

Between 4 November, 2008, and 11 November, 2009, 923 patients who had a positive FOBT or who had been referred for surveillance colonoscopy were scheduled to undergo colonoscopy in our endoscopy unit. Three hundred and sixty-two patients were excluded from enrolment for the following reasons: (1) a history of colorectomy or major abdominal surgery; (2) symptoms suspicious of colorectal stenosis or cancer; (3) inflammatory bowel disease, familial polyposis or known colorectal cancer; (4) severe organ failure, non-correctable coagulopathy, or receiving anticoagulant therapy; or (5) when the colonoscopist judged that the patient was unable to comprehend and give true consent to the process of random allocation. This left 561 patients to be randomly assigned to the different groups. One thousand one hundred and five lesions were detected in 380 patients. Specimens were not obtained from 13 lesions, thus histological diagnosis was available for 1092 lesions. Eight hundred and seventy-five lesions were diagnosed as neoplasms and 217 as non-neoplastic. There were 383 (69%) patients in whom lesions were detected and 329 (59%) with neoplasms.

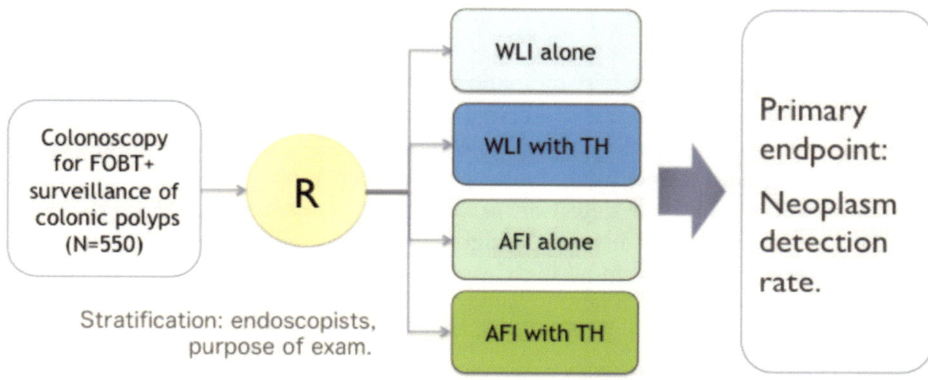

Fig. 6. Study design of a 2 × 2 factorial designed randomized controlled trial for investigation the impact of autofluorescence imaging and a transparent hood. (R; randomization.)

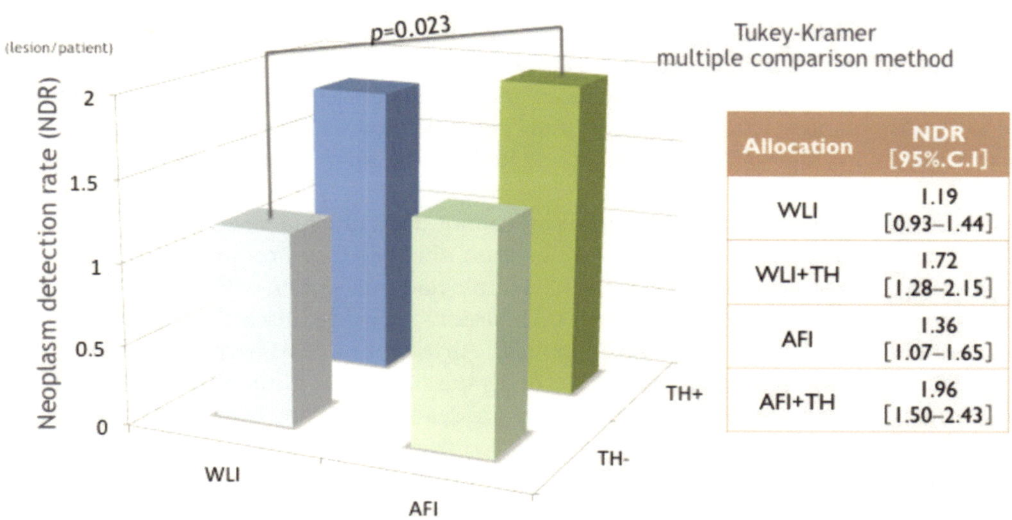

Fig. 7. Primary endpoint of the randomized controlled trial. Neoplastic lesion detection rate in the AFI + TH group was significantly higher than in the WLI group. (AFI; Autofluorescence imaging, TH; transparent hood, WLI; white light imaging)

The primary endpoint, neoplasm detection rate (number of detected neoplasms per patient [95% CI]) in the AFI + TH group was significantly higher than in the WLI alone group (1.96 [1.50–2.43] vs 1.19 [0.93–1.44], $P = 0.023$ [Tukey-Kramer multiple comparison method]). AFI with a TH detected more neoplasms than did conventional colonoscopy (Fig. 7). Subgroup analysis revealed that mounting a TH resulted in a higher detection rate for polypoid neoplasms than did not mounting a TH, and that AFI observation resulted in a higher detection rate for flat neoplasms than did WLI observation. It was concluded that a combination of the different complementary mechanisms of AFI and a TH would be efficacious in the detection of colorectal neoplasms.

3. New problems caused by accurate colonoscopy and the key to a solution to these problems

It has here been reported that a combination of AFI and a TH detects more colorectal neoplasms than does conventional WLI colonoscopy, however most of the lesions detected in the trial were small, low-grade adenomas. Although detection and resection of colorectal adenomas is an efficacious and basic strategy for prevention of colorectal cancer, such an accurate diagnostic method for detection of colorectal neoplasms increases the cost, time and labor required for formal histopathological diagnosis of the resected small indolent neoplasms. Because it results in a high yield of colorectal neoplasms, more accurate colonoscopy can, in itself, cause a new problem.

The 'DISCARD' (Detect InSpect ChAracterize Resect and Discard) policy (Ignjatovic et al., 2009), which is supported by 'optical diagnosis' using NBI without magnification, can lead to substantial savings in cost, time and labor for formal histopathology, making it a really impressive proposal. In the 'DISCARD' trial, it was reported that the capability to correctly diagnose polyps during screening colonoscopy (optical diagnosis) allows recto-sigmoid hyperplastic polyps to be left *in situ* and small adenomas to be resected and discarded without the need for formal histopathology. This policy could be key to a solution to the new problems created by the high yields of the new colonoscopic techniques.

However, small polypoid invasive cancer, though uncommon, does actually exist. The present authors have detected an 8 mm polypoid carcinoma that had invaded the submucosa in the sigmoid colon (Fig. 8). It looked like a small adenoma in the sigmoid colon.

We suppose that NBI without magnification cannot distinguish a small polypoid invasive cancer from a small indolent adenoma because their shapes are so similar. Although invasive cancer requires colorectomy with lymph node dissection after estimation of the possibility of lymph node metastasis, such lesions may be discarded without formal histopathology under the 'DISCARD' policy. Furthermore, NBI without magnification does not allow assessment of the degree of dysplasia. In the United States, the interval between surveillance colonoscopies is determined according not only to the number of detected adenomas and their size, but also to the degree of dysplasia and the presence of villous components. Therefore, the 'DISCARD' policy cannot be adopted in countries supporting the US guidelines. An alternative endoscopic technique is proposed here, one that, while decreasing the number of formal histopathological examinations required, is expected to provide information about the histopathological dysplasia of any lesions detected.

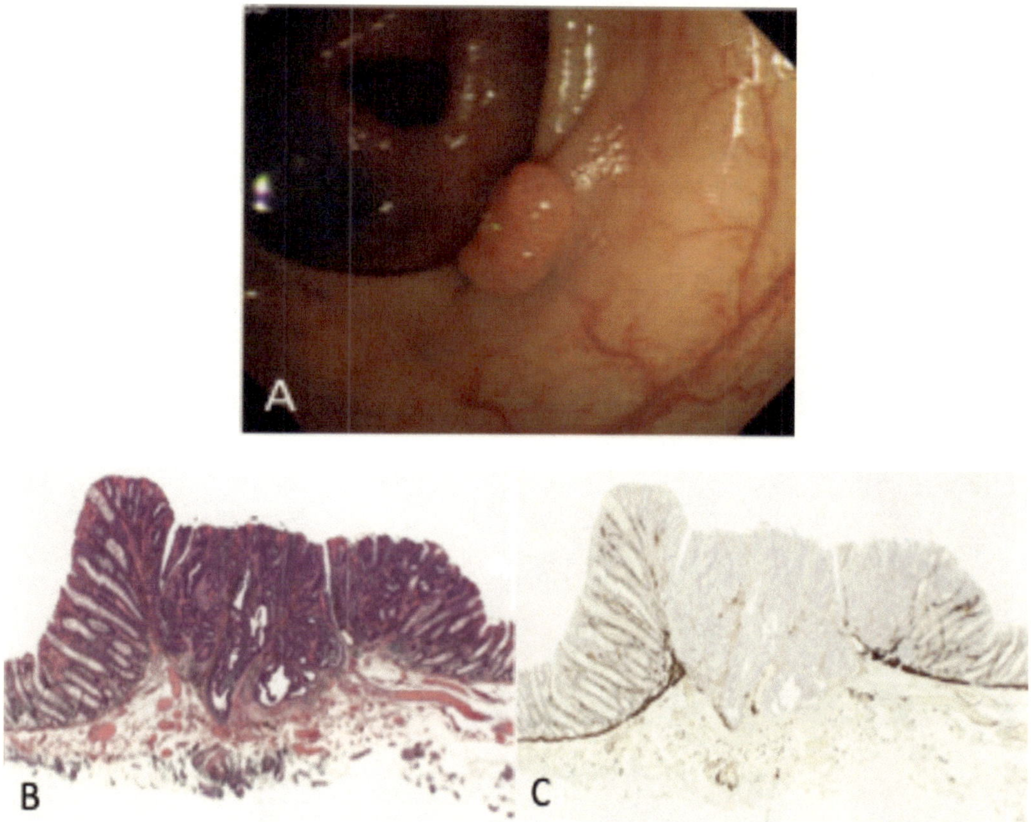

Fig. 8. Small (8 mm) submucosally invasive, polypoid colon cancer. (A) Endoscopic image of a small polypoid (Paris classification, 0-Is) lesion in the sigmoid colon. (B) Microscopic image of endoscopically resected specimen (hematoxylin and eosin stain). The lesion has invaded the submucosal layer. (C) Microscopic image of endoscopically resected specimen (Desmin stain). The muscularis mucosa has been disrupted by the invading carcinoma

4. 'DISCARD with magnifying endoscopy (DISCARD-ME)' policy

Magnifying endoscopy is one method for obtaining histopathological findings by endoscopy *in vivo*. It has been reported that the capillary patterns observed by using NBI with magnifying endoscopy (NBI-ME) can help in assessing the degree of dysplasia in early colorectal neoplasia (Katagiri et al., 2008). Therefore, the present authors believe that NBI-ME provides a more accurate strategy than the conventional 'DISCARD' policy in which NBI is used without ME. Here, a new policy for management of small polyps using NBI-ME; namely the 'DISCARD-ME' policy, is proposed.

4.1 Diagnostic criteria for the 'DISCARD-ME' policy

The diagnostic criteria in the 'DISCARD-ME' policy are basically according to the capillary pattern (CP) classification (Fig. 9), which has been reported to be useful for assessing the degree of dysplasia in early colorectal neoplasia (Katagiri et al., 2008). Lesions with invisible or faintly visible micro-capillary (MC) vessels are categorized as non-neoplastic (CP Type I), and lesions with clearly visible MC vessels are categorized as neoplastic. Neoplastic lesions are subdivided into low-grade dysplasia (CP Type II) and high-grade dysplasia or carcinoma (CP Type III). In CP type II, the MC vessels is arranged in a round or oval, honeycomb-like pattern. In CP type III, the MC vessels is not arranged regularly in a honeycomb-like pattern and exhibits at least one of the following features: irregular size, complex branching, disruption, or irregular winding.

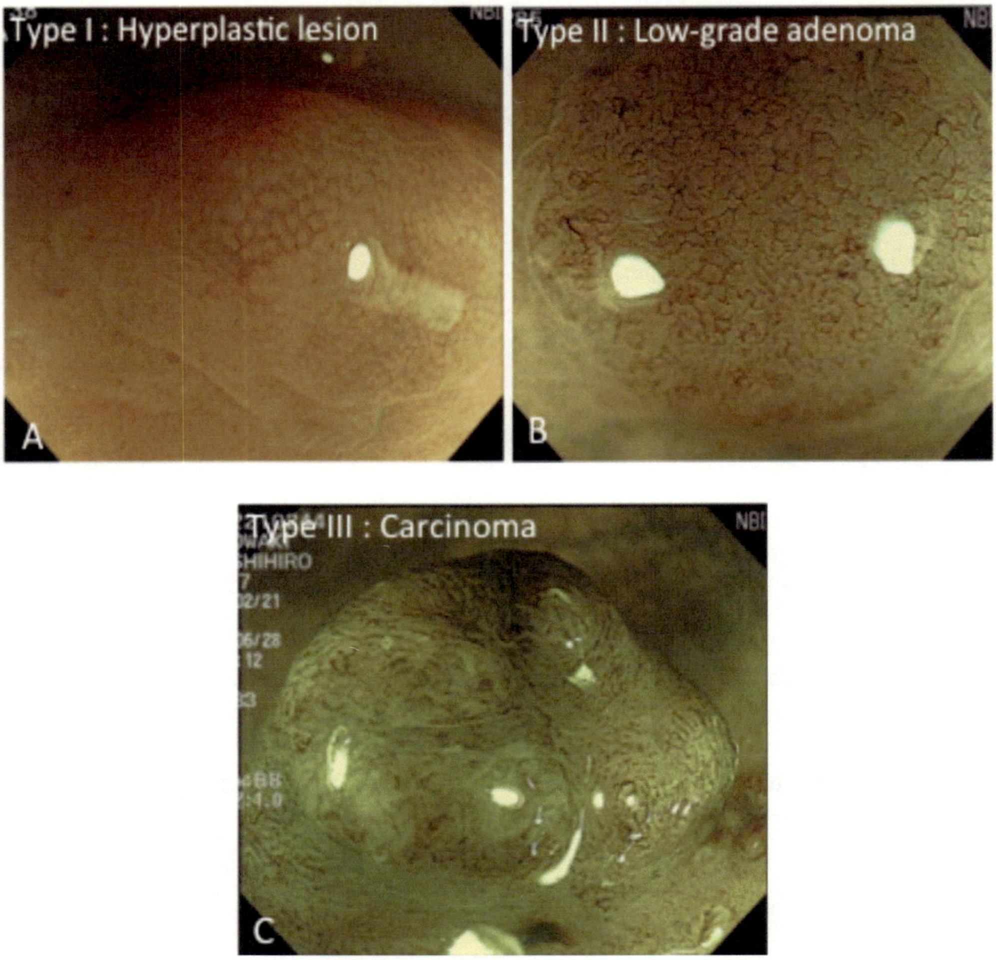

Fig. 9. Capillary pattern (CP) classification using narrow band imaging with magnifying endoscopy (NBI-ME). (A) Type I: NBI-ME image of hyperplastic polyp. The microcapillary (MC) vessels are invisible or faintly visible. (B) Type II: NBI-ME image of low-grade adenoma. The MC vessels are arranged in a round or oval, honeycomb-like pattern. (C) Type III: NBI-ME image of invasive carcinoma. The MC vessels are not arranged regularly in a honeycomb-like pattern and exhibit at least one of the following features: irregular size, complex branching, disruption, or irregular winding

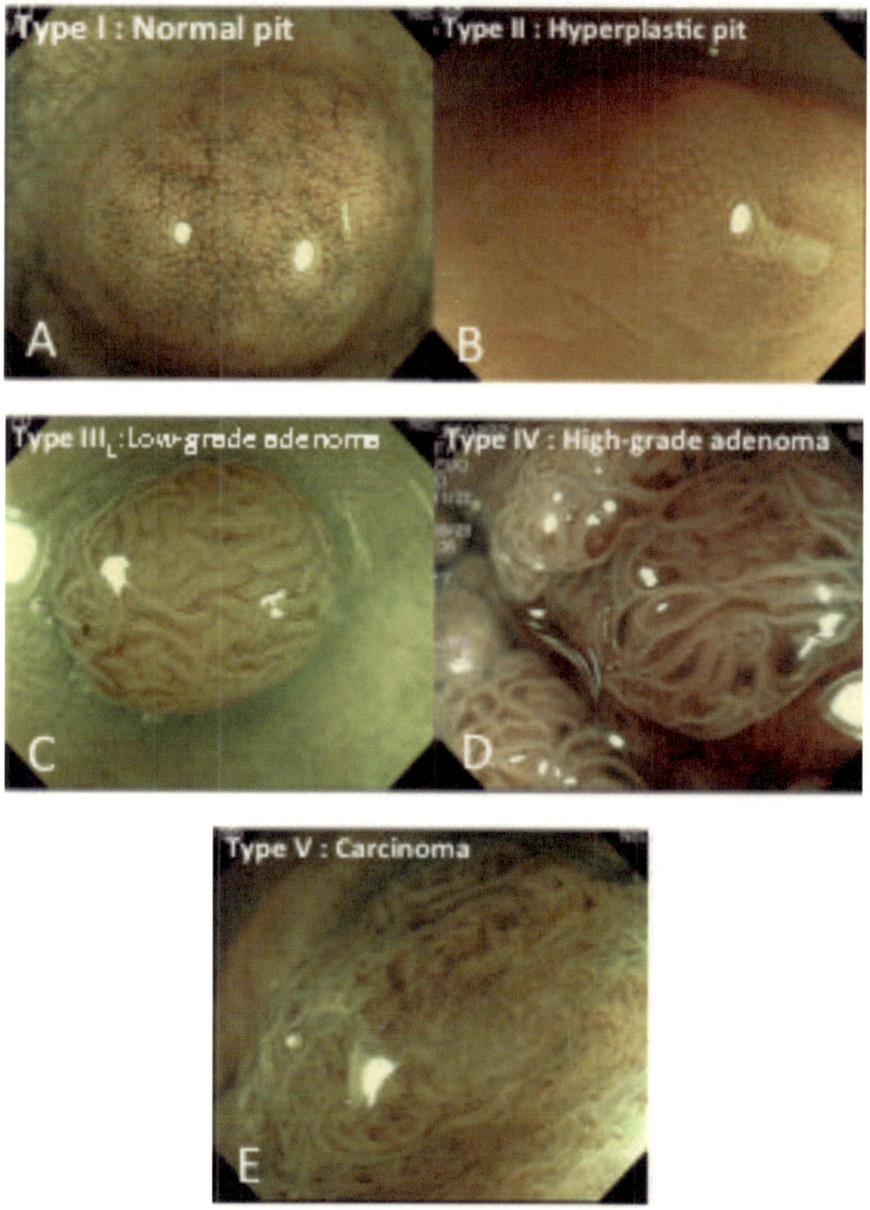

Fig. 10. Pit pattern classification of surface pattern observed by narrow band imaging with magnifying endoscopy (NBI-ME). (A) Type I: NBI-ME image of submucosal tumor (granular cell tumor). The surface pattern is normal, round and regular. (B) Type II: NBI-ME image of hyperplastic polyp. The surface pattern is star-like, slightly dilated and regular. (C) Type III: NBI-ME image of low-grade adenoma. The surface pattern is tubular, long and narrow, not branched and regular. (D) Type IV: NBI-ME image of villous high-grade adenoma. The surface pattern is branched, dendritic, villous or gyrus-like. (E) Type V: NBI-ME image of invasive carcinoma. The surface pattern is irregularly arranged and shaped

When the microvascular architecture cannot be assessed, the pit pattern classification of surface pattern is applied, because Hirata et al. have reported that determination of the pit patterns of colorectal neoplasia by NBI-ME is almost the same as that achieved by standard magnification with chromo-endoscopy (Hirata, et al., 2007, Fig. 10). According to the pit pattern classification, lesions with Type I and II pit patterns are categorized as non-neoplastic, and lesions with Type III, IV and V pit patterns as neoplastic (Kudo, et al., 1994). Neoplastic lesions with a Type III pit pattern are categorized as low-grade adenomas and lesions with Type IV and V pit pattern as high-grade adenomas, villous adenomas or carcinomas. In cases where different histologic categories have been assigned by the CP and pit pattern classifications, the more severe category is adopted.

4.2 Strategy of 'DISCARD-ME' policy

Where the 'DISCARD-ME' policy has been adopted, when colonoscopists have detected a colorectal polyp during a screening colonoscopy, they can predict the polyp type (non-neoplastic, low grade adenoma, suspicious of high grade adenoma or carcinoma) by careful observation using NBI-ME and the above-described criteria. In addition to predicting histopathology, colonoscopists can make the following decisions for polyp management on the basis of the optical diagnosis using NBI-ME (Fig. 11): (1) whether to 'resect and discard' polyps (for serrated lesions in the proximal colon or low-grade adenomas; no formal histopathology required); (2) whether to 'resect and send' them for histopathology (if they cannot decide on the type of polyp or are concerned about high-grade adenoma or carcinoma), or (3) whether to 'leave it *in situ*' (for diminutive recto-sigmoid non-neoplastic lesions).

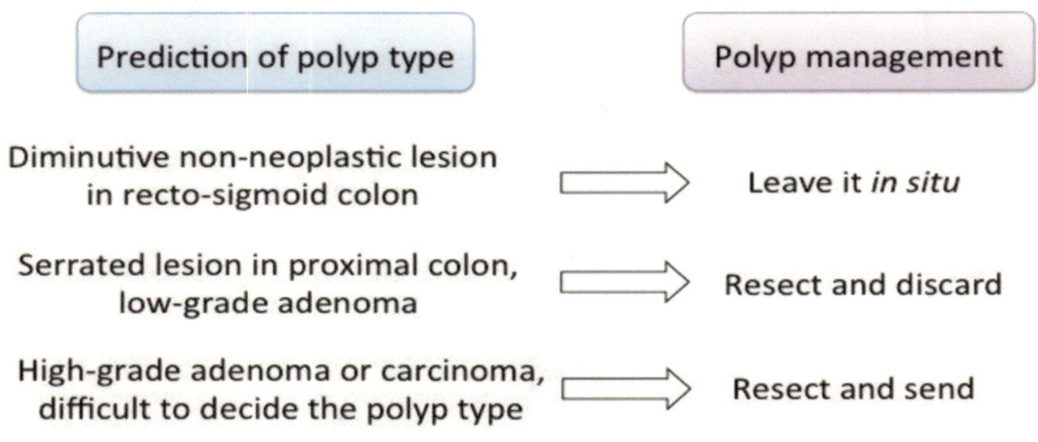

Fig. 11. Strategy of the 'DISCARD-ME' policy

4.3 A 'proof of principle' pilot study for the 'DISCARD-ME' policy

A prospective 'proof-of-principle' pilot study was conducted by the present authors to investigate the feasibility of the 'DISCARD-ME' policy. Forty-one patients undergoing colonoscopy for investigation of a positive screening FOBT, or who had been referred for surveillance colonoscopy after endoscopic resection of colorectal neoplasms, were enrolled.

In this pilot study, 105 lesions were detected. The histopathological diagnoses of two lesions were not obtained, histological diagnosis being available for the other 103 lesions (24 non-neoplastic lesions, 77 low grade adenomas, 1 high-grade adenoma, and 1 non-invasive carcinoma).

In 13 lesions (13%) which were endoscopically diagnosed as suspicious for high-grade adenoma or carcinoma, a decision was made to 'resect and send'. Of these 13 lesions, one was histopathologically diagnosed as high-grade adenoma and one as intramucosal carcinoma. Among the lesions for which the endoscopically made decisions were to 'resect and discard' or 'leave *in situ*', there were no high-grade adenomas or carcinomas. Therefore, it was concluded that decisions for management without formal histopathology could safely be made in 88% of small polyps (Fig. 12). The sensitivity of 'resect and send' for high-grade adenoma and carcinoma was 100%, and its specificity was 90%.

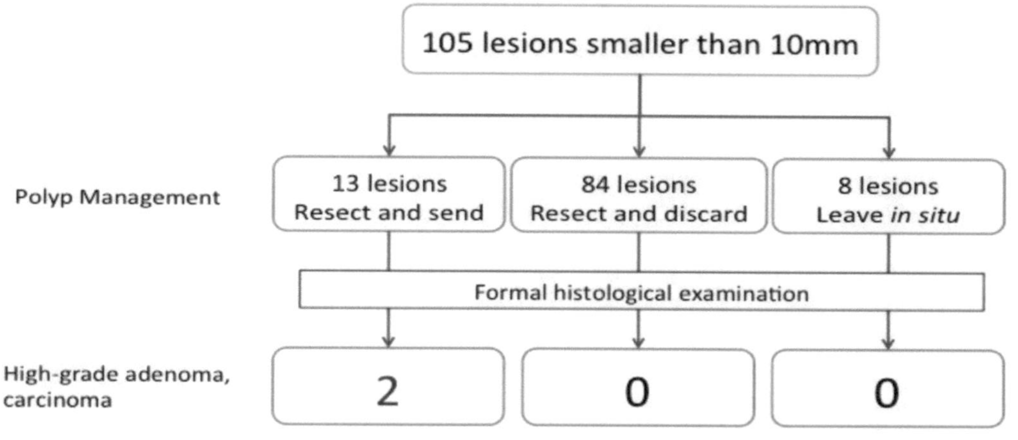

Fig. 12. Flow diagram of the pilot study. In this pilot study, 'resect and send' could safely have been selected for the 13 lesions that included the 2 high-risk lesions, and histopathological examination was omitted for the remaining 88% of lesions

Minimally invasive submucosal cancer is morphologically similar to intramucosal carcinoma, from which it is sometimes difficult to distinguish. Submucosal cancer should be assessed by histopathological examination for lymphovascular involvement and the vertical margin of the resected specimen to determine the need for additional surgery to prevent lymph node metastasis. With the 'DISCARD' policy without NBI-ME, there is a risk of small submucosal carcinomas being discarded, whereas the 'DISCARD-ME' policy could prevent inappropriate discarding. Furthermore, the 'DISCARD-ME' policy could be adopted in countries supporting the US guidelines, because these countries do not discard high-risk lesions.

5. Conclusion

The combination of AFI and TH results in more accurate detection of colorectal neoplasms. These new modalities lead to high yield colonoscopy, and the increase in detected lesions, resulting in more time, labor and cost being expended on the histopathological diagnosis of small indolent low-grade adenomas. The 'DISCARD-ME' policy using NBI-ME may decrease the time, labor and cost of histopathological diagnosis without running the risk of discarding lesions that require formal histopathological diagnosis for assessment of the possibility of lymph node metastasis. These new diagnostic technologies may contribute to a new 'high yield and discard' era in surveillance colonoscopy.

6. References

Adler A., Pohl H., Papanikolaou I., Abou-Rebyeh H., Schachschal G., Veltzke-Schlieker W., Khalifa A., Setka E., Koch M., Wiedenmann B., & Rösch T. (2008) A prospective randomized study on narrow-band imaging versus conventional colonoscopy for adenoma detection: does narrow-band imaging induce a leaning effect? *Gut,* Vol. 57, No. 1, pp. 5964. ISSN 0017-5749

Adler A., Aschenbeck J., Yenerim T., Mayr M., Aminalai A., Drossel R., Schröder A., Scheel M., Wiedenmann B., & Rösch T. (2009) Narrow-band versus whitelight high definition television endoscopic imaging for screening colonoscopy: a prospective randomized trial. *Gastroenterology,* Vol. 136, No. 2, pp. 410416. ISSN 0002-9270.

Aminalai A., Rösch T., Aschenbeck J., Mayr M., Drossel R., Schröder A., Scheel M., Treytnar D., Gauger U., Stange G., Simon F., & Adler A. (2010) Live image processing does not increase adenoma detection rate during colonoscopy: a randomized comparison between FICE and conventional imaging (Berlin Colonoscopy Project 5, BECOP-5) *American Journal of Gastroenterology,* Vol. 105, No. 11, pp. 23832388. ISSN 0002-9270.

Brooker J., Saunders B., Shah S., Thapar C., Thomas H., Atkin W., Cardwell C., & Williams C. (2002) Total colonic dye-spray increases the detection of diminutive adenomas during routine colonoscopy: a randomized controlled trial. *Gastrointestinal Endoscopy,* Vol.56, No.3, pp. 333338. ISSN 0016-5107.

Chung S., Kim D., Song J., Park M., Kim YS, Kim J., Jung H., & Song I. (2010) Efficacy of computed virtual chromoendoscopy on colorectal cancer screening: a prospective, randomized, back-to-back trial of Fuji Intelligent Color Enhancement versus conventional colonoscopy to compare adenoma miss rates. *Gastrointestinal Endoscopy,* Vol.72, No.1, pp. 136142. ISSN 0016-5107.

Hewett D. & Rex D. (2010) Cap-fitted colonoscopy: a randomized, tandem colonoscopy study of adenoma miss rates. *Gastrointestinal Endoscopy,* Vol.72, No.4, pp. 775781. ISSN 0016-5107.

Hirata M., Tanaka S., Oka S., Kaneko I., Yoshida S., Yoshihara M., & Chayama K. (2007) Magnifying endoscopy with narrow band imaging for diagnosis of colorectal tumors. *Gastrointestinal Endoscopy,* Vol.65, No. 7, pp. 988995. ISSN 0016-5107.

Ignjatovic A., East J., Suzuki N., Vance M., Guenther T., & Saunders B.. (2009) Optical diagnosis of small colorectal polyps at routine colonoscopy (Detect InSpect ChAracterise Resect and Discard; DISCARD trial): a prospective cohort study. *Lancet Oncology,* Vol. 10, No. 12, pp. 11711178. ISSN 1470-2045.

Inoue T., Murano M., Murano N., Kuramoto T., Kawakami K., Abe Y., Morita E., Toshina K., Hoshiro H., Egashira Y., Umegaki E, & Higuchi K. (2008) *Journal of Gastroenterology,* Vol. 43, No. 1. pp. 4550. ISSN 0944-1174.

Jemal A., Siegel R., Ward E., Hao Y., Xu J., & Thun M. (2009) Cancer statistics, 2009. *CA: A Cancer Journal for Clinicians,* Vol. 59, No. 4, pp. 22549. ISSN 0007-9235.

Kaltenbach T., Saon Y., Friedland S., & Soetikno R. American Gastroenterological Association. (2008) American Gastroenterological Association (AGA) Institute technology assessment on image-enhanced endoscopy. *Gastroenterology,* Vol. 134, No. 1, pp. 327340. ISSN 0016-5085.

Katagiri A., Fu K., Sano Y., Ikematsu H., Horimatsu T., Kaneko K., Muto M., & Yoshida S. (2008) Narrow band imaging with magnifying colonoscopy as diagnostic tool for predicting histology of early colorectal neoplasia. *Alimentary Pharmacology & Therapeutics,* Vol. 27, No. 12, 12691274. Online ISSN 1365-2036.

Kudo S., Hirota S., Nakajima T., Hosobe S., Kusaka H., Kobayashi T., Himori M., & Yagyuu A. (1994) Colorectal tumors and pit pattern. *Journal of Clinical Pathology,* Vol. 47, No. 10, pp. 880885. ISSN 0021-9746.

Leufkens A., DeMarco D., Rastogi A., Akerman P., Azzouzi K., Rothstein R., Vleggaar F., Repici A., Rando G., Okolo P., Dewit O., Ignjatovic A., Odstrcil E., East J., Deprez P., Saunders B., Kalloo A., Creel B., Singh V., Lennon A., & Siersema P (The Third Eye Retroscope Randomized Clinical Evaluation [TERRACE] Study Group) (2011) Effect of a retrograde-viewing device on adenoma detection rate during colonoscopy: the TERRACE study. *Gastrointestinal Endoscopy,* Vol. 73, No. 3, pp. 480489. ISSN 0016-5107.

Matsuda T., Saito Y., Fu K.I, Uraoka T., Kobayashi N., Nakajima T., Ikehara H., Mashimo Y., Shimoda T., Murakami Y., Parra-Blanco A., Fujimori T., & Saito D. (2008) Does autofluorescence imaging videoendoscopy system improve the colonoscopic polyp detection rate?--a pilot study. *American Journal of Gastroenterology,* Vol. 103, No. 8, pp. 19261932. ISSN 0002-9270.

Matsushita M., Hajiro K., Okazaki K., Takakuwa H., & Tominaga M. (1998) Efficacy of total colonoscopy with a transparent cap in comparison with colonoscopy without the Cap. *Endoscopy,* Vol. 30, No. 5, pp. 444447. ISSN 0013726X.

Morson B. (1974) President's address: the polyp-cancer sequence in the large bowel. *Proceedings of the Royal Society of Medicine,* Vol. 67, No. 6, pp. 45157. ISSN 0035-9157.

Rex D., Cutler C., Lemmel G., Eahmani E., Clark D., Helper D., Lehman G., & Mark D.. (1997) Colonoscopic miss rates of adenomas determined by back-to-back colonoscopies. *Gastroenterology,* Vol. 112, No. 1, pp. 2428. ISSN 0016-5085.

Triadafilopoulos G., Watts H., Higgins J., & Van Dam J. (2007) A novel retrograde-viewing auxiliary imaging device (Third Eye Retroscope) improves the detection of simulated polyps in anatomic models of the colon. *Gastrointestinal Endoscopy,* Vol. 65, No. 1, pp. 139144. ISSN 0016-5107.

Uraoka T., Saito Y., Matsuda T., Sano Y, Ikehara H., Mashimo Y., Kikuchi T., Saito D., & Saito H. (2008) Detectability of colorectal neoplastic lesions using a narrow-band imaging system: a pilot study. *Journal of Gastroenteroogy and Hepatology,* Vol. 21, No. 12, pp. 18101815. ISSN 0815-9319.

Vucelic B., Rex D., Pulanic R., Pfefer J., Hrstic I., Levin B., Halpern Z., & Arber N. (2006) The Aer-O-Scope: Proof of concept of a pneumatic, skill-independent, self-propelling, self-navigating colonoscope. *Gastroenterology,* Vol. 130, No. 3, pp. 672677. ISSN 0016-5085.

Winawer S., Zauber A., Ho M., O'Brien M., Gottlieb L., Sternberg S., Waye J., Schapiro M., Bond J., Panish J., Ackroyd F., Shike M., Kurtz R., Lewis L., Gerdes H., Stewart E., & the National Polyp Study Workgroup. (1993) Prevention of colorectal cancer by colonoscopic polypectomy. *New England Journal of Medicine,* Vol. 329, No. 27, pp. 19771981. ISSN 0028-4793.

16

Efficacy of the Pediatric Colonoscope Used as a Push Enteroscope

Francisco Pérez-Roldán,
Pedro González-Carro and María Concepción Villafáñez-García
Hospital General La Mancha-Centro; Alcázar de San Juan
Spain

1. Introduction

Numerous advances have recently been made in endoscopy for both diagnosis and treatment of gastrointestinal diseases. However, these advances have taken little account of the small bowel, as access by endoscopy is often difficult. With the advent of push endoscopy in 1971, the proximal jejunum could be examined to about 50 cm from the ligament of Treitz. The subsequent introduction of videoendoscopy combined with an overtube enabled us to examine the whole jejunum. The most recent discoveries—capsule endoscopy and double-balloon enteroscopy—have improved our ability to examine the small intestine. Capsule endoscopy has provided us with a new challenge, namely, how to diagnose and treat the lesions found. Hospitals with a small bowel unit in which double-balloon enteroscopy and push endoscopy are available can provide an effective solution in a large percentage of cases. In hospitals where these techniques are not available, lesions identified in the jejunum must be resolved using non-balloon enteroscopy. Colonoscopy is a well-known alternative, although its rigidity and caliber prevent it from advancing smoothly through the jejunum. An intermediate solution could be found in the pediatric colonoscope, which is smaller in cross-section and more flexible and has a working channel that enables therapy to be administered.

In this chapter, we describe the different diagnostic therapeutic approaches to lesions of the small bowel. We also examine the application of endoscopy, including the possibilities offered by the pediatric colonoscope in the diagnosis and treatment of lesions found using capsule endoscopy.

2. Radiological examination of the small bowel

The small bowel is the longest part of the digestive tract; however, it is the least examined using radiological techniques. Although simple in structure—it is a tube of regular caliber with fairly constant folds—examination is problematic due to its length and motility, the lower incidence of small bowel disease, frequent overlapping between loops, and the difficulty in differentiating between a healthy bowel and a diseased one.

Originally, the small bowel could only be examined using radiological techniques, some of which were barium-based. These techniques have improved over the years. Below we describe the methods used to date.

1. *Intestinal transit.* Today, barium-based examination of the small intestine is limited by the huge advances made in enteroscopy, especially capsule endoscopy, which has made it possible to examine sections of the digestive tract that were previously inaccessible. Nevertheless, intestinal transit can sometimes provide us with important information. It is used exclusively for diagnosis, and findings must be confirmed by histology or other techniques.

   Contrast can be administered in 2 ways:

   - Orally, with a single contrast.
   - Using enteroclysis: Contrast is introduced via a tube in the distal duodenum to obtain faster and more uniform opacification, thus increasing the technique's sensitivity (Figure 1). The contrast may be single or double (barium and methylcellulose or air). The latter has been of little use in the small intestine due to its poor diagnostic yield.

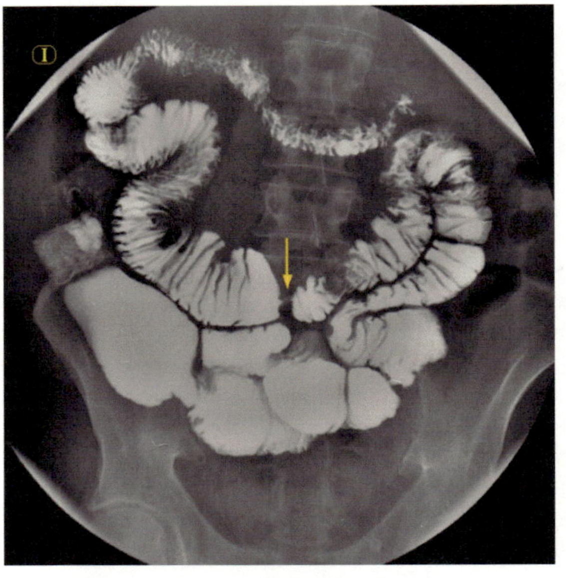

Fig. 1. Jejunal stenosis (arrow) in a patient with Crohn disease

Currently, the indications for a contrast study of the small intestine are as follows:

- Before capsule endoscopy (only if stenosis is suspected)
- Diagnosis of extension and follow-up of inflammatory diseases (especially Crohn disease)
- Monitoring of celiac disease
- Obstructive disease of the small intestine, including volvulus and stenosis
- Examination of the anatomy of the small intestine after resection
- Diagnosis of diverticula, hernias, or intestinal tumors
- Study of enteral fistulas
- Other less well-defined indications, such as undiagnosed abdominal pain and malabsorption. The contraindications for barium-based techniques are those of any radiologic study, namely, pregnancy, lack of patient cooperation, and allergy to contrasts.

2. *Computed tomography enterography and computed tomography enteroclysis.* These techniques are dedicated examinations of the small bowel that allow the detection of both vascular lesions and tumors. Computed tomography-based techniques optimize luminal distension by enabling larger volumes of neutral oral contrast to be administered via a peroral or nasojejunal tube, thereby providing optimal visualization of mucosal detail and vasculature. It is also possible to evaluate wall thickness. In addition, uptake of intravenous contrast enables us to characterize tissues and lesions. An additional advantage of computed tomography enterography is that it can identify small bowel strictures/obstruction prior to capsule endoscopy and provide important information on luminal and extraluminal findings that cannot be detected on capsule endoscopy.
   Moreover, computed tomography enables us to perform invasive diagnostic and therapeutic procedures such as fine-needle aspiration, biopsy, and percutaneous drainage.
3. *Magnetic resonance imaging.* Magnetic resonance imaging is based on the magnetic properties of the protons of water molecules and lipids, which act as small magnets that line up in the magnetic field of the device when a radiofrequency pulse is applied, thus generating 2 signals of differing intensity (T1 and T2). As the images take some time to be acquired, movement, including respiration, can produce artifacts. The lumen must be well distended, either by direct enteral infusion of contrast (magnetic resonance-enteroclysis) or ingestion of large volumes of contrast. Interest in magnetic resonance imaging for evaluation of the small bowel is growing, due to the absence of ionizing radiation, the excellent contrast resolution, direct multiplanar acquisition, and the use of non-nephrotoxic intravenous contrast. Nevertheless, magnetic resonance imaging does not provide clear advantages in most diseases of the digestive tract.
4. *Abdominal angiography.* The use of arteriography for the study of digestive disorders has been partly superseded by advances in other, less invasive imaging techniques, such as computed tomography angiography or magnetic resonance angiography. However, it continues to be indicated and is difficult to replace, especially for therapeutic purposes. The current indications in the small bowel are as follows:
   - Uncontrollable gastrointestinal bleeding due to therapeutic failure or failure to locate the bleeding source or impossibility of applying endoscopy. Angiography enables hemostatic therapy to be administered (vasoactive substances, particle embolization, balloon-catheter occlusion)
   - Acute mesenteric ischemia. Therapy can also be administered, namely, embolectomy, fibrinolysis, and perfusion of substances to treat vascular spasm.

   The contraindications for this technique are those which are typical of radiologic examinations, as well as allergy to iodine contrast and the risk of severe shock.
5. *Abdominal ultrasound.* Ultrasound represents a huge advance in the diagnosis and treatment of digestive diseases. The technique is harmless, fast, inexpensive, and examiner-dependent. It is indicated mainly for examination of solid organs involved in digestive disorders, especially the liver, biliary tract, spleen, and pancreas.
   In the digestive tract, ultrasound provides scant and indirect information on extrinsic and wall disorders. However, it does enable us to evaluate wall morphology and thickness, caliber, compressibility, and peristalsis. The most characteristic ultrasound sign in gastrointestinal disease is the so-called pseudokidney sign or target sign, which is composed of an echogenic center (intestinal content) surrounded by a hypoechoic halo corresponding to a thickened intestinal wall. This sign is specific and can result

from inflammatory abnormalities (neoplastic or other). In pediatric patients, the technique reveals conditions such as concentric pyloric stenosis and intussusception, in which ultrasound findings alone are characteristic and diagnostic.

3. Video capsule endoscopy

Video capsule endoscopy is a noninvasive technique that has proven effective for the evaluation of patients with suspected small bowel bleeding. It enables the whole small bowel to be examined. Several studies have shown its superiority over more conventional methods, including barium x-ray. Capsule endoscopy is currently considered the procedure of choice in small bowel diseases. However, this technique has a series of limitations that have yet to be resolved, namely, the real significance of findings and false negatives, and that it is only diagnostic (Figure 2).

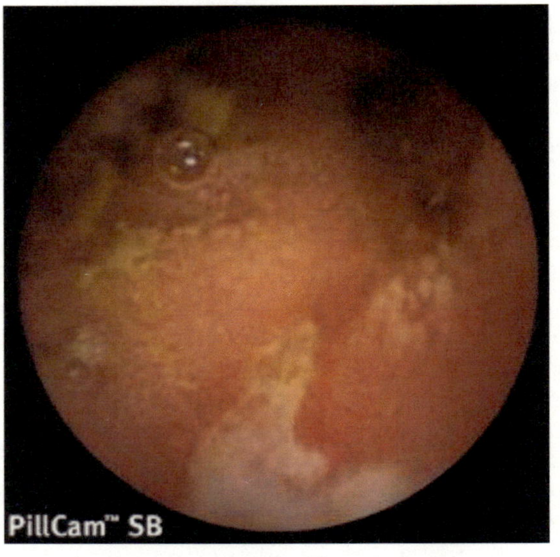

Fig. 2. Geographic ulcer in the ileum surrounded by edema suggestive of Crohn disease

As the diagnostic potential of this technique and treatment options have become clearer, its indications have varied and now include the following:

- Gastrointestinal hemorrhage of unknown origin
- Tumors
- Crohn disease
- Polyposis and polyps (Peutz-Jeghers syndrome and familial adenomatous polyposis)
- Malabsorption, celiac disease, and lymphoma
- Further study of findings in other imaging techniques
- Gastroenteropathy induced by nonsteroidal anti-inflammatory drugs

The patient must be well prepared in order to ensure good image quality: 8 hours' fasting, low-residue diet during the days before the procedure, and antifoam solutions and bowel cleansing solutions (increasingly recommended). Complications are exceptional and no deaths have been reported. The main complications include inability to swallow the capsule (in which case it must be inserted using an endoscope), contact with pyriform sinuses, contact with the esophagus or a bronchus, delay in evacuating the stomach, retention in an afferent loop, retention in lesions of the small intestine (stenosis, diverticula, tumors), or malfunctioning capsule (short recording time, interference by magnetic sources, or error in the images due to disconnection of a sensor).

Capsule endoscopy makes it possible to examine the whole small bowel, and several studies have shown its superiority over other more conventional modalities, including barium x-ray. However, this technique is not completely reliable, and a series of limitations have yet to be resolved, including the real significance of specific findings and false negatives attributable to the presence of food and liquid residue, the lack of distension or propulsion, and rapid passage through large segments. The main drawback of capsule endoscopy is that it exclusively diagnostic, with limited capacity for locating the lesion accurately and no options for biopsy or therapeutic procedures.

4. Endoscopic methods for examination of the small intestine

Although numerous advances have recently been made in endoscopy for diagnosis and treatment of gastrointestinal diseases, they have taken little account of the small bowel, as access by endoscopy is often difficult. The most recent discoveries—capsule endoscopy, double-balloon enteroscopy, and spiral enteroscopy—have improved our ability to examine the small bowel. Capsule endoscopy has given rise to a new challenge, namely, how to diagnose and treat the lesions found. In this section, we describe the different methods used to perform enteroscopy, from the earliest to the most recent.

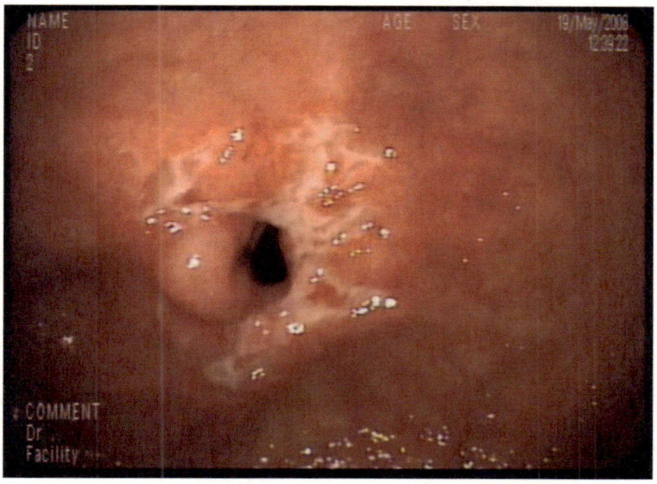

Fig. 3. Jejunal stenosis in a patient with Crohn disease. Geographic ulcers at the level of the stenosis

Push Enteroscopy. For several years, push enteroscopy has been the most widely used and effective procedure for direct examination of the intestinal mucosa. It comprises a 200-cm-long endoscope and a 2.8-mm working channel. One of its limitations is that is only allows us to visualize the proximal and medial jejunum, leaving much of the small intestine unexplored. In order to progress, smooth and intermittent aspiration maneuvers are necessary to avoid suction artifacts on the mucosa. Minimal insufflation should be applied due to the risk of overdistension and greater formation of loops. The technique identifies fewer lesions than upper and lower endoscopy, as the small bowel is less commonly affected by disease (Figure 3); therefore, the indications should be carefully selected in order to achieve diagnostic yield, and more importantly, therapeutic yield. The mucosa is usually more visible on withdrawal, during which the distance reached relative to the angle of Treitz is better appreciated.

Balloon-assisted enteroscopy.

a. *Double-balloon enteroscopy.* Double-balloon enteroscopy represents a huge advance. In theory, the whole small bowel can be examined, biopsies taken, and treatment administered, or, if this is not possible, the lesion can be marked. The technique comprises a thin enteroscope with a special flexible overtube, at the distal end of which 2 balloons are attached. These balloons are inflated and deflated by continuous pressure control, and both instruments can be pushed forward or withdrawn. The technique makes it possible to reach more distal sections of the small bowel, although it rarely manages to reach the terminal ileum; therefore, enteroscopy requires the combination of the antegrade and retrograde approaches for an examination of the whole bowel. Double-balloon enteroscopy is considered a safe and well-tolerated technique for the diagnosis and treatment of small bowel diseases, with a working channel ranging in size from 2.2 mm to 2.8 mm.

   The technique is contraindicated in patients who have recently undergone digestive surgery and in those with perforated viscus, life-threatening hemodynamic instability, and severe respiratory insufficiency. The most common complications are cardiopulmonary abnormalities, bacteremia, hemorrhage, pancreatitis, dissected aortic aneurysm, volvulus, and incarcerated inguinal hernia. At present, double-balloon enteroscopy is used mainly to administer therapy after capsule endoscopy, except when it is contraindicated.

b. *Single-balloon enteroscopy.* Single-balloon enteroscopy is the latest balloon-assisted endoscopic technique for the evaluation and management of small bowel disorders. It involves inserting a balloon catheter through the working channel of a colonoscope and moving the endoscope progressively along the small intestine by inflating and deflating the balloon. This technique has proven safe and effective, and in some cases (up to 25%) has made it possible to perform a complete enteroscopy. The earliest versions involved an enteroscope with a 2.8-mm working channel; however, more recently, a pediatric colonoscope with a wider working channel (3.2 mm) has been used, with no reduction in insertion depth. Compared with double-balloon enteroscopy, this technique presents fewer complications, enables a complete enteroscopy to be performed in a lower percentage of patients, and has a similar or wider working channel.

Spiral enteroscopy. Spiral enteroscopy allows for advancement and withdrawal of the enteroscope through the small bowel by using clockwise and counterclockwise movements, respectively. The distal end of the overtube is positioned 25 cm from the tip of the enteroscope and locked into place. The system is then advanced to the ligament of Treitz with gentle rotation. The collar is subsequently unlocked, and the enteroscope is advanced past the ligament of Treitz. The overtube is then advanced using clockwise rotation until pleating of the small bowel no longer occurs over the enteroscope. The enteroscope is then unlocked and advanced to facilitate further advancement into the small bowel. In order to ease withdrawal of the enteroscope, the overtube is rotated in a counterclockwise direction.

Insertion depth is 262±57 cm and the examination takes an average of 35 minutes. This endoscopic modality also allows the use of therapeutics, including biopsy, hemostatic agents, and polypectomy (working channel of 2.8 mm). Only minor complications of sore throat and minimal mucosal trauma have been reported to date and no perforations. Some studies compare this approach with double-balloon enteroscopy and show that the latter has a higher diagnostic yield. In addition, this technique requires 2 endoscopists, one to turn the overtube and the other to push the endoscope. It is important to remember that the overtube contains latex—as do the balloons in balloon-assisted enteroscopy—and therefore represents an added risk in patients with latex allergy.

Intraoperative enteroscopy. Intraoperative enteroscopy by insertion of an endoscope through 1 or more enterotomies to examine the whole small bowel has a high diagnostic yield, identifying lesions in 70-100% of patients. The technique commences once the surgeon has performed a laparotomy to gain access to the small bowel. Once the small bowel is exposed, 2 or more enterotomies are made and the colonoscope is inserted with the surgeon's help. Intraoperative enteroscopy makes it possible to examine the whole small bowel, although the assistance of a surgeon is necessary. It is limited by its high morbidity (intestinal wall hematoma, mesenteric hemorrhage, prolonged ileus, intestinal ischemia, and perforation) and is therefore reserved for patients with persistent bleeding and high transfusional requirements in whom diagnosis cannot be established by other means (Figure 4). A variation of the technique involves oral insertion of the enteroscope during surgery, which makes it possible to visualize 93% of the ileum and establish a diagnosis in almost 60% of cases. Its drawback is the considerable operative morbidity in a relatively high proportion of cases (serosal tear or mesenteric vein avulsion).

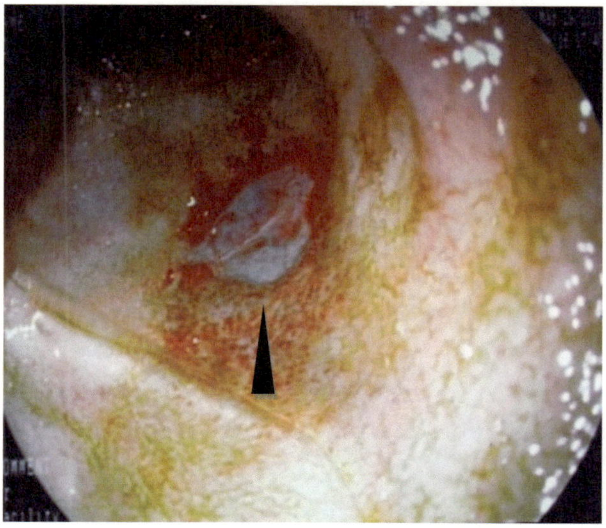

Fig. 4. Ileal ulcer (arrow) with completely denuded submucosa

5. Push enteroscopy performed using a pediatric colonoscope

Capsule endoscopy can be used to examine the small bowel for the indications presented above. However, it is exclusively a diagnostic technique; therapy must be administered using single-balloon or double-balloon enteroscopy or spiral enteroscopy. These new endoscopes are flexible and generally have a 2.8-mm working channel that partially collapses after passing through several loops, thus making it difficult to insert commercially available catheters. In addition, they are not universally available. An alternative in the case of proximal lesions of the small bowel (mainly the jejunum) is to use a pediatric colonoscope with a 3.2-mm channel, which makes it easy to insert even metal prostheses or the catheters habitually used in colonoscopy. The caliber of the standard working channel is 2.8 mm (2.2 mm in the diagnostic double-balloon enteroscope). Another advantage of this type of colonoscope is that it is more flexible and manageable than a standard colonoscope, enabling us to reach more distal parts of the jejunum.

Therefore, a pediatric colonoscope with a 3.2-mm working channel can be used as a push enteroscope to treat jejunal lesions. We can use any type of catheter applied in colonoscopy (this does not need to be longer, as is the case with standard push enteroscopy) and we can insert sclerotherapy needles to mark the lesions identified and the furthest point reached. Hemoclips can also be used for this purpose. If necessary, ink marks can be visualized using capsule endoscopy, and clips are easily identified on a plain radiograph (Figure 5) or can be palpated by the surgeon.

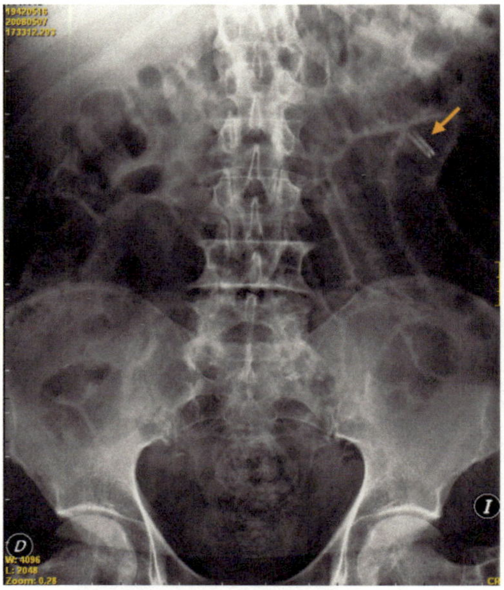

Fig. 5. Note the 2 hemoclips (arrow) marking the distance reached with the pediatric colonoscope

Our experience shows that diagnosis is not always consistent: capsule endoscopy did not reveal the lesions we expected to find in the section examined or there were no identifiable lesions. Push endoscopy using a pediatric colonoscope, on the other hand, made it possible to identify the lesions to be treated (argon plasma, hydropneumatic dilation), take biopsy specimens to provide an accurate diagnosis (stenosis caused by Crohn disease, jejunal carcinoma in patients with celiac disease), and, importantly, mark the bowel (hemoclips or Indian ink) in order to locate lesions or the most distal point reached.

6. Summary

Capsule endoscopy is the technique of choice for examination of the small bowel. Several options are available for treatment, including balloon-assisted enteroscopy or spiral enteroscopy. A pediatric colonoscope enables us to perform the examination using conventional push enteroscopy (50 cm from the angle of Treitz), take biopsy specimens, administer endoscopic treatment of the lesions found, and mark lesions using standard clinical techniques. It has the advantages that it can be performed in selected patients at any hospital without the need for advanced technology and enables metallic prostheses to be inserted.

7. References

Hiratsuka H. Endoscopic diagnosis in the small intestine. Stomach Intestine 1972; 7: 1679-85.

Yamamoto H, Kita H. Enteroscopy. J Gastroenterol 2005; 40:555-562.

Nolan DJ. The true yield of small-intestinal barium study. Endoscopy 1997; 29: 447-53.

Dixon PM, Roulston ME, Nolan DJ. The small bowel enema: a ten year review. Clin Radiol 1993; 47: 46-8.

Zamboni GA, Raptopoulos V. CT Enterography. Gastrointest Endosc Clin N Am 2010; 20: 347-66.

Dave-Verma H, Moore S, Singh A, Martins N, Zawacki J. Computed tomographic enterography and enteroclysis: pearls and pitfalls. Curr Probl Diagn 2008; 37: 279-87.

Baker ME, Einstein MD, Veniero JC. Computed tomography enterography and magnetic resonance enterography: the future of small bowel imaging. Clin Colon Rectal Surg 2008; 21: 193-212.

Filder JL, Guimaraes L, Einstein DM. MR imaging of small bowel. Radiographics 2009; 29: 1811-25.

Geboes K, Geboes KP, Maleux G. Vascular anatomy of the gastrointestinal tract. Best Pract Res Clin Gastroenterol 2001; 15: 1-14.

Scheible W, Goldberger LE. Diagnosis of small bowel obstruction: the contribution of diagnostic ultrasound. Am J Roentgenol 1979; 133: 685-8.

Liao Z, Gao R, Xu C, Li ZS. Indicactions and detection, completion, and retention rates of small-bowel capsule endoscopy: a systematic review. Gastrointest Endosc 2010; 71: 280-6.

Van Gossum A, Ibrahim M. Video capsule endoscopy: what is the future?. Gastroenterol Clin North Am 2010; 39: 807-26.

Hayat M, Axon AT, O'Mahony S. Diagnostic yield and effect on clinical outcomes of push enteroscopy in suspected small-bowel bleeding. Endoscopy 2000; 32: 369-72.

Gómez Rodríguez BJ, Ortiz Moyano C, Romero Castro R, Caunedo Álvarez A, Hernández Durán MD, Hergueta Delgado P, et al. Diagnostic yield of 335 push video-enteroscopies. Rev Esp Enferm Dig 2006; 98(2): 82-92.

Pérez-Cuadrado E, Más P, Hallal H, Shanabo J, Muñoz E, Ortega I, et al. Double-balloon enteroscopy: a descriptive study of 50 explorations. Rev Esp Enferm Dig 2006; 98(2): 73-81.

Ross A, Mehdizadeh S, Tokar J, Leighton JA, Kamal A, Chen A, et al. Double balloon enteroscopy detects small bowel mass lesions missed by capsule endoscopy. Dig Dis Sci 2008; 53: 2140-3.

Lo SK, Mehdizadeh S. Therapeutic uses of double-balloon enteroscopy. Gastrointest Endosc Clin N Am 2006; 16: 363-76.

Matsumoto T, Moriyama T, Esaki M, Nakamura S, Iida M. Performance of antegrade double-balloon enteroscopy: comparison with push enteroscopy. Gastrointest Endosc 2005; 62: 392-8.

Tsujikawa T, Saitoh Y, Andoh A, Imaeda H, Hata K, Minematsu H, et al. Novel single-balloon enteroscopy for diagnosis and treatment of small intestine : preliminary experiences. Endoscopy 2008; 40: 11-5.

Kawamura T, Yasuda K, Tanaka K, Uno K, Ueda M, Sanada K, et al. Clinical evaluation of a newly developed single-balloon enteroscope. Gastrointest Endosc 2008; 68: 1112-6.

Akerman PA, Agrawal D, Chen W, Cantero D, Avila J, Pangtay J. Spiral enteroscopy: a novel method of enteroscopy by using the Endo-Ease discovery SB overtube and a pediatric colonoscope. Gastrointest Endosc 2009; 69: 327-32.

Frieling T, Heise J, Sassenrath W, Hülsdonk A, Kreysel C. Prospecctive comparison between double-balloon enteroscopy and spiral enteroscopy. Endoscopy 2010; 42: 885-8.

Schulz HJ, Schmidt H. Intraoperative enteroscopy. Gastrointest Endosc Clin N Am 2009; 19: 371-9.

Kopácová M, Bures J, Vykouril L, Hladík P, Simkovic D, Jon B, Ferko A, Tachecí I, Rejchrt S. Intraoperative enteroscopy: ten years' experience at a single tertiary center. Surg Endosc 2007; 21: 1111-6.

Pérez Roldán F, González Carro P, Legaz Huidobro ML, Roncero García-Escribano O, Ynfante Ferrús M, Aoufi S, Sánchez-Manjavacas Muñoz N, Ruiz Carrillo F. Efficacy of pediatric colonoscopy used as push enteroscopy in the management of capsule endoscopy findings . Rev Esp Enferm Dig 2009; 101:468-576.

17

Endoscopy in Paediatric Inflammatory Bowel Disease (IBD)

Marco Gasparetto and Graziella Guariso
Department of Paediatrics,
Unit of Gastroenterology, Hepatology,
Digestive Endoscopy and Care of the Liver Transplanted Child,
University of Padua,
Italy

1. Introduction

Endoscopic investigation has become more and more important for diagnosis, follow-up and management of Inflammatory Bowel Disease (IBD) affected patients in the last decades [1].

In fact it allows us to evaluate the grade and extension of bowel inflammation, thus the severity of disease, its prognosis, and the response to therapy as well as the possible indication to a surgical intervention [1]. An endoscopic treatment of several complications (i.e. stenosis) also represents a useful possibility being available.

Moreover, the advent of techniques such as capsule and both single and double-balloon-assisted enteroscopy is revolutionizing small-bowel imaging and has major implications for diagnosis, classification, therapeutic decision making and outcomes in the management of IBD [2].

The last available Consensus document reached by a group of international experts in the fields of endoscopy and IBD at a meeting held in Brussels (organised jointly by the European Crohn's and Colitis Organisation ECCO and the Organisation Mondiale d'Endoscopie Digestive OMED) dates back to 12–13th December 2008 [2]. The statements included in this document with the relative levels of evidence and grades of recommendation will be reported as a referral along the chapter.

Endoscopy is able to differentiate Crohn's Disease (CD) and Ulcerative Colitis (UC) in 89% of cases. Essentially it is nowadays the most efficacious and diffused technique to evaluate CD localisation and activity at the level of terminal ileum and colon; its accuracy for results are therefore significantly superior with respect to bowel enema [1].

An immediate diagnosis with excellent accuracy is obtainable when endoscopy is associated to the histological examination of biopsy samples [3].

The endoscopic procedure for paediatric patients with IBD differs significantly from the modalities in use for adults, especially in regards of the use of sedation-analgesia, and the number and localisation of the mucosal biopsies effectuated and the regular inclusion of terminal ileum intubation within a complete investigation. [4-6].

In the paediatric age, assistance with anesthesia allows one to perform a complete endoscopic examination with visualisation of terminal ileum in 90% of cases [3].

Limitations of endoscopy are however the impossibility to completely evaluate the small bowel, just the first 2-3 loops of small-bowel and the last 20-30 cm of terminal ileum, as well as the necessity of profound sedation-analgesia in the paediatric age [3].
The endoscopic evaluation of mucosal healing is important to identify the efficacy of a specific therapeutic regimen: a significant correlation has been observed, for instance, among administration of new drugs such as anti TNF –α (infliximab, natalizumab and adalimumab), azathioprine and methotrexate, clinical improvement and disappearance of endoscopic lesions; mucosal healing has not been shown, but instead to be predictive for response to orally administered corticosteroids [1].
Determinant is the role of endoscopy for the prediction of a possible post-surgical relapse (endoscopic relapse is reported in 60- 70% of cases at 6- 12 months whereas a clinical relapse is observed in 50% of cases at 3 years follow-up for Crohn's disease); for those patients with an endoscopic remission, a significant reduction of hospitalization and surgical intervention has also been observed [1].

2. Upper gastrointestinal tract endoscopy: General aspects

The presence of symptoms related to the upper gastrointestinal tract such as disphagia, odinophagia, nausea and/or vomit, oral ulcers, represents a typical indication to an upper-tract endoscopy in the phases of diagnosis and staging of IBD [4-5].
It should also be noted that even in the absence of symptoms, the upper gastrointestinal tract involvement appears more and more frequently present at the endoscopic and histological evaluation of patients with CD. The importance of taking biopsies at this level has to be considered, even with an endoscopically normal mucosa [4-5].
'Small-bowel endoscopy' is defined as any endoluminal examination of the small bowel, including capsule endoscopy, push enteroscopy and balloon- or other device-assisted endoscopy [2].
A gastroscope with a diameter of 9 mm is used for children weighing more than 15 Kg and a probe with a diameter of 8 mm is used for body weights between 5 and 15 Kg. A diameter of 5-7 mm is used for newborns weighing 2.5-4 Kg whereas a probe with a diameter of 5-6 mm is used for newborn weighing less than 2.5 Kg [7-8].
The endoscopic lesions that are typically observed in oesophagus include erythema, ulcerations, strictures and mucosal bridges. The histological finding of non caseating granulomata in oesophagus is observed in 20-30% of patients [4-5].
At the gastric and duodenal levels, typical endoscopic lesions include ulcerations (which can be linear, curve-shaped, diffuse, superficial or aphtous), nodularities, cobble-stone mucosa, bowel wall rigidity and luminal strictures [4-5].
A focal antral gastritis, negative for Helicobacter Pylori, has been observed in 84% of CD affected patients.
UC was not traditionally associated to an extension involving more than colon and ileum.
However, inflammatory lesions at the level of the upper gastrointestinal tract have recently been frequently observed also in UC patients (up to 70%) [4-5].

3. Ileum – colonoscopy: General aspects

A video – colonoscope with adulthood-dimensioned size can be used for patients aged from 3-4 years and/or with body weight of at least 12-15 Kg [4-5-8]. This colonoscope for adults is more rigid and diminishes the risk of loops formation; it requires, however, a peculiar attention of the operator for the risk of perforations, mainly for smaller children. Moreover its larger diameter can determine limitations in manoeuvrability in the more restricted lumen of the child.

A colonscope with a diameter of 11.1-11.7 mm is therefore more indicated for the whole pediatric age [7-8].

Before any colonoscopy, it's good practice to perform a digital anal exploration and, subsequently, a rectal exploration in order to detect any possible lesion being localized at the lower segments; the retroversion of the colonoscope is also important for this purpose [4-5].

An adequate lubrication allows an easier transit through into the rectum, which can also be helped by the guide of the index finger of the operator [4-5].

As for inflation, CO2 can represent an alternative to air since it is more rapidly absorbed thus produces minor discomfort, as well as a minor theoretical risk of perforation [4-5].

The patient is usually placed in lateral security position [4-5].

If during the procedure a difficulty in overcoming the splenyc flexure is observed, the patient can be replaced in the supine position as well as on the opposite side. An assistant located on the left of the operator exercises an abdominal pressure in order to check and prevent any loop formation at the sigma or traverse colon. A moderate air inflation is preferable in the Sigma to avoid that an excessive volume increases any risk of loop formation [4-5].

When the operator needs to increase the penetration pressure of the instrument, a loop formation may have been produced [4-5].

The length of the colonoscope at the splenyc flexure in the absence of loops is of 40 cm for older children whereas it can decrease to 20-25 cm in children aged 3-4 years old. At the hepatic flexure, instead, it is of 60 cm in the absence of loops for the older children and 40 cm for 3-4 year old children. At the cecum, the length from the anus is about 80 cm for the older children and 40-60 cm for the younger ones. The ileum-cecal valve is localized at about 1-4 cm distally in respect to the appendix orifice and opens perpendicularly to the colon axis [4-5].

In order to prevent any tension of the bowel wall, the aspiration of the air inside the cecum is suggested before ileum intubation. Ileum intubation allows its evaluation up to 40 cm. At this level, therapeutic dilations of the terminal ileum can be effectuated through a perendoscopic balloon [4-5].

Bioptic samples should be performed on each area, including segments of apparently normal mucosa [4-5].

4. Morphology of lesions

Typical endoscopic lesions in **CD** are [3-5] (Fig. 1-4):

- aphthous ulcerations (generally multiple, focal, with small diameter and surrounded by normal erythematous mucosa)
- mucosal nodularities
- mucosal aspect of cobblestone (resulting from interception of long ulcerative lesions and large tortuous ones including areas of thickened mucosa within)
- flattening of ileal mucosa
- pseudomembranous formations

- mucosal bridges
- stenosis (mild to severe, more frequently localized at the Bauhin valve) [1][3].

Inflammatory pseudopolips are less frequent in CD with respect to UC [3].

According to the mucosal and phenotypical characteristics at onset, CD is classified into inflammatory, stenosing and fistulizing.

Since CD can potentially involve the whole gastrointestinal tract, the intubation of ileum and upper gastrointestinal endoscopy are always indicated for a complete stadiation of the disease.

At the level of the strictures, the intestinal mucosa usually appears actively inflamed, frequently ulcerated and bleeding.

In the fistulizing CD phenotype, the internal orifice of the fistula can be observed on the bowel wall, generally in correspondance of inflamed areas.

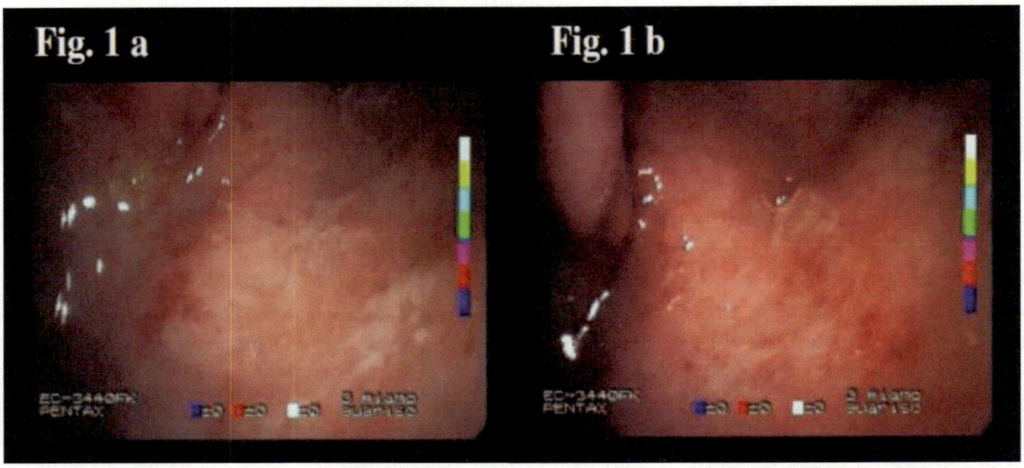

Fig. 1. Gastric mucosa with focal aphthous ulcerations (a) surrounded by herythematous mucosa (b) in Crohn's Disease

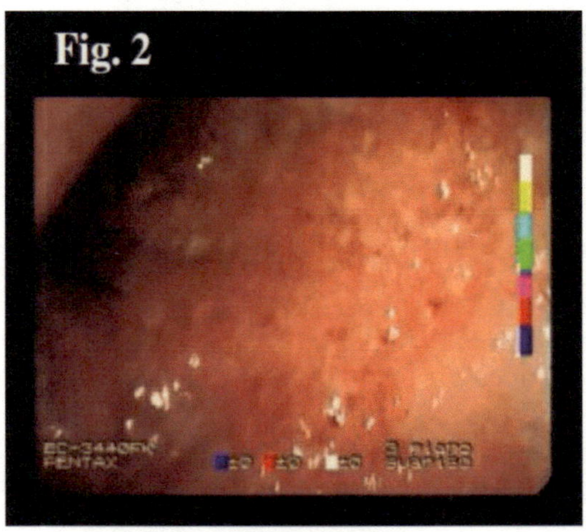

Fig. 2. Gastric mucosal nodularities and cobblestone pattern in Crohn's Disease

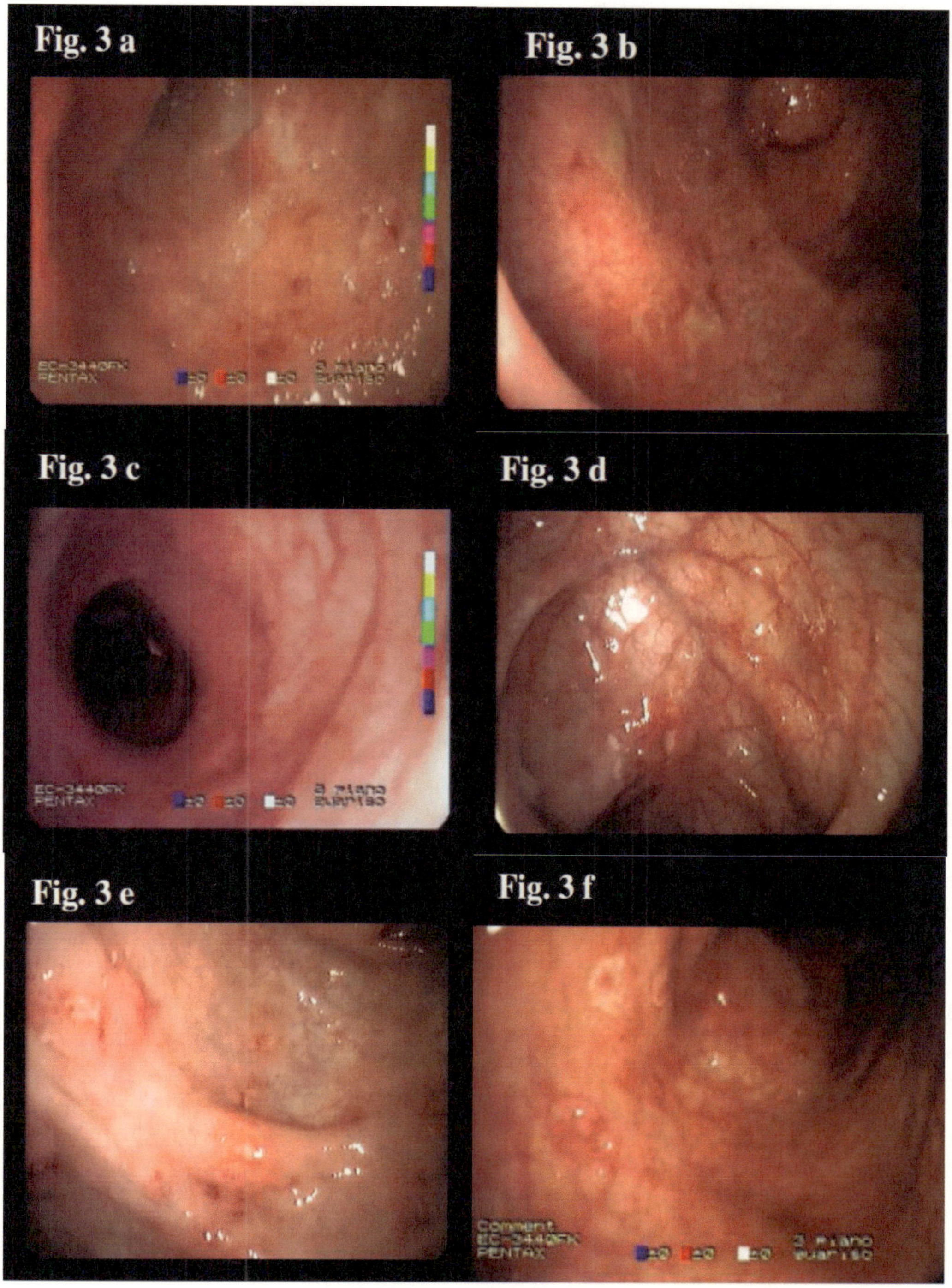

Fig. 3. Colonic mucosa with focal aphthous ulcerations (a-b) surrounded by herythematous mucosa (c-d-e-f) in Crohn's Disease

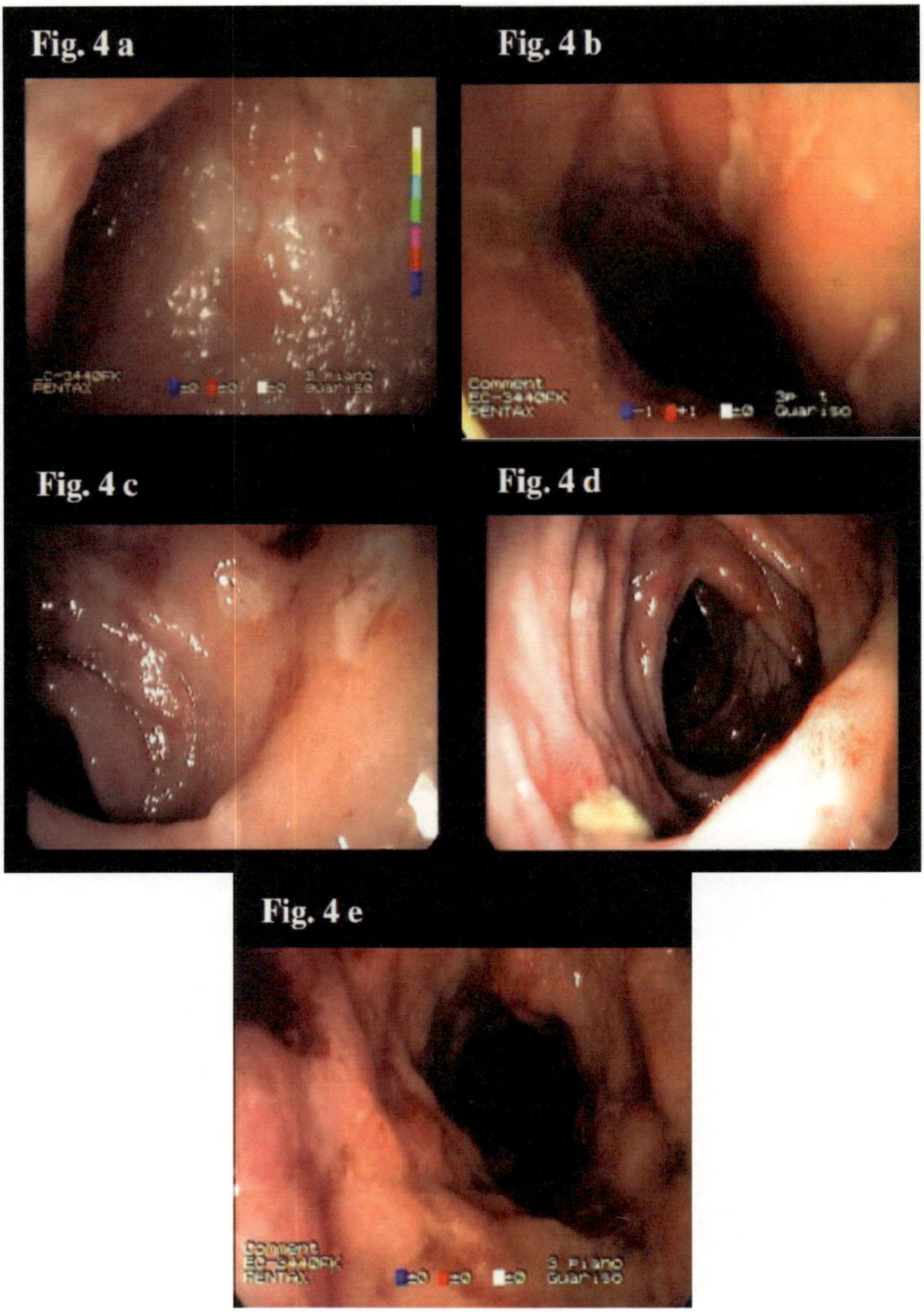

Fig. 4. Colonic mucosa with extensive deep ulcerations (a, b, c, d) and cobblestone pattern (e) in Crohn's Disease

The histological findings which are more characteristic of CD are: trans-mural inflammation with infiltration and fibrosis; dilatation and sclerosis of lymphatic vessels; lymphatic aggregates; the typical non - caseating granulomata. Other possible findings include eccess of histiocytes, giant perinucleated cells (Langhan's like), mucous gland cells hyperplasia, focal criptitis, pseudopyloric metaplasia of colocites and decrease of inflammation grade from the upper to the lower colon [9].
Even though the macroscopic and hystological characteristics are frequently discriminating for UC and MC, in those cases in which a differential diagnosis cannot be set, the disease is identified as Unclassified IBD, presenting intermediate characteristics between CD and UC. Infective colitis can also present a macroscopic pattern being similar to that of IBD [3].
For this reason, multiple biopsies should always be suggested at each segment for diagnosis [3].
In UC the inflammatory process is limited to mucosa and submucosa and it spreads for continuity from rectum to the whole colon [3].
Instead in CD inflammation is trans-mural and "patchy" lesions can be found throughout the whole gastrointestinal tract; an involvement of adjacent lymphonodes and mesenther as well as the formation of fistula and abscesses can be observed [3].

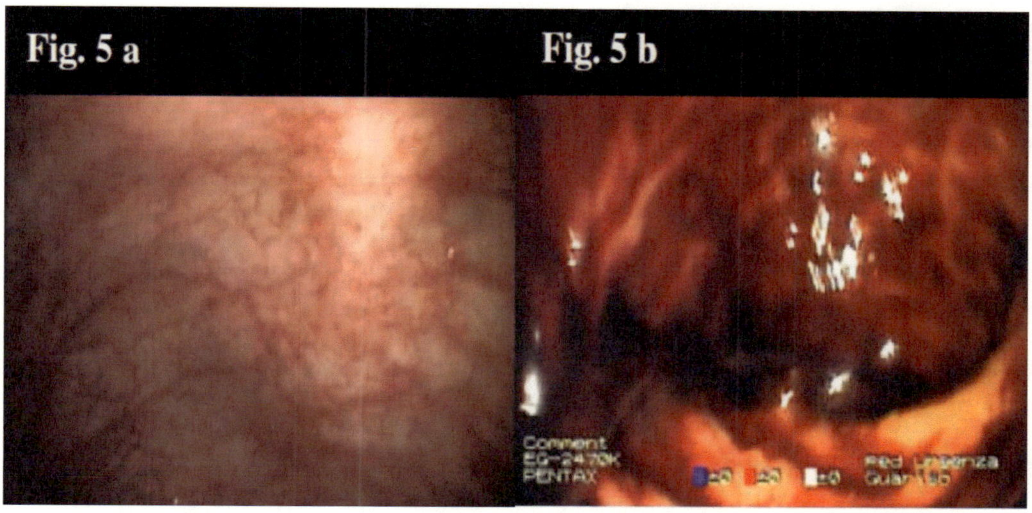

Fig. 5. Colonic herythematous mucosa with crispness (a) and mucosal bleeding (b) in Ulcerative Colitis

Endoscopic characteristics in **UC** [3-5] (Fig. 5):
- loss of vascularization
- diffuse hyperemia
- edema
- mucosal crispness and/or bleeding at the contact of the endoscope
- mucous – suppurative secretion
- diffuse erosions covered by fibrine

Other possible findings:
- ulcerations of variable diameter and number, surrounded by actively inflamed and potentially bleeding mucosa

- aphthous ulcerations
- inflammatory pseudopolips, generally parietal, consequence of the regeneration of previously ulcerated areas
- mucosal granularity
- nodules with erosions above
- loss of colonic haustrae with aspect of "rigid tube"
- backwash ileitis: ileal extension of lesions in pancolitis
- patchy colitis
- relative rectal sparing

Baron and Mayo scores are the two principle indexes for the endoscopic grading of UC [3].
As regards the major histological alterations in UC, they are distorted with the disappearance of mucous glandular architecture and inflammatory infiltration of the crypts. They also have a villi-like profile of the mucosal surface, a high grade alteration of the mucosal architecture, Paneth cells metaplasia and a decrease of the inflammation and mucosal alteration grade from the upper to the lower colonic tract are seen [9].

5. Contraindications to endoscopic procedure

Absolute: toxic megacolon, suspect of intestinal perforation, shock [3]
Relative: hyperacute situations with associated risk of severe complications such as perforation and abundant bleeding.
The risk of complications is equal to 0.3% per procedure and decreases to 0.05% in the absence of polipectomy [4].
Conservative therapy is used in cases of asymptomatic perforations or in localized peritonitis, in the absence of signs and symptoms of sepsis. In any more severe situations, the operating approach consists in the resection of the intestinal segment and anastomosis [4-5].
Splenyc rupture is a very rare complication, that manifests with hypovolemia, pain at the shoulder or abdominal pain appearing within 24 hours after the performance of ileum-colonoscopy.
Equally rare is also pancreatitis caused by the rupture of the pancreas within the procedure [4-5].

6. SES – CD score for Crohn's Disease

Being mucosal healing a fundamental end-point for treatment of CD, the necessity to define a simple score for the endoscopic activity of disease has emerged in the last few years [1].
Such a score results from the addition of single evaluations: ulcer's dimension, extension of the ulcerated surface, presence and severity of stricture [1].
From the validation studies, SES - CD comes out to be simple, reproducible and easy to be used for CD; a strong relation among the score value, the clinical parameters of the disease (pCDAI) and blood levels of CRP have been identified [1].
The correlation between SES -CD and pCDAI is statistically significant, despite the limitation due to the fact that many extra intestinal manifestations are clinically manifested but are not necessarily accompanied by any mucosal involvement [1].
Other possible limitations of SES-CD are the presence of fistulas (for the evaluation of which endoscopy does not represent the best diagnostic tool), underestimation of strictures (due to the functional nature of the classification being used; what is considered is, in fact, the

capacity of the endoscope to overcome the stricturing tract) and overestimation of non-specific lesions (at this level the endoscopic experience of the operator is determinant) [1].

The addition prefigures the evaluation of 5 pre-determined ileum-colonic segments: ileum (explorable portion), right colon (comprehending the ileum-cecal valve, cecum, ascendant colon, hepatic flexure), transverse colon, left colon (comprehending descendant colon, sigma, rectum-sigmoid junction), rectum. For each segment, the evaluation of four endoscopic variables is prefigured: presence of ulcers, extension of ulcerated surface, extension of the surface with lesions, presence of stenosis. For each variable, a score ranging from 0 to 3 is assigned to each segment [1].

The classification of the ulcers for the SES-CD addition is based on their dimensions; therefore the extension of the ulcerated segment is evaluated attributing a score of 3 to those cases with a surface involvement exceeding 30%: such a proportion of extension is thus considered as the most severe pattern, since a major extension has no additional effect on the severity of symptoms [1].

The classification of strictures for SES-CD is both descriptive and functional; in fact it is based on the capacity of the endoscope to overcome a segmental luminal narrowing [1].

7. Further diagnostic applications of the endoscopic examination

Device-assisted enteroscopy (DAE) is a generic term for endoluminal examination of the small bowel by any endoscopic technique that includes assisted progression (e. g. by a balloon, overtube, or other stiffening device) [2]. DAE can be used to diagnose Crohn's disease, because histological corroboration is available.

A fundamental endoscopic application in the follow-up of IBD affected patients is the endoscopic surveillance for any dysplasia (a high-grade dysplasia evolve to invasive carcinoma in 33-100% of cases) [1]. As reported by the American Gastroenterology Society guidelines, the risk of neoplasia increases in cases of a long lasting disease with early onset, severe extension of disease, familiarity for cancer of colon-rectum, presence of backwash ileitis and history of sclerosing cholangitis [3]. Furthermore carcinogenesis correlates with the activity of inflammation [4-5].

Aiming to the surveillance and early diagnosis of any arising neoplasia, the ideal number of biopsies to be taken during an endoscopic examination is 2-4 every 10 cm (and on 4 quadrants). For the paediatric age, such a surveillance schedule is indicated for cases with disease duration > 8 years [4].

Techniques like chromoendoscopy and AFI (auto-florescence imaging) increase from 2 to 5 times the sensitivity for the identification of any neoplastic lesion; on the contrary no significant advantages have been observed with NBI (narrow binding imaging) technique, with respect to traditional endoscopy [1].

An endoscopic examination is recommended, after 2-3 months since the beginning of treatment in patients with a new diagnosis, in order to evaluate the efficacy of the ongoing therapy to get mucosal healing.

Another major role of the endoscopic examination involves those patients with IBD that undergo a surgical intervention with confectioning of ileal-pouch [3][10]. A post-surgical pouchitis is- in fact- common: it can be mild to severe and generally does not involve the last ileal oxbow (23-46% of cases at 10-11 years of age). A surveillance of the macro- and microscopic inflammation is possible through scheduled post-operative controls.

The *push enteroscopy*, per os or laparoscopic, is an evolving technique which is useful for diagnostic evaluation of the small bowel [4-5]. It consists in an endoluminal examination of the proximal jejunum using a long, flexible endoscope [2]. At present, endoscopes with length up to 230 cm, diameter of 10 mm and deflexion grades up to 160-180^ are used. Per os, it is possible to reach a length of 120-180 cm beyond Treitz ligament; with laparoscopic assistance, also the terminal ileum is reached.

Push enteroscopy allows tissue sampling, polypectomy, and treatment of bleeding lesions [2].

In recent years, balloon-assisted endoscopic techniques have largely replaced push enteroscopy in examination of the small bowel.

More recently, advanced endoscopic techniques of *balloon-assisted* and *spiral enteroscopy* have allowed direct tissue sampling for histopathology and therapeutic procedures in the small bowel. However the role of these investigations in the diagnosis and management of IBD is unclear [2][3].

Balloon-assisted enteroscopy (BAE) is a generic term for endoluminal examination of the small bowel by any endoscopic technique that includes balloon-assisted progression [2].

Single-balloon enteroscopy (SBE) is defined as endoluminal examination of the small bowel using a single-balloon endoscope [2].

Double-balloon enteroscopy (DBE) is defined as endoluminal examination of the small bowel using a double-balloon endoscope [2]. DBE, first described by Yamamoto and colleagues in 2001, allows deep (even complete) intubation of the small bowel by pleating the bowel onto a long, flexible endoscope fitted with an overtube [2].

DBE needs to be performed under deep sedation or general anesthesia which allows the execution of biopsies as well as of therapeutical procedures such as emostasis and dilatations [4]. The DBE system consists in a video-enteroscope (length of 200 cm, diameter of 8.5 mm), with overtube and elevate resolution. On the overtube as well as on the extremity of the instrument, two balloons are placed; these can be inflated and deflated with air, throughout a pressure-regulated control system (P max 45 mmHg). Both are deflated at the beginning of the procedure. Once duodenum is reached, the balloon on the overtube is inflated to stabilize the tube which is pushed foreword as much as possible. Subsequently, the balloon on the enteroscope is inflated while the one on the overtube is deflated, so that the overtube can be pushed foreword to the tip of the instrument. By repeating the procedure with the same order, the instrument progressively advances visualizing the entire small bowel.

DBE is particularly useful for patients with obscure gastrointestinal bleeding as well as for those with suspicion of CD but with negative ileoscopy and imaging. It allows us to identify early lesions like aphthae, erosions and small ulcers. Large portions of the small bowel can be visualized directly; oral and anal routes, alone or in combination, are used to achieve complete small-bowel examination [2].

Endosonography uses a colonoscope with frontal vision and with a transducer (emitting sound waves with a frequency of 7.5 Hz) placed on the rigid extremity or being introduced through the operative tube. A fluid of interface is necessary and can be obtained through filling the balloon with water as well as in the intestinal segment to be examined [4]. In the paediatric age, indications to this technique can include suspicion of neoplasia (early identification of adenoma), evaluation of the extension and depth of lesions (in particular perirectal and pericolonic abscesses), strictures, fistula and anastomosis [4-5].

Characteristic findings of IBD from endosonography are bowel wall thickening with loss of the normal structure, which is secondary to progressive inflammation. Although the differentiation between CD (with transparietal involvement) and UC may be set through echoendoscopy, UC in phase of activity can in certain cases manifest with findings which are referable to CD [4-5].

Other useful parameters which can be evaluated through echoendoscopic doppler are velocity of maximal flux in the superior mesentheric artery and the increase in transparietal vascularisation [4-5].

The high magnification endoscopy (HMCC) allows a magnification of up to 100 times. The images obtained close in on the histological findings both for the segments of normal mucosa and for those with clearly evident lesions; it is not possible, however, to identify those mild mucosal alterations, which are-on the contrary-recognizable at histology [4]. This technique is particularly useful for the execution of targeted biopsies and can be taken into consideration also for the surveillance of the development of neoplasia in IBD affected patients.

Confocal Laser Endomicroscopy (CLE) is a technology developed in the last 5 years which focalises on a single point of a laser illumination at a low power [4-5]. The distal extremity of the endoscope contains a channel for air and water, two guide lights, an operating channel with diameter 2.8 mm and an auxiliary channel for water. The sodium-fluorescein administered i.v. at the beginning of the procedure is used as a mean of contrast. Cellular and subcellular microscopic images are obtained. This technique allows the execution of targeted biopsies in IBD affected patients, reducing the number of bioptic samples to be taken [4-5].

Intraoperative enteroscopy (IOE) is defined as an endoluminal examination of the small bowel during abdominal surgery with manual external assistance for endoscope progression. By definition, IOE is an exploration of the small intestine with an endoscope (gastroscope, colonoscope, pediatric colonoscope, or enteroscope) during a surgical procedure [2].

Spiral enteroscopy is a recently developed technique. An enteroscope, introduced orally, is passed through a single-use overtube, which has helical spirals at its distal end and rotates independently from the enteroscope. The enteroscope can be locked in the overtube allowing the option of spiral enteroscopy, or unlocked and advanced through the overtube [2].

8. Operative endoscopy

Beside diagnostic endoscopy, operative endoscopy also has a determinant role in the practical management of IBD affected patients [3].

In particular, CD patients have an elevated risk of relapses in the sites of surgical anastomosis where strictures can appear [3]. At this level, pneumatic endoscopic dilatations (balloons of 12-18 mm with pressures of 25-50 psi are used) as well as the placement of coated stents are techniques of important efficacy for the rechanneling of severe strictures (early efficacy in 86% of cases; late efficacy in 55% of cases) [1].

Before the advent of pneumatic perendoscopic dilators, patients with significant strictures necessary underwent a surgical intervention of resection of intestinal segments, with a risk of short bowel syndrome [3].

The response to operative endoscopy techniques has been demonstrated significantly higher, observing a minor risk of surgical intervention in those cases with extension of the stricture being ≤ 4 cm [1]. A recent study by Stienecker K [11], examined 31 strictures in a group of CD affected patients: in 30 of them balloon dilatation was successful in a single endoscopic session, so that eventually the strictures could be passed easily with the standard colonoscope. Sufficient dilatation was not possible in one patient with a long stricture of the ileum involving the Bauhin valve and an additional stricture of the ileum which were 15 cm apart. This patient therefore required surgery. Available follow-up was in the range of 54-118 months (mean 81). The relapse rate over this period was 46%, but 64% of relapsing strictures could be successfully dilated again. Only in four patients was surgery required during this follow-up period. These initial results support endoscopic balloon dilatation, especially for short strictures in Crohn's disease, perforation a rare complication. In the long-term, the relapse rate is probably higher than after surgery, but usually a second endoscopic treatment can be performed successfully, leading to a considerable success rate of the endoscopic procedure. The overall technical success rate, defined as achieving an endoscopically passable residual stricture, is between 70% and 90 %, independent of the balloon's diameter having being used.

Indications to endoscopic dilatation of the strictures are [3]:

- severe strictures, with proximal bowel dilatation
- length of stenosis being < 2-3 cm
- endoscopic accessibility
- CD in remission or with low inflammatory activity

The dilatation is effectuated under deep sedation by insertion of the dilator across the stenosis and by inflation of the associated balloon with water and gastrographin in order to render it radio-opaque, therefore subjected to control [3]. Once the targeted diameter is reached, the balloon remains in loco for 1-2 minutes. An endoscopic control is usually performed one month later, in order to evaluate the diameter at the level of the precedent stenosis: if it is normal, a following endoscopic control is performed after 6 months whereas if the luminal diameter remains lower than 50% of the normal size, a new dilatation is programmed. The procedure should always be performed in a secure setting, in order to prevent the arousal of any complications [3].

The principle limitations to the use of endoscopy in paediatric age are mainly determined by the dimensions of the instrument [1].

Other frequently used endoscopic applications are: intra-operative ileoscopy (for the study of ileum during laparotomy), the removal of videocapsule (in cases when it is retained into the small bowel) and mucosal marking with china blue (to consent a major accuracy of the histological analysis) [1].

9. Small bowel capsule endoscopy (SBCE)

"Small-bowel capsule endoscopy (SBCE)" or "video capsule endoscopy" is a method of endoluminal examination of the small bowel using a wireless capsule shaped tool which is usually swallowed and then propelled through the gastrointestinal tract by gut motility.

Until a decade ago, mucosal visualization of the small bowel was limited to the reach of the push enteroscope as well as of the invasive and expensive intraoperative enteroscopy [2].

Even though push-enteroscopy has allowed us to access the visualization of the proximal jejunum extending the diagnostic potentialities of EGDS, it incidentally results in a relatively invasive technique [12]. Even more invasive is intra-operatory enteroscopy which in effect requires laparotomy and laparoscopy. Double-balloon enteroscopy allows a visualization of the entire bowel without necessity of surgical access, but requires a long time for manipulation.

Before the advent of video capsule endoscopy, the small bowel remained a "black box", being almost inaccessible to the paediatric endoscopists.
The advent of small-bowel capsule endoscopy (SBCE) allowed for the first time direct visualisation of the entire small bowel, albeit without the ability for tissue sampling [2].
This new technique has actually revolutionised the field of enteroscopy, offering a method for the complete evaluation of the small bowel. It is a non invasive technique, secure both for the paediatric and the adult patient, that overcomes the limitations of barium contrasted enteroscopy (low specificity for initial inflammatory lesions) and of ileum-colonoscopy (which can at its best evaluate the terminal ileum) [13].
The lens with extremely short focus (1 mm) allows a very high precision of image, without requiring inflation with air and with a resolution of 0.1 mm [14].
A recent metanalysis demonstrated the accuracy of video capsule endoscopy for the evaluation of the small bowel to be significantly superior to the one of enteroscopy and ileum-colonoscopy (63% vs 23% and 46% respectively); such a superiority is observed also with respect of other traditional techniques of imaging (i.e. TAC). Furthermore SBCE, can be useful for diagnosis of diseases involving the right colon [13].
This technique is therefore efficacious for the identification of superficial lesions which are not radiologically visible and the localisation of which can not be explored through endoscopy.
It is important for the study of the small bowel diseases (particularly for CD and U-IBD) in which the localisation at the small bowel can represent the unique site of disease, with consequent difficulty for a correct diagnosis [12].
The 2008 ECCO and OMED Consensus Statement [2] indicated that ileocolonoscopy must be performed prior to SBCE for the diagnosis of Crohn's disease. Small-bowel cross-sectional imaging should generally precede SBCE. The choice of radiographic imaging depends on local availability and expertise.
SBCE should be performed in children or adolescents with a high suspicion of Crohn's disease, when conventional endoscopy and small-bowel imaging are normal.
Younger children, under 9 years in particular, cannot generally assume and swallow the capsule. Determinants are the dimensions of the child, in terms of compatibility between capsular dimensions and the oesophageal sphincters, pylorus and ileum-cecal valve. It is important to ascertain the swallowing capacity of the child through simulations, i.e. vitaminic capsules with comparable dimensions, before performing SBCE. A valid alternative is the insertion of the capsule (length 25,3 mm, diameter 11 mm, weight 3.7 g) directly in the duodenum, using a dedicated device to perform the insertion [12-13].
This technique is particularly efficacious for the identification of paediatric patients with suspicion of Crohn's disease manifesting a protein-loosing enteropathy and/or growth deficit, gastro-duodenal bleeding, malabsorption, chronic abdominal pain, chronic diarrhoea, anorexia, anemia, hypoalbuminemia, positive serology for ASCA (being negative or poorly significant the other exams of the diagnostic flow-chart i.e. EGDS, ileum-colonoscopy, abdominal radiography); in these cases, moreover, capular endoscopy results economic as a test to be performed as a first-line indication [11] [14].
Other applications of SBCE comprehend [2][14][15]:

- Non invasive evaluation of the small bowel in patients with diagnosed CD but manifesting unexplained signs and symptoms (i.e. anemia)
- Assessment of postoperative recurrence of Crohn's disease (SBCE should only be considered if ileocolonoscopy is contraindicated or unsuccessful)

- The discrimination between CD and UC in patients with U-IBD (video capsule endoscopy allows a diagnostic redefinition in 29-40% of patients with diagnosis of IBD-U)
- Evaluation of mucosal healing after treatment

The fotographic objective, with angle of vision of 140^, permits an adequate visualization of the small bowel - considering the relative small diameter [12]. A complete evaluation of the gastrointestinal segments with major diameters, such as stomach and colon is in stead not possible.

Inside the capsule a coloured miniaturized camera, a battery and a transmission device are placed. Two images per second are acquired and sent, in form of radio waves, to 8 detection electrodes being placed on the abdominal surface of the patient and, from them, to an external recorder. The film on a monitor is then analyzed by the specialist. The duration of the test is of about 8 hours.

An adequate intestinal preparation to be effectuated the day before through assumption of iso-osmolar solutions at a dosage of 25-30 ml/Kg is recommended. It is in fact critically important for a good visualization of the small bowel mucosa [14]. Oral preparations of sodium-phosphate or poliethilenglicole (PEG) are used.

The administration of prokinetics may reduce transit times, increasing the complete evaluation of the small bowel. Randomized studies are nevertheless necessary to confirm their efficacy [14].

Patients should fast for at least 8 hours before the procedure and can start consuming liquids 1-2 hours after its begun; they can have light meals 2 hours after the ingestion of the capsule [14].

By the way, there is no available evidence to support a particular bowel preparation for SBCE in the subset of patients with suspected Crohn's disease [2]. The technique was approved by the American FDA in 2001 for adults and in 2003 for patients aging 10 to 18 years and presents a very low risk of complications. It can be performed for outpatients and does not expose to ionizing radiations, as it happens with the more common radiological techniques such as small bowel enema and abdominal TAC [8]. Also, small bowel lesions identified through capsular endoscopy are observed in 13% of normal asymptomatic adults, so they are not sufficient for a diagnosis of IBD. More importantly similar lesions are, identified in patients affected by Celiac Disease, allergic–infective-ischemic-rheumatic-autoimmune enteropathy, in immunodeficiencies and in NSAD enteropathy [14-15].

Video capsule endoscopy is the most efficacious test for diagnosis of patients with symptomatic "occult" CD but it is unspecific and does not allow itself the differential diagnosis among the above-mentioned patterns [14].

In summary, as it is stated in the 2008 ECCO and OMED Consensus, SBCE is able to identify mucosal lesions compatible with Crohn's disease in some patients in whom conventional endoscopic and small-bowel radiographic imaging modalities have been non diagnostic. As with other imaging modalities, a diagnosis of Crohn's disease should not be based on the appearances at capsule endoscopy alone. A normal capsule endoscopy has a high negative predictive value for active small-bowel Crohn's disease [2].

Principle limitations of SBCE [2]:

- Difficulties in swallowing of the younger child (Diameter 25.3 mm)
- Poor quality of the intestinal preparation
- Poor standardization of diagnostic reports
- Elevate costs

- A specificity of lesions (10% of patients can present IBD like lesions)
- Risk of capsule retention (5% of CD affected patients)

Principal contraindications to capsular endoscopy are suspected or known obstructions of the gastrointestinal tract because of an increased risk of retention of the capsule (incidence of 0,75 -5%), recent surgical interventions and patients with pace-maker [14][16].

Causes of obstruction and consequent retention of the capsule can be primitive lesions of IBD, drug induced lesions (es. NSAD), radiation induced lesions and neoplastic lesions (mainly in the young adults with a longer follow-up) [14].

In the majority of cases, retentions are temporary and asymptomatic [14].

In order to minimize the risk of capsule retention, an accurate anamnesis and clinical examination are fundamental. Any symptom possibly related to obstruction has to be identified, even though in most cases the capsule retention results asymptomatic [14].

Since the preliminary performance of enteroscopy for the evaluation of any possible stenosis does not exclude afterwards a capsule retention, the "patency capsule" appears, in stead, a more useful opportunity. It is made of lactose and barium, and begins to break up after the thirtieth hour: if its passage does not determine complications (the patient eliminates the capsule unbroken or the radio-frequencies emitted give out within thirty hours), then the video capsule endoscopy can be safely performed [14][16].

Extremely rare side effects of the patency capsule are abdominal pain and occasional temporary episodes of bowel occlusion.

When the capsule is actually retained, an orally administered corticosteroid therapy generally permits the progression of the capsule through the stricture [14].

The incidence of capsule retention among patients with suspected CD is of 10% whereas it is of 4-7% among those with diagnosis of CD [14].

In summary, as reported in the 2008 ECCO and OMED Consensus Statement [2]:

- In patients with suspected Crohn's disease the risk of small-bowel capsule retention is low and comparable to that when the indication for SBCE is bleeding.
- In patients with an established diagnosis of Crohn's disease the risk of small-bowel capsule retention is increased, particularly in those with known intestinal stenosis. It is essential to attempt to exclude small-bowel strictures by a thorough clinical history and radiographic imaging before SBCE [2]. However, normal radiographic studies cannot entirely exclude the potential for small-bowel capsule retention [2].

A patency (biodegradable, 'dummy') capsule to reduce the risk of retention should be considered, or DAE, if strictures are identified [2].

Passage of an intact patency capsule predicts safe transit of a small-bowel capsule of identical or lesser size. A patency capsule may itself cause obstruction at tight strictures, but this is usually transient. A retained small-bowel capsule can often be retrieved by DAE [2].

10. References

[1] Daperno M, D'Haens G, Van Assche G, Baert F, Bulois P, Maunoury V, Sostegni R, Rocca R, Pera A, Gevers A, Mary JY, Colombel JF, Rutgeerts P: Development and validation of a new, simplified endoscopic activity score for Crohn's disease: the SES -CD. *Gastrointestinal Endoscopy* 2004; 60: 505-12.

[2] Bourreille A et al. Role of small-bowel endoscopy in IBD: international OMED–ECCO consensus. *Endoscopy 2009*; 41: 618–637

[3] De Angelis GL, Bizzarri B, De Angelis N, Borrelli O: The endoscopic diagnosis. In: SIGENP Consensus Statement (Italian Society of Gastroenterology Hepatology and Nutrition): Inflammatory Bowel Disease in the paediatric age. Eds Area Pediatrica Publ Milan Italy 2008, pp 23-26.

[4] Venkatesh K, Thomson M. Endoscopic Modalities in Pediatric Inflammatory Bowel Disease. In: Pediatric Inflammatory Bowel Diseases. Mamula P, Markowitz JE, Baldassano RN eds Springer Publ New York 2008, pp 211-35.

[5] Venkatesh K, Thomson M. Endoscopic Modalities in Pediatric Inflammatory Bowel Disease. In: Pediatric Inflammatory Bowel Diseases. Perspectives and Consequences. Walker-Smith JA, Lebenthal E, Branski D eds Karger Publ Basel Switzerland 2009, pp 100-122.

[6] Guariso G, Gasparetto M, Visonà Dalla Pozza L, D'Incà R, Zancan L, Sturniolo G, Brotto F, Facchin P. Inflammatory bowel disease developing in paediatric and adult age. *J Pediatr Gastroenterol Nutr.* 2010 Dec;51(6):698-707.

[7] Boyle JT. Esophagogastroduodenoscopy in the pediatric patient. In: Gastroenterologic Endoscopy. Sivak MV eds Saunders Company Publ, Philadelphia, London, Toronto, Montreal, Sydney, Tokyo, 2000, pp 783-98.

[8] Mougenot JF, Bontems P, Cadranel S. Endoscopic Equipment. In: Pediatric Gastrointestinal Endoscopy. Textbook and Atlas. Winter SH, Murphy MS, Mougenot JF, Cadranel S edsBC Decker Inc Publ Hamilton Ontario 2006, pp 6-33.

[9] Girardin M, Seidman EG. Video Capsule Endoscopy in Pediatric Inflammatory Bowel Disease. In: Pediatric Inflammatory Bowel Diseases. Mamula P, Markowitz JE, Baldassano RN eds Springer Publ New York 2008, pp 275-87.

[10] Miele E: Pouchitis. In: SIGENP Consensus Statement (Italian Society of Gastroenterology Hepatology and Nutrition): Inflammatory Bowel Disease in the paediatric age. Eds Area Pediatrica Publ Milan Italy 2008, pp 27-30.

[11] Stienecker K, Gleichmann D, Neumayer U, Joachim Glaser H, Tonus Long V. Term results of endoscopic balloon dilatation of lower gastrointestinal tract strictures in Crohn's disease: a prospective study. *World J Gastroenterol* 2009 June 7; 15(21): 2623-2627.

[12] De Angelis GL, Bizzarri B, Vincenti F: Video capsule endoscopy. In: SIGENP Consensus Statement (Italian Society of Gastroenterology Hepatology and Nutrition): Inflammatory Bowel Disease in the paediatric age. Eds Area Pediatrica Publ Milan Italy 2008, pp 25-27.

[13] Seidman SG, Dirks MH: Wireless Capsule Endoscopy in IBD: State of The Art and Image of the Future. *Journal of Pediatric Gastroenterology and Nutrition* 2006; 43, suppl. 2.

[14] Mescoli C, Rugge M. Histology in Inflammatory Bowel Disease. In: SIGENP Consensus Statement (Italian Society of Gastroenterology Hepatology and Nutrition): Inflammatory Bowel Disease in the paediatric age. Eds Area Pediatrica Publ Milan Italy 2008, pp 37-41.

[15] Dirks MH, Costea F, Sant'Anna, Peretti N, Seidman EG: Videocapsule Endoscopy in Pediatric Crohn's Disease: a 4 -year experience. *Journal of Pediatric Gastroenterology and Nutrition* 2006; 43, suppl. 2.

[16] Role of the Wireless Capsule Endoscopy in Diagnosis of Undetermined Colitis and Suspect IBD in Paediatric Patients. *Journal of Pediatric Gastroenterology and Nutrition* 2006; 43, suppl. 2.

Part 5

Gastrointestinal Bleeding

18

Rare and Emergency Gastric Bleeding Cause – Dieulafoy's Lesion

Baki Ekçi[1], Can Aktas[2], Sezgin Sarikaya[2], Asli Cetin Celik[2] and Didem Ay[2]
[1]*Yeditepe University Hospital, Department of General Surgery, Istanbul,*
[2]*Yeditepe University Hospital, Department of Emergency Medicine, Istanbul*
Turkey

1. Introduction

Gastrointestinal bleeding is among the most common causes of emergency admissions. Having high mortality rates, high diagnosis and treatment costs, this condition constitutes a clinical problem that requires a multidisciplinary approach. Extra-varicose bleeding of the upper gastrointestinal system has still been frequent and it usually stops spontaneously. However, recurrent bleeding is the most important cause of mortality and morbidity. (Erickson & Glick, 1986; Rivkin & Lyakhovetskiy, 2005; Pfau et al., 2004)

Any remarkable cause could not be demonstrated in approximately 4-9% of massive upper gastrointestinal hemorrhage. (Cotton et al., 1973; Palmer, 1969). Bleeding and anemia might be associated with gastrointestinal vascular malformations. Some epidemiological studies suggest that symptomatic vascular anomalies may be present in approximately 1/10000 individuals (Hodgson et al., 2001). Dieulafoy's lesion is a rarely found vascular malformation in symptomatic vascular anomalies group of disease. It is commonly located in the proximal aspect of the stomach. Dieulafoy's lesion constitutes 1% to 5.8% of nonvariceal bleeds and is more common in men than in women (2:1) (Garg, 2007). Pathogenesis is still unknown, but it is assumed that it might be a congenital lesion (Regula et al.,2008). The typical lesion is generally located in the submucosa and described as a large tortuous vessel and a small defect in the overlying mucosal surface (Ekci et al., 2010; Vats et al., 2006). (Fig 1 & 2 & 3).

In 1884, Gallard first described this lesion, but it was attributed to a French surgeon Dieulafoy in literature (Alva et al., 2006). This medical condition usually presents with a large tortuous arteriole in the stomach wall that erodes and bleeds. In addition, this lesion is generally located at the lesser curvature of the stomach within 6 to 10 cm of the esophagogastric junction (Stojakov et al., 2007). It consists of a single large tortuous arteriole that does not exert normal branching or has a branch 1–5 mm in diameter(Fig 2 & 3). This size is more than the normal diameter of mucosal capillaries. The most common location of the lesion is the body of stomach, followed by the cardia and the esophagus, but they have also been reported in the esophagus, small and large bowel (Ekci et al., 2010; Turan et al., 2008).

This condition is commonly seen in elder males (Schmulewitz & Baillie, 2001; Stark et al, 1992). Large majority of patients having Dieulafoy's lesion might present with comorbidity including cardiovascular diseases, diabetes, chronic renal failure and hypertension (Norton et al., 1999). However, in a study no association with concomitant disease was found (Veldhuyzen van Zanten et al, 1986)

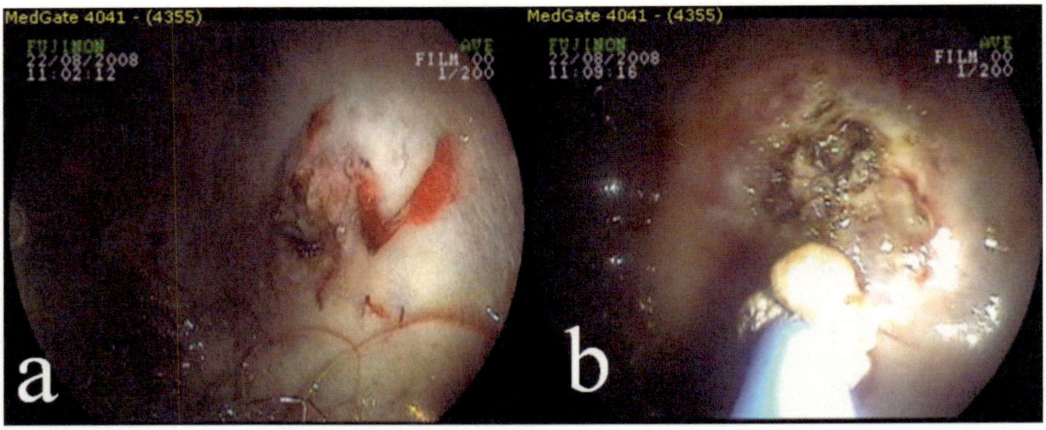

Fig. 1. **a**- Dieulafoy's lesion **b**: After heater probe application (Ekci et al., 2010)

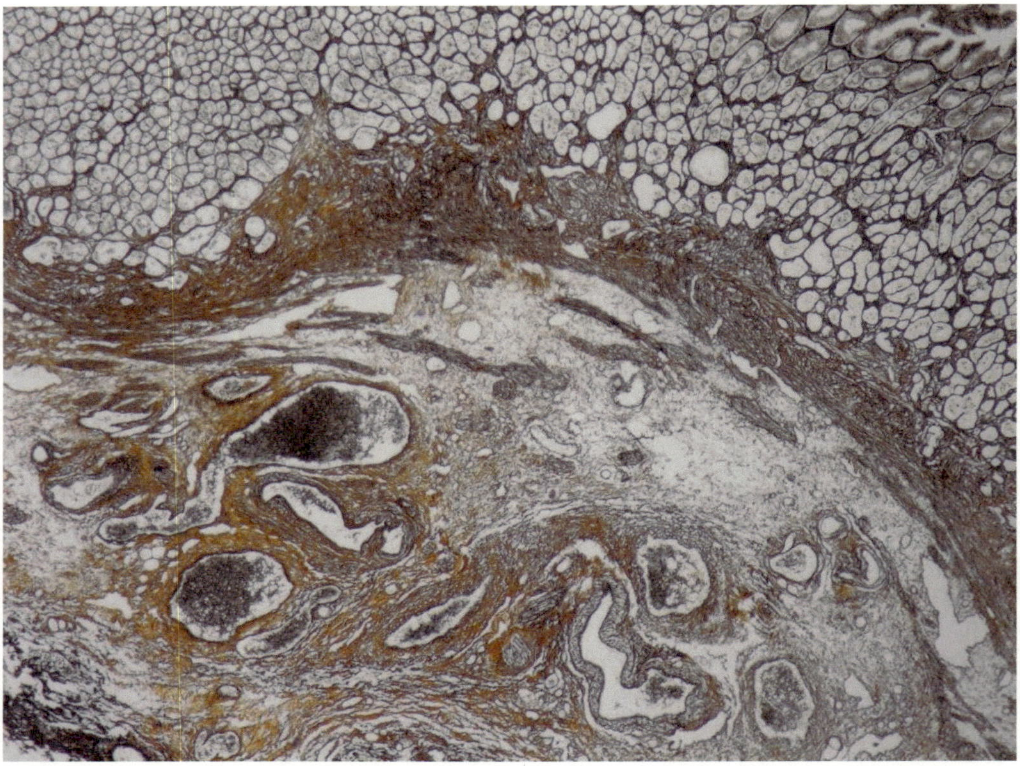

Fig. 2. Large tortuous malformed vessels in the gastric submucosa (Reticulin stain; x100) (Ekci et al., 2010)

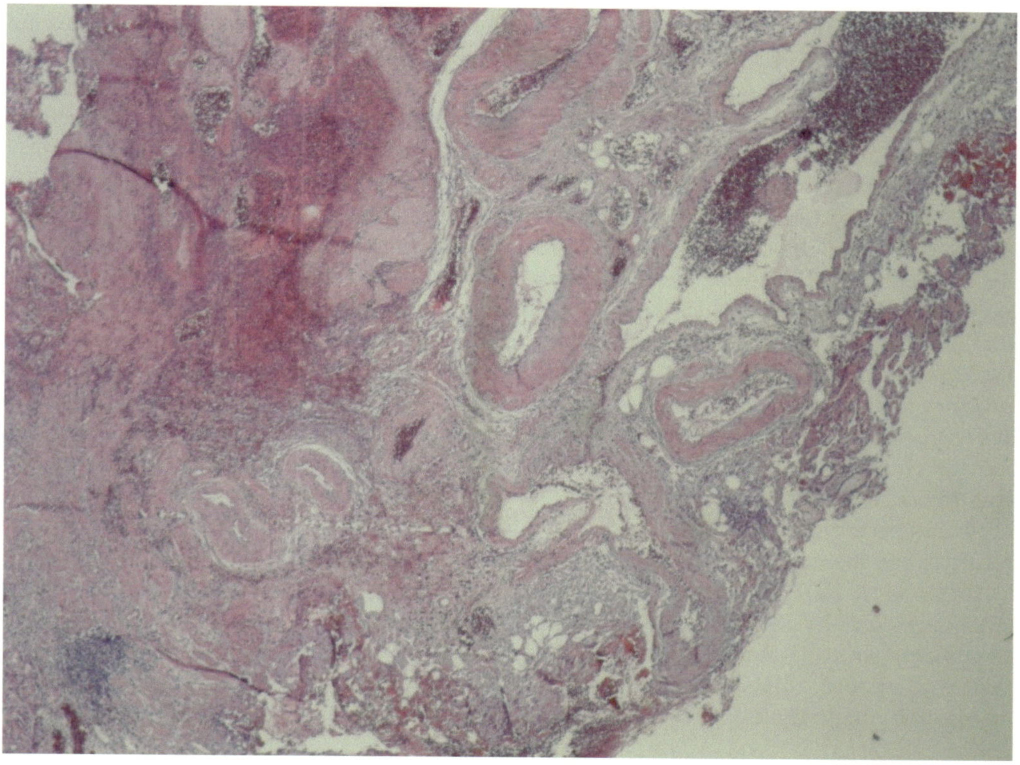

Fig. 3. Large tortuous vessels in the gastric submucosa and overlying eroded, necrotic mucosal surface could be seen (Hematoxylen and Eosin; x100) (Ekci et al., 2010)

The location of the Dieulafoy's lesion usually influences the variety of symptoms. It may rupture spontaneously and lead to massive bleeding. Therefore, the most common clinical symptom is recurrent, often massive, haematemesis associated with melaena (Ekci et al., 2010). However, lesion may present with haematemesis alone, or melaena alone. When this lesion occurs in the duodenum and proximal jejunum, patients often present with symptoms similar with gastric lesions. However, lesions in middle or distal jejunum as well as right colon and rectum are associated with massive rectal bleeding(Boix et al 1988 ; McClave et al 1988). Nearly all patients with this lesion may have hemodynamic instability. (Stark et al.,1992). In physical examination, hemodynamic instability and postural hypotension can be found. When gastrointestinal bleeding increases, hypotension and tachycardia become prominent. In such cases, transfusion for the initial resuscitation is usually necessary (Baettig et al., 1993; Reilly & Al-Kawas, 1991).

Occasionally, amyloid deposition may be found on the vessel wall (Rosai, 2004). In contrast, the histopathologic examination of large tortuous malformed vessels revealed no amyloid deposition in vessel walls (fig 2). The pathology in extragastric locations is essentially the same as that of the more common gastric lesion (Fig 3).

The standard treatment of Dieulafoy's lesion was surgical wedge resection in the past, but today the diagnosis of this lesion is made by endoscopy. Endoscopic methods should be the first choice of treatment in bleeding Dieulafoy's lesions (Yanar et al., 2007). In times when surgical resection was the choice of treatment, mortality and morbidity rates were high

(Goodman 1964). For the lesions located at colon, colonoscopy may be helpful in defining the source of bleeding (Barbier et al., 1985). Sometimes, multiple endoscopies may be necessary. Endoscopic evaluation reveals tiny ulcer, the protruding vessels, surrounding inflammatory reaction and occasionally a clot on this lesion. Since this lesion is small and the bleeding in stomach might interfere with the endoscopic visualization, the aspiration of intragastric blood and good air insufflation is necessary. If the visualization can not be enhanced with these interventions, endoscopy should be ended and restarted after the hemodynamic stabilization is achieved. Endoscopy is used for both diagnosis and treatment (Fig 1) Successful hemostasis has been reported with many different endoscopic techniques. Endoscopic hemoclip application, endoscopic band ligation, heater probe application, Nd:YAG, with or without epinephrine injection therapy have all been shown to be effective in various studies(Al-mıshlab et al., 1999; Ekci et al., 2010). An experienced endoscopist and appropriate therapeutic instruments are essential to achieve a high success rate. Reilly et al. (Reilly & Al-Kawas, 1991) achieved permanent haemostasis in 85% of cases with endoscopic therapy. The authors concluded that of the remaining 15% in whom re-bleeding occurs, 10% can successfully be treated by repeat endoscopic therapy and 5% may ultimately require surgical intervention.

If endoscopic therapy fails, angiography with embolization or surgery is indicated (Alva et al., 2006; Garg, 2007; Reilly & Al-Kawas, 1991; Regula et al., 2008). While the bleeding is active, angiography might be helpful with cases in which initial endoscopy failed to show the bleeding source(Katz & Salas., 1993). It should be kept in mind that angiography can not make a diagnose unless there is active bleeding, and therefore, it is of little value. Angiography may also be used therapeutically by gelfoam embolisation (Helliwell & Irving, 1981).

In cases where endoscopic therapy is not effective, surgical therapy is necessary. After a gastrotomy and identification of the lesion, the bleeding vessel can be ligated. Furthermore, proximal gastric resection, or a large wedge resection might be performed. Limited wedge resection is most commonly employed surgical procedure (Turan et al., 2008; Ekci et al., 2010 ; Yanar et al., 2007). During surgery, intra-operative endoscopy might be helpful with the identification of the lesion, thereby unnecessary bowel resection is avoided.

In conclusion, for patients with Dieulafoy's disease, early diagnosis through emergency endoscopy and endoscopic therapy might be very effective and life saving. But if these techniques are not successful, surgical management should be the treatment choice.

2. References

Al-mıshlab T, Amin AM, Ellul JPM. (1999) Dieulafoy's lesion: an obscure cause of GI bleeding. *J. R. Coll. Surg. Edinb.* 44, 222-5

Alva. S, Abir F, Tran DD. (2006) Laparoscopic Gastric Wedge Resection for Dieulafoy's Disease Following Preoperative Endoscopic Localization With India Ink and Endoscopic Clips. *JSLS* 10: 244–246

Baettig B, Haecki W, Lammer F, Jost R. (1993) Dieulafoy's disease: endoscopic treatment and follow up. *Gut* 34: 1418-21

Barbier P, Luder P, Triller J, Ruchti CH, Hassler H, Stafford A. (1985) Colonic haemorrhage from a solitary minute ulcer. Report of three cases. *Gastroenterology* 88: 1065-8

Boix J, Humbert P, Fernandez-Llamazares J, Planas R, Ojanguren I, Salva JA.(1988) Dieulafoy malformation. *Dig Dis Sci* 33: 1496-7

Cotton, PB. Rosenberg MT, Waldram RPL, Axon ATR. (1973) Early endoscopy of oesophagus, stomach, and duodenal bulb in patients with haematemesis and melaena. *Br Med J* 2: 505-9

Ekci B, Gokce O, Ekici I, Akyuz U. (2010). A dangerous gastric bleeding cause: Dieulafoy's lesion. Hong Kong J Emerg Med 17:177-79

Erickson RA, Glick ME. (1986) Why have controlled trials failed to demonstrate a benefit of esophagogastroduodenoscopy in acute upper gastrointestinal bleeding? A probability model analysis. *Dig Dis Sci* 31: 760-8.

Garg, R. (2007) Bleeding from a gastric Dieulafoy lesion. *Emerg.Med.J.* 24: 520

Goodman RL. (1964) Mucosal arterial malformation ("aneurysm") of the stomach with fatal hemorrhage. *Gastroenterology* 46: 589-94.

Helliwell M, Irving JD. (1981) Haemorrhage from gastric artery aneurysms. *Br Med J* 282: 460-1

Hodgson, H. Watkinson A, Gordon FH. (2001) Vascular malformations of the gastrointestinal tract. *Best Practice & Research Clinical Gastroenterology*. 15: 41-58.

Katz, PO. (1993) Salas L. Less frequent causes of upper gastrointestinal bleeding. *Gastroenterol Clin Nor Amer* 22: 875-89

McClave SA, Goldschmid S, Cunningham JT, Boyd W Jr. (1988) Dieulafoy cirsoid aneurysm of the duodenum. *Dig Dis Sci* 33: 801-5

Norton ID, Petersen BT, Sorbi D, Balm RK, Alexander GL, Gostout CJ. (1999) Management and long–term prognosis of Dieulafoy lesion. *Gastrointest Endosc* 50: 762-767

Palmer, ED. (1969) The vigorous diagnostic approach to upper gastrointestinal tract haemorrhage. *JAMA* 207: 1477-80

Pfau PR, Cooper GS, Carlson MD, Chak A, Sivak MV Jr, Gonet JA, Boyd KK, Wong RC. (2004) Success and shortcomings of a clinical care pathway in the management of acute nonvariceal upper gastrointestinal bleeding. *Am J Gastroenterol* 99: 425-31.

Regula, J. Wronska E, Pachlewski J. (2008) Vascular lesions of the gastrointestinal tract . *Best Practice & Research Clinical Gastroenterology* 22: 313–28

Reilly HF, Al-Kawas FH.(1991) Dieulafoy lesion: Diagnosis and management. *Dig Dis Sci* 36:1702-7

Rivkin K, Lyakhovetskiy A. (2005) Treatment of nonvariceal upper gastrointestinal bleeding. *Am J Health Syst Pharm* 62: 1159-70.

Rosai, J. (2004) in Rosai and Ackerman's Surgical Pathology. Mosby press, New York, Volume 1, Chapter 11 (Stomach); p:656

Schmulewitz N, Baillie J. (2001) Dieulafoy lesion: A review of 6 years of experience at a tertiary referral center. *Am J Gastroenterol* 96: 1688-1694

Stark ME, Gostout CJ, Balm RK. (1992) Clinical features and endoscopic management of Dieulafoy's disease. *Gastrointest Endosc* 38: 545-50.

Stojakov, D. Velicković D, Sabljak P, Bjelović M, Ebrahimi K, Spica B, Sljukić V, Pesko P. (2007) Dieulafoy's lesion: rare cause of massive upper gastrointestinal bleeding. *Acta Chir Iugosl.* 54:125-9

Turan, I. (2008) Ozturk A, Akarca U, Ozutemiz O. An unusual cause of massive upper gastrointestinal bleeding: Dieulafoy's lesion within a giant midesophageal diverticulum.*Endoscopy* 40: 177

Vats, HS. Wengert TJ, Torbey CF. (2006) Gastrointestinal Stromal Tumor with Dieulafoy Lesion:A Novel Association. *Clinical Medicine & Research* 4: 228-9

Veldhuyzen van Zanten SJ, Bartelsman JF, Schipper ME, Tytgat GN. (1986) Recurrent massive hematemesis from Dieulafoy vascular malformations- a review of 101 cases. *Gut* 27: 213-222

Yanar, H. (2007) Dolay K, Ertekin C, Taviloglu K, Ozcinar B, Guloglu R, Barbaros U. An infrequent cause of upper gastrointestinal tract bleeding: "Dieulafoy's lesion". Hepatogastroenterology. 54: 1013-7

19

Pharmacological Therapy for Recurrent Obscure Gastrointestinal Bleeding

Javier Molina-Infante,
Gema Vinagre-Rodriguez and Miguel Fernandez-Bermejo
*Department of Gastroenterology,
Hospital San Pedro de Alcantara, Caceres,
Spain*

1. Introduction

Obscure gastrointestinal bleeding (OGIB) is defined as occult or overt bleeding of unknown origin that persists or recurs despite negative primary radiological and endoscopic studies. It can be classified into two different clinical forms: obscure-overt OGIB, defined as visible passage of blood (ie, melena or hematochezia) and obscure-occult OGIB, manifested by iron-deficiency anemia or positive fecal occult blood test without other evidence of bleeding.[1]

Since the source of bleeding is not readily identifiable by upper GI endoscopy and colonoscopy, OGIB is therefore, by definition, recurrent. Approximately, 5% of GI bleeding occurs between the ligament of Treitz and the ileocecal valve. Angiodysplasias of the small bowel account for 30% to 40% of OGIB and are the most common source of bleeding in patients over 60 years.[1,2] They can be found as a primary disease or a gastrointestinal manifestation of systemic diseases such as hereditary haemorrhagic telangiectasia (HHT), von Willebrand (vW) disease, cardiac valvular disease, radiation enteritis, end-stage renal disease, portal hypertension, connective tissue diseases or vasculitis. Other causes include non-steroidal anti-inflammatory drugs enteropathy, inflammatory bowel disease, small bowel tumors (ie, leiomyomas, carcinoid, lymphomas, adenocarcinomas), Meckel´s diverticulum or Dieulafoy´s lesion.

Over the last decade, the diagnostic yield and therapeutic capabilities of small bowel endoscopy have dramatically changed with the development of video capsule endoscopy and deep enteroscopy systems (single balloon, double balloon or spiral). Nonetheless, the diagnostic yield is 75% at best combining both techniques, so a quarter of patients lack a diagnosis of the source of bleeding despite exhaustive evaluation and may be at high risk of rebleeding.[1] Additionally, a variable percentage of patients with a diagnosis may not respond to endoscopic therapy or may not be tributary to aggressive endoscopic or surgical management due to severe comorbidities or diffuse distribution of lesions throughout the GI tract. In this particular subset of patients, medical therapy is commonly required to stop, or at least, ameliorate bleeding, which usually leads to high transfusional requirements, exacerbations of medical conditions and subsequent hospital admissions. Indications for medical therapy in OGIB, as approved in the latest American Gastroenterology Association technical review, are listed in Table 1.[2]

1.	Patients who are not candidates or do not respond to endoscopic, surgical or interventional radiological therapy.
2.	Diffuse vascular lesions in the small bowel or extended to upper or lower segments.
3.	Relative unaccesible location of lesions for endoscopy.
4.	Unknown source of bleeding.

Table 1. Indications for pharmacological therapy in OGIB

The aim of this chapter is to give an overview of current scientific evidence supporting the use of pharmacological therapy in these, often difficult to treat, OGIB patients. The standard diagnostic and therapeutic approach involving endoscopic and radiological techniques, the management of concomitant antiplatelet and anticoagulant drugs and the supportive care of anemia in OGIB patients, are described elsewhere. Up to date, data regarding pharmacological agents for OGIB are scarce and exclusively based on case reports and small uncontrolled studies. The available evidence suggests a potential role for pharmacological therapy as an adjunctive measure in patients with either multiple comorbidities or in whom lesions are inaccessible or refractory to endoscopic therapy. However, their clinical utility remains to be proven in randomized controlled trials. Similarly, the appropriate dose and schedule required for long-term therapy are also unknown. The different pharmacological agents used for OGIB reported in the literature are listed in Table 2.

Hormonal therapy
Somatostatin analogues
Octreotide
Long acting release (LAR) octreotide
Lanreotide
Antiangiogenic drugs
Thalidomide
Lenalidomide
Bevacizumab
Miscellaneous
Antifibrinolytics (aminocaproic acid, tranexamic acid)
Danazol
Desmopressin
Recombinant activated factor VII
Tamoxifen
Non selective beta-blockers

Table 2. Pharmacological agents used in OGIB

Depending on the type of bleeding
Life-threatening: vasoactive medication, rFVIIa
Depending on the source of bleeding
Angiodysplasias: long-acting somatostatin analogues, antiangiogenic drugs (thalidomide, lenalidomide)
Hereditary hemorrhagic telangiectasia: antifibrinolytics, tamoxifen, antiangiogenic drugs (thalidomide, bevacizumab)
Portal hypertension: beta-blockers
von Willebrand disease: desmopressin, vW factor, antifibrinolytics

Table 3. Suggested therapeutic algoritham for pharmacological therapy in OGIB

2. Hormonal therapy

Estrogen-progesterone combination was proposed for OGIB because of preliminary reports of improvement of epistaxis in patients with HHT during pregnancy and further relapse in the puerperium.[3] Its effect, which is not immediate, seems to be estrogen dose-dependent and acts by enhancing microvascular circulation, coagulation, and vascular endothelial integrity. The most common combination schedule has been ethynil estradiol 0.01-0.05 mg and noresthisterone 1-3 mg.[4] This therapy should be used over six-month periods with pauses to reduce the incidence of adverse effects, mostly due to the estrogen component (vascular thrombosis, gynecomastia and loss of libido in men, breast tenderness and vaginal bleeding in women). However, the two largest placebo-controlled studies addressing the impact of hormonal therapy on GI bleeding from angiodysplasias failed to demonstrate any significant benefit. In the first study, patients with out-of-reach bleeding small-bowel angiodysplasias were treated using high-dose estrogens, estrogen-progesterone or placebo, but no statistical improvement of transfusion requirements was observed amongst the groups.[5] Additionally, in the second study, the authors failed to identify any significant effect of hormonal therapy compared to placebo in 72 non-cirrhotic patients bleeding from documented angiodysplasia[6]. This latter study, however, has setbacks such as the use of low doses of ethynil estradiol and the exclusion of patients with vascular ectasia associated to cirrhosis and HHT. Overall, the effectiveness of hormonal therapy remains unclear and both negative controlled trial results and serious and frequent side effects strongly limit its use in OGIB. Recent reports on the effectiveness of other agents with an improved safety profile displace hormonal therapy as first-line therapeutic option for OGIB.

3. Somatostatin analogues

In 1993, octreotide was first reported for the treatment of bleeding small bowel angiodysplasias, in a small series of three patients successfully treated for 10 to 40 months.[7] The rationale for the use of somatostatin analogues is based on its effects on splanchnic circulation, as they induce a marked reduction of portal and mesenteric blood flow mediated through inhibition of vasodilator peptides. Additionally, experimental studies have shown that octreotide has antiangiogenic effects, by downregulation of vascular

endothelial growth factor (VEGF).[8] In fact, a study reported endoscopic resolution of angiodysplastic lesions after treatment with octreotide, albeit the effect was not quantified.[9] Interestingly, a more recent study showed that a 3-month-treatment of long-acting release (LAR) octreotide 20 mg once a month in cirrhotic patients decreased significantly both the hepatic venous pressure gradient and VEGF in hepatic venous blood.[10] Other potential mechanisms of action of somatostatin analogues in OGIB, although more controversial, are by increasing vascular resistance and improving platelet aggregation.
Octreotide is, by far, the most studied somatostatin analogue in OGIB. However, recent studies are focusing on long-acting intramuscular (LAR octreotide) or subcutaneous (lanreotide) formulations, which have the great advantage of a once monthly administration. A recent meta-analysis, which included three prospective studies, aimed at evaluating the effectiveness of conventional and depot somatostatin analogues for bleeding vascular malformations, showed an average clinical response rate of 76%.[11] Despite the small sample size of the studies included and the heterogeneity in the dose and molecular forms of the medication, these results are encouraging and a trial of somatostatin analogues is warranted, especially in patients in whom endoscopic therapy has failed, with unaccessible lesions or unknown source of bleeding. Its good safety profile, when compared with other pharmacological agents such as hormonal therapy or thalidomide, is another meaningful advantage. Nonetheless, randomized controlled trials are needed to confirm this data.

3.1 Octreotide

Octreotide can be administered intravenously (50 µg per hour) or subcutaneously (50-100 µg b.i.d or t.i.d). Its main disadvantage for long-term therapy is the need of parenteral administration several times a day, owing to its short half-life (90-120 minutes). Octreotide has been reported successful in stopping GI bleeding from angiodysplasia in multiple case reports and small series, both in acute and chronic bleeding.
To date, the most solid evidence is obtained in two prospective cohort studies, the latter comparing the results to historical controls. The former included 17 patients, (of whom 6 were cirrhotic), with chronic bleeding from angiodysplasias. 7 patients had isolated angiodysplasias, whereas other 7 had diffuse lesions in upper and lower segments of the GI tract and 3 watermelon stomach.[9] Octreotide was given subcutaneously (100 µg t.i.d) for 6 months. More than half of the patients (10/17) achieved complete remission without further iron or transfusion requirements, whereas a transient improvement was observed in another 4 patients. Of note, octreotide lead subjectively to disappearance or reduction of the number, size and colour of the vascular malformations on follow-up endoscopy. The second study included 32 patients with acute or chronic bleeding due to GI angiodysplasias, which were treated with octreotide 50 µg b.i.d for a 1-2 yr period.[12] Cirrhotic patients were excluded. Treatment failure (rebleeding or iron deficiency anemia during follow-up) was significantly higher in the controls cohort (48%) in comparison with the octreotide cohort (23%). A significant decrease in iron requirements, but not in hemoglobin or transfusion requirements, was also observed in the octreotide arm. Adverse effects in both studies were uncommon and mild, including diarrhea, constipation, hyperglycemia or gallbladder stones.

3.2 Long-acting release (LAR) octreotide

Several case reports and small series have recently revealed the efficacy of a depot formulation of octreotide (LAR octreotide) for severe OGIB, either of unknown origin or related to diffuse small bowel angiodysplasias.[13-18] LAR octreotide is administered intramuscularly monthly, which makes it an attractive and comfortable therapy on an outpatient basis.

Two small prospective uncontrolled series have been published using LAR octreotide. In the first study, 13 patients with chronic GI bleeding due to angiodysplasias were treated with octreotide LAR 10 mg per month and followed for at least 1 year.[19] Nine out of the thirteen patients (69%) did not require further blood or iron supplementation, and partial improvement was also observed in another patient. The second study addressed the response to octreotide LAR 20 mg per month in a cohort of 11 elderly patients with multiple comorbidities and severe OGIB, mostly related to small-bowel diffuse angiodysplasia (72%).[20] Median follow-up was 15 months (5-48). Only 2 out of 11 patients (18%) remained free of transfusions. However, a significant decrease in the need of red cell packets (14 (9-49) vs 4 (0-9), p 0.002) and in hospital stay due to GI bleeding (27 days (10-99) vs 7 days (0-23), p<0.001) during the first year of treatment was observed. These less promising results were perhaps due to a higher proportion of patients on anticoagulation or antiplatelet therapy, which was not withdrawn at study inclusion. Furthermore, the patients included in this study had more severe GI bleeding as shown by higher transfusional requirements.

The main disadvantage of this drug formulation is its high cost, ranging from 785 euros (10mg) to 1300 euros (30 mg) monthly. However, it may be cost-effective in very specific difficult to treat patients, only tributary to conservative management, with higher transfusional requirements and repeat admissions.

3.3 Lanreotide

The main advantage of lanreotide over LAR octreotide is its subcutaneous administration, avoiding painful intramuscular injections and their inherent risk for complication in anticoagulated or cirrhotic patients. Up to date, there is only a case report on the successful use of lanreotide in a patient with severe OGIB due to universal portal hypertension stigmata in stomach, small bowel and colon.[21] After a successful response to octreotide at a dose of 100 µg twice a day, the patient was given lanreotide, administered at dose of 60 mg, subcutaneously, on a monthly basis. This drug achieved complete remission of bleeding during 15 months of follow-up.

4. Antiangiogenic drugs

4.1 Thalidomide

Thalidomide is a drug with powerful immunomodulatory, anti-inflammatory and antiangiogenic effects, banned in the 1960s because of its teragenocity. However, it has been recently reintroduced for the treatment of leprosy, multiple myeloma and a variety of tumors. Over the last decade, thalidomide has gained interest as a therapeutic tool for OGIB. The rationale for its use in bleeding GI angiodysplasias is based on the inhibition of VEGF-dependent angiogenesis. It is administered orally at a variable dose of 100-300 mg per day, usually during a 3-month course due to adverse effects.

Thalidomide has been reported to be effective in controlling refractory severe bleeding from small bowel angiodysplasia, bleeding portal hypertensive gastropathy and enteropathy, radiation-induced proctitis and Crohn´s disease.[22-29] Thalidomide, at a dose of 100 mg per day for three months, controlled OGIB in a case series of 3 patients with chronic bleeding from small-bowel angiodysplasia evidenced by capsule endoscopy.[30] Repeat capsule

endoscopy after therapy revealed a substantial reduction in lesion number, size and colour intensity. Of note, the response was sustained for a median of 34 months despite discontinuation of the drug. Due to its antiangiogenic property, thalidomide may not only lead to cessation of bleeding but also to prevention of further angiodysplasia formation. More recently, two small prospective series, involving 3 and 7 patients, respectively, have confirmed the utility of thalidomide for bleeding small-bowel angiodysplasia.[31,32] However, a high rate of discontinuation was observed in these series (1/3 and 4/7, respectively), owing to intolerable side effects (fatigue, peripheral neuropathy, dizziness, urticarial rash).
The main drawback of thalidomide is it frequent side effects, although these are mostly minor (fatigue, somnolence, constipation, dizziness, peripheral neuropathy). Nonetheless, fatal complications such as acute liver failure have been reported.[33] In addition, the risk of thromboembolic events associated with thalidomide should be considered in OGIB patients. Overall, thalidomide is an effective drug for refractory bleeding GI angiodysplasia. Taking into account its numerous side effects, it seems cautious to save thalidomide for OGIB refractory to both endoscopic therapy and a trial of somatostatin analogues, albeit a head-to-head comparison is required to validate this algorithm.

4.2 Lenalidomide

Lenalidomide is an antiangiogenic drug commonly used for multiple myeloma. It has two mayor advantages over thalidomide: a more powerful antiangiogenic effect and a lower toxicity profile. Its use in the context of life-threatening bleeding due to gastrointestinal angiodysplasia in a patient suffering from HHT, in whom thalidomide was effective but had to be stopped because of severe neuropathy has been recently reported[34]. Lenalidomide successfully controlled bleeding and the patient remained free of either gastrointestinal bleeding or drug symptoms. However, although lenalidomide is more effective and better tolerated than thalidomide, further studies are warranted to evaluate its role in refractory OGIB. On the other hand, lenalidomide is 10 times more expensive than thalidomide and dosing should be carefully titrated owing to severe bone marrow suppression, much higher than that described for thalidomide.

4.3 Bevacizumab

Recently, a growing number of reports on the use of VEGF antagonist bevacizumab in HHT have lead to outstanding improvement in GI bleeding episodes, reductions in cardiac output and liver size, even obviating the need for liver transplantation in a single patient.[35,36] This benefit has been also proven for recurrent epistaxis, administering bevacizumab intravenously, injected locally or sprayed topically to the nasal mucosa.[37,38]

5. Miscellaneous drugs

5.1 Antifibrinolytics

Aminocaproic acid is a powerful inhibitor of the fibrinolytic system that blocks conversion of plasminogen to plasmin when used at low doses. There is only one isolated report in which it was effective in the management of epistaxis from arteriovenous malformations in two patients with HHT at a dose of 1.5 g twice a day, although it was not clear whether concomitant gastrointestinal bleeding was present.[39]
Tranexamic acid is a synthetic lysine analog that inhibits the conversion of plasmin to fibrinogen, with less antifibrinolytic power than aminocaproic acid. Tranexamic acid has

been proven useful for chronic bleeding from angiodysplasias in patients with end-stage renal failure and bleeding gastric antral vascular ectasia in cirrhosis.[40-42] A systematic review on the use of tranexamic acid for upper GI bleeding was recently published.[43] Although it seemed to reduce overall mortality, there were no significant differences regarding bleeding, surgery or transfusion requirements. Of note, tranexamic acid did not increase thromboembolic risk. Therefore, the current evidence does not support routine use of tranexamic acid in clinical practice. The main risk derived from the use of antifibrinolytics is thrombosis, so thrombophilia should be ruled out before prescribing them. Adverse events associated to ACA and tranexamic acid may be frequent, and the use of these drugs is not supported by randomized controlled trials, which makes antifibrinolytics a last option for OGIH.

5.2 Danazol

Danazol is an anti-gonadotropin drug with weak androgenic activity that blocks pituitary secretion of FSH and LH, leading to ectopic and normal endometrial tissue atrophy. It has been widely used for endometriosis and uterine bleeding disorders. Anecdotal reports suggest a partial improvement with danazol in patients with gastrointestinal bleeding and HHT,[44-46] although cosmetic stigmata (acne, hair loss, mild hirsutism) and uncommon but severe adverse effects (intracranial hypertension, peliosis hepatitis, thrombosis, seizures) leave danazol to a secondary role in OGIH, when other therapies have failed.

5.3 Desmopressin

Desmopressin is a synthetic analog of the antidiuretic hormone vasopressin that lacks vasopressor activity. It increases vW factor and factor VIII levels, and also enhances hemostasis in patients with defective platelet function. It is indicated as a hemostatic therapy for patients with hemophilia A and von Willebrand's disease, and can be administered intravenously, subcutaneously, or by intranasal spray. An isolated report showed a benefit of intravenous desmopressin for life-threatening gastrointestinal bleeding in a patient with HHT and vW factor deficiency, allowing elective colectomy and bleeding resolution[47].

5.4 Recombinant activated factor VIIa

Recombinant activated human factor VII (rFVIIa) is a drug that strongly promotes hemostasis, and is currently indicated for hemophiliac A and B patients with antibody inhibitors to coagulation factors VIII or IX, congenital deficiency of factor VII, and Glanzmann's thromboasthenia. This drug has been used anecdoctically for stopping hemorrhage, with or without hematological disorders, in massive or uncontrollable bleeding at multiple GI and non GI locations. Its short half-life of 2 hours requires frequent boluses or continuous infusion to achieve hemostasis, and it can induce definite control of bleeding or be a bridge until a causal therapy can be provided. It has been mainly used in cirrhotic patients with acquired coagulation factor deficiencies, especially in variceal and non-variceal upper GI hemorrhage related to cirrhosis or acute liver failure.[48,49] Albeit preliminary results showed that it might have a beneficial effect for advanced cirrhotic patients with variceal bleeding, a randomized placebo controlled trial failed to demonstrate a significant benefit of rFVIIa for controlling variceal bleeding or preventing rebleeding in these patients.[50] Thus, the use of rFVIIa should be carefully individualized in cirrhotic patients and it is not recommended in the routine clinical practice.

This drug has been proven useful in other settings as well. In a series of 11 unselected patients with upper GI haemorrhage, half of them related to liver disease, rFVIIa stopped the bleeding in 7 patients and markedly reduced it in other 2 patients.[51] Other successful indications relating severe GI bleeding have been refractory bleeding after endoscopic sphincterotomy in patients with preexisting coagulopathy,[52] severe recurrent GI bleeding due to multiple GI angiodysplasias in a patient with vW disease,[53] massive colonic bleeding[54] or exsanguinating bleeding due to Mallory-Weiss tear.[55] Of note, no thromboembolic events were reported in the aforementioned trials or series. However, secondary myocardial and cerebrovascular infarctions have been described while using factor VIIa.[56,57] As such, it is important to stress once more that the use of this drug should always be carefully individualized.

5.5 Tamoxifen

In a recent randomized, double-blind placebo controlled trial, the efficacy of antiestrogen therapy (Tamoxifen) was evaluated in patients with epistaxis due to HHT.[58] There was a significant reduction in the frequency of epistaxis in the tamoxifen-treated group, frequently associated to a rise in haemoglobin or a reduction in transfusion requirements. As previously mentioned in the case of bevacizumab, a potential therapeutic role for GI bleeding in HHT patients warrants further research.

5.6 Non-selective beta-blockers

These drugs aim to control hemorrhage by reducing gastrointestinal blood flow due to splanchnic vasoconstriction and reduction of cardiac output in cirrhotic patients with portal hypertension. Its proven benefit for secondary prophylaxis of bleeding portal hypertensive gastropathy in two randomized controlled trials led to the consensus recommendation that beta-blockers should be used for chronic bleeding once the acute episode of bleeding is controlled.[59,60]

6. References

[1] ASGE Standards of Practice Committee, Fisher L, Lee Krinsky M, Anderson MA, et al. The role of endoscopy in the management of obscure GI bleeding. Gastrointest Endosc 2010;72:471-9.

[2] Zuckerman GR, Prakash C, Ashkin MP, et al AGA technical review: evaluation and management of occult and obscure gastrointestinal bleeding. Gastroenterology 2000;118:20.

[3] Harrison DF. Use of estrogen in treatment of familial hemorrhagic telangiectasia. Laryngoscope 1982;92: 314-20.

[4] Van Cutsem E, Rutgeerts P, Vantrappen G. Treatment of bleeding gastrointestinal vascular malformations with oestrogen-progesterone. Lancet 1990;335:953-5.

[5] Lewis B, Salomon P, Rivera-MacMurray S, et al. Does hormonal therapy have any benefit for bleeding angiodysplasia?. J Clin Gastroenterol 1992;15: 99–103.

[6] Junquera F, Feu F, Papo M, et al. A multicenter, randomized, clinical trial of hormonal therapy in the prevention of rebleeding from gastrointestinal angiodysplasia. Gastroenterology 2001; 121:1073-9.

[7] Rossini FP, Arrigoni A, Pennazio M. Octreotide in the treatment of bleeding due to angiodysplasia of the small intestine. Am J Gastroenterology 1993;88:1424-7.

[8] Lurosaki M, Saeger W, Abe T, et al. Expression of vascular endothelial gowth factor in growth hormone-secreting pituitary adenomas: special reference to the octreotide management. Neurol Res 2008;30:518-2.

[9] Nardone G, Rocco A, Balzano T, et al. The efficacy of octreotide therapy in crhonic bleeding due to vascular abnormalities of the gastrointestinal tract. Aliment Pharmacol Ther 1999;13: 1429-36.

[10] Spahr L, Giostra E, Frossard JL, et al. A 3-month course of long-acting repeatable octreotide (Sandostatin LAR) improves portal hypertension in patients with cirrhosis: a randomized controlled study. Am J Gastroenterol 2007;102:1397-405.

[11] Brown C, Subramanian V, Wilcox CM, et al. Somatostatin analogues in the treatment of recurrent bleeding from gastrointestinal vascular malformations: an overview and systematic review of prospective observational studies. Dig Dis Sci 2010;55:2129-34.

[12] Junquera F, Saperas S, Videla S, et al. Long-term efficacy of octreotide in the prevention of recurrent bleeding from gastrointestinal angiodysplasia. Am J Gastroenterol 2007; 102:254-60.

[13] Orsi P, Guatti-Zuliani C, Okolicsanyi L. Long-acting octreotide is effective in controlling rebleeding angiodysplasia of the gastrointestinal tract. Dig Liver Dis 2001;33:330-4.

[14] Tamagno G, Mioni R, De Carlo E, et al. Effects of a somatostatin analogue in occult gastrointestinal bleeding: a case report. Dig Liver Dis 2004;36:843-6.

[15] Krikis N, Tziolamos K, Perifanis V, et al. Treatment of recurrent gastrointestinal haemorhage in a patient with von Willebrand´s disease with octreotide LAR and propanolol. Gut 2005;54: 171.

[16] Molina-Infante J, Perez-Gallardo B, González-García G, et al. Octreotide LAR for severe obscure-overt gastrointestinal haemorrhage in high-risk patients on anticoagulation therapy. Gut 2007;56:447.

[17] Boesby L, Christensen NJ, Kristensen LO. Somatostatin analogues in the treatment of bleeding GI-angiodysplasias. Ugeskr Laeger 2008;170:958.

[18] Almadi M, Ghali PM, Constantin A, et al. Recurrent obscure gastrointestinal bleeding: dilemmas and success with pharmacological therapies. Case series and review. Can J Gastroenterol 2009; 23:625-31.

[19] Scaglione G, Pietrini L, Russo F, et al. Long-acting octreotide as rescue therapy in chronic bleeding from gastrointestinal angiodysplasia. Aliment Pharmacol Ther 2007;26:935-42.

[20] Molina-Infante J, Perez-Gallardo B. Hernandez-Alonso M, et al. Octreotide long acting release for severe obscure gastrointestinal haemorrhage in elderly patients with serious comorbidities. Med Clin (Barc) 2009;133:667-70.

[21] Hutchinson JM, Jennings JS, Jones RL. Long-acting somatostatin therapy in obscure-overt gastrointestinal bleeding in noncirrhotic portal hypertension: a case report and literature review. Eur J Gastroenterol Hepatol 2010;22:754-8.

[22] Shurafa M, Kamboj G. Thalidomide for the treatment of bleeding angiodysplasias. Am J Gastroenterol 2003;98:221-2.

[23] Bauditz J, Schachschal G, Wedel S, et al. Thalidomide for treatment of severe intestinal bleeding. Gut 2004;53:609-12.

[24] Karajeh MA, Hurlstone DP, Stephenson TJ, et al. Refractory bleeding from portal hypertensive gastropathy: a further novel role for thalidomide therapy?. Eur J Gastroenterol Hepatol 2006;18:545-8.

[25] Craanen ME, van Triest B, Verjeihen RH, et al. Thalidomide in refractory haemorrhagic radiation induced proctitis. Gut 2006;55:1371-2.

[26] Hirri HM, Green PJ, Lindsay J. Von Willebrand's disease and angiodysplasia treated with thalidomide. Haemophilia 2006;12:285-6.

[27] De Konig DB, Drenth JP, Friederich P, et al. Thalidomide for the treatment of recurrent gastrointestinal blood loss due to intestinal angiodysplasias. Ned Tijdschr Geneeskd 2006;150:1994-7.

[28] Kirhkam SA, Lindley KJ, Elawad MA, et al. Treatment of multiple small bowel angiodysplasias causing severe life-threatening bleeding with thalidomide. J Pediatr Gastroenterol Nutr 2006;42:585-7.

[29] Jimenez-Saenz M, Romero-Vazquez J, Caunedo-Alvarez J, et al. Benefitial effects and reversi6n of vascular lesions by thalidomide in a patient with bleeding portal hypertensive enteropathy. Dig Liver Dis 2010;42:232-3.

[30] Bauditz J, Lochs H, Voderholzer W. Macroscopic appearance of intestinal angiodysplasias under antiangiogenic treatment with thalidomide. Endoscopy 2006;38:1036-9.

[31] Dabak V, Kuriakose P, Kamboj G, et al. A pilot study of thalidomide in recurrent GI bleeding due to angiodysplasias. Dig Dis Sci 2008;53:1632-5.

[32] Kamalaporn P Saravanan R, Cirocco M, et al. Thalidomide for the treatment of chronic gastrointestinal bleeding from angiodysplasias: a case series. Eur J Gastroenterol Hepatol 2009;21:1347-50.

[33] Hamadani M, Benson DM Jr, Copelan EA. Thalidomide-induced fulminant hepatic failure. Mayo Clin Proc 2007;82:638.

[34] Bowcock SJ, Patrick HE. Lenalidomide to control gastrointestinal bleeding n hereditary haemorrhagic telangiectasia: potential implications for angiodysplasias?. Br J Haematol 2009;146:220-2.

[35] Flieger D, Hainke S, Fischbach W. Dramatic improvement in hereditary hemorrhagic telangiectasia after treatment with the vascular endothelial growth factor (VEGF) antagonist bevacizumab. Ann Hematol 2006;85:631.

[36] Mitchell A, Adams LA, MacQuillan G, et al. Bevacizumab reverses need for liver transplantation in hereditary hemorrhagic telangiectasia. Liver Transpl 2008;14:210-3.

[37] Bose P, Holter JL, Selby GB. Bevacizumab in hereditary hemorrhagic telangiectasia. N Eng J Med 2009;361:931.

[38] Karnezis TT, Davidson TM. Efficacy of intranasal bevacizumab (Avastin) treatment in patients with hereditary hemorrhagic telangiectasia-associated epistaxis. Laryngoscope 2011;121:636-8.

[39] Saba HI, Morelli GA, Logrono LA. Brief report: Treatment of bleeding in hereditary hemorrhagic telangiectasia vith aminocaproic acid. N Engl J Med 1994; 330:1789.

[40] Philips MD. Stopping bleeding in hereditary telangiectasia. N Engl J Med 1994; 330:1822-1823.

[41] Vujkovac B, Lavre J, Sabovic M. Successful treatment of bleeding from colonic angiodysplasias with tranexamic acid in a hemodialisis patient. Am J Kidney Diseases 1998;3:536-538.

[42] McCormick PA, Ooi H, Crosbie O. Tranexamic acid for severe bleeding gastric antral vascular ectasia in cirrhosis. Gut 1998;42:750-2.

[43] Gluud LL, Klingenberg SL, Langholz SE. Systematic review: tranexamic acid for upper gastrointestinal bleeding. Aliment Pharmacol Ther 2008;27:752-8.

[44] Haq AU, Glass J, Netchvolodoff CV, et al. Hereditary hemorrhagic telangiectasia and danazol. Ann Intern Med 1988; 109:171.

[45] Korzenik J, Topazian M, Burdge C, et al. Danazol in the treatment of GI hemorrhage secondary to hereditary hemorrhagic telangiectasia (abstract). Gastroenterology 1995; 108:A297.

[46] Longacre AV, Gross CP, Gallitelli M, et al. Diagnosis and management of gastrointestinal bleeding in patients with haemorrhagic hereditary telangiectasia. Am J Gastroenterol 2003;98:59-63.

[47] Quitt M, Froom P, Veisler A, et al. The effect of desmopressin on masive gastrointestinal bleeding in hereditary telangiectasia unresponsive to treatment with cryoprecipitate. Arch Intern Med 1990;150:1744-6.

[48] Romero-Castro R, Jimenez-Saenz M, Pellicer-Bautista M, et al. Recombinant-activated factor VII as hemostatic therapy in eight cases of severe hemorrhage from esophageal varices. Clin Gastroenterol Hepatol 2004;2:78-84.

[49] Bosch J, Thabut D, Bendtsen F, et al. Recombinant factor VIIa for upper gastrointestinal bleeding in patients with cirrhosis: a randomized, double-blind trial. Gastroenterology 2004; 127:1123-30.

[50] Bosch J, Thabut D, Albillos A, et al. Recombinant factor VIIa for varicela bleeding in patients with advanced cirrosis: a randomized, controlled trial. Hepatology 2008;47:1604-14.

[51] Vilstrup H, Markiewicz M, Biesma D, et al. Recombinant activated factor VIIa in an unselected series of cases with upper gastrointestinal bleeding. Thromb Res 2006;118:595-601.

[52] Romero-Castro R, Jimenez-Saenz M, Pellicer-Bautista F, et al. Refractory bleeding after endoscopic sphincterotomy: a new indication for recombinant factor VII therapy?. Am J Gastroenterol 2004;99:2063-5.

[53] Meijer K, Peters FT, van der Meer J. Recurrent severe bleeding from gastrointestinal angiodysplasia in a patient with von Willebrand's disease, controlled with recombinant factor VIIa. Blood Coagul Fybrinolisis 2001;12:211-3.

[54] Mitchell JG, Speake WJ, Russell NK, et al. Recombinant factor VIIa: a useful tool for life-threatening colonic bleeding: a case report. Dis Colon Rectum 2007;50:2238-40.

[55] Shah K, Banerjee D, Gambhir RP, et al. Mallory-Weiss tear: use of recombinant factor VII for exsanguinating bleed. Trop Gastroenterol 2009;30:226-7.

[56] Basso IN, Keeling D. Myocardial infarction following recombinant activated factor VII in a patient with type 2A von Willebrand disease. Blood Coagul Fybrinolisis 2005; 15: 503-4.

[57] Alkyldiz M, Turan I, Ozutemiz O, et al. A cerebrovascular event after single-dose administration of recombinant factor VIIa in a patient with esophageal variceal bleeding. Dig Dis Sci 2006;51:1647-9.
[58] Yaniv E, Preis M, Hadar T, et al. Antiestrogen therapy for hemorrhagic hereditary telangiectasia: a double-blind placebo controlled trial. Laryngoscope 2009;119:284-8.
[59] de Francis R. Evolving consensus in portal hypertension. Report of the Baveno IV consensus workshop on methodology of diagnosis and therapy in portal hypertension. J Hepatol 2005; 43:167-76.
[60] Ripoll C, Garcia-Tsao G. The management of portal hypertensive gastropathy and gastric antral vascular ectasia. Dig Liver Dis 2011;43:345-51.